ERNEST AMORY CODMAN

The End Result of a Life in Medicine

BILL MALLON, M.D.

CONTENTS

FOREWORD

This biography of Ernest Amory Codman, a distinguished Harvard orthopaedic surgeon, is exceedingly well written and thoroughly documented. Moreover, it is quite timely, as he was a pioneer in the field of outcomes research which has assumed increasing significance in the recent past.

Codman was born in Boston and graduated from Harvard in 1891 and then entered Harvard Medical School. This was followed by a surgical internship at the Massachusetts General Hospital and later by appointment as an instructor in anatomy at Harvard. It is interesting that in the same year that Codman began his internship, Wilhelm Conrad Röntgen discovered X-rays, which greatly expanded the potential of all fields of medicine and especially orthopaedics, a discipline in which Codman was to become internationally famous. With the use of the X-ray, he was one of the early writers emphasizing its role and significance in diagnosing diseases of the bone and in following many disorders.

While they were interns at the Massachusetts General Hospital, Codman and Harvey Cushing introduced an anesthesia chart that was used in many hospitals. In 1910, Codman made an innovative recommendation that there should be a follow-up system to record the course of diseases and document the methods of treatment with attention to the outcome. He was quite influential on the Committee on Hospital Standardization of the Society of Clinical Surgery, which had been founded by Harvey Cushing. Codman's participation in this very select group reflects his stature in the eyes of his colleagues, since membership in the society was restricted to the leading surgeons in the

United States and limited to fifty active members. Their meetings were held in major medical centers in the United States with intermittent visits to Europe. This society established the Committee on Hospital Standardization, which later became a part of the American College of Surgeons. Dr. Codman was invited to be the first chairman of this committee. It is clear that he was a pioneer in the field of outcomes research, with detailed an objective follow-up of patients in a fully documented manner. As Mallon emphasizes, Codman's approach was "methodical, complete, and precise." As is thoroughly recorded in this biography, Codman also became a towering figure in the field of orthopaedics and made many distinctive contributions. He gave primary effort to two major activities, his monograph entitled *The Shoulder*, published in 1934, and his introduction of the Registry of Bone Sarcoma.

Bill Mallon has produced a very readable and carefully referenced biography. Of considerable interest is the fact that he has previously received literary distinction by publishing his excellent text entitled *Quest for Gold: The Encyclopedia of American Olympians*. It is apparent that this engaging author clearly admires and deeply respects Codman for his many contributions and unflagging commitment to his ideals and principles. This important work is one that will predictably be read and appreciated by a wide circle of interested readers. It is indeed a masterwork that quite predictably will be frequently quoted in the future. The author has drawn upon an immense base of documentaries and family records for this work. With obvious attention to every detail, this biography is thoroughly deserving of a glowing review.

David C. Sabiston, Jr., M.D.
James B. Duke Professor of Surgery
Director of International Programs
Duke University Medical Center
Durham, NC 27710

FOREWORD

What a wonderful treat it was to read Bill Mallon's captivating biography of E. A. Codman. Codman has long been a personal hero of mine and I, like many other orthopaedists, have always claimed him as "one of us." I know he was a general surgeon, but with Codman's Paradox, Codman's Triangle, Codman's Tumor, and Codman's great work leading to his book on the shoulder, wasn't he really an orthopaedist?

Later I became aware of his seminal works on outcome assessment. During my training in the Massachusetts General Hospital (MGH) fracture clinic, we still did end result analysis on every patient, following Codman's precepts. As I became more involved in the orthopaedic outcomes movement, first as president of the Hip Society trying to create a uniform set of outcome measures for hip surgery and later as chair of the American Academy of Orthopaedic Surgery's Task Force on Outcome Studies, I realized how prescient E. A. Codman had been. What we think of as a very modern concept is no more and no less than Codman's "End Result Idea."

Bill Mallon's passion for the person and the work of E. A. Codman breathes life and excitement into the story of one of the most colorful, innovative, and controversial American surgeons. Before this scholarly work, those of us who have come to admire Codman could glean bits and pieces here and there about this remarkable man; however, Mallon has woven these threads into a rich and exciting tapestry, bringing to life this remarkable man, his times and accomplishments. He leads from early studies on the anatomy of the shoulder through the first applications of X-rays to study joint motion and fractures, through his collaborative work with Harvey Cushing in creating the first anesthesia charts, and his original work on the treatment of duodenal ulcers. Through it all there is Codman's passion for following every patient treated until the results of that treatment are known, and furthermore, for making that knowledge available to both physicians and patients to guide their choice—a revolutionary idea 100 years ago and still controversial in some circles today. Bill Mallon's scholarly and readable book clearly establishes Ernest Amory Codman as father of outcome studies as well as the father of study of the shoulder.

Clement B Sledge, M.D.
John B. and Buckminster Brown
Professor of Orthopaedic Surgery
Harvard Medical School
Boston, MA 02115

PREFACE

For interns and junior residents in general surgery, Monday afternoons were always devoted to a teaching conference known to us all as "Man Rounds." The teaching conference was led by Dr. David C. Sabiston, the Chairman of Surgery at Duke University Medical Center, renowned as perhaps the best-known teacher of academic surgeons in the country. To all of us he was known, for what we considered obvious reasons, as "The Man," a nickname we never used to his face, but which he knew and understood well.

"Man Rounds" could be intimidating. With an imperious, foreboding manner, Dr. Sabiston spent 1½ hours grilling us on some topic of surgery, asking us pertinent questions on any aspect of some surgical problems, and we were always expected to know everything. Dr. Sabiston placed especial pressure on his chief residents, who were expected to prepare all of the lower-level residents for this conference and, if we were found wanting, although he would be upset with us, his chief residents would also slink a bit lower in their seats, as we stumbled or mumbled through some obviously less than adequate explanation of the problem at hand.

He was an excellent teacher, and this conference was very valuable. We did not wish to fail, and our preparations for this conference in trying to figure out which questions would be asked on which topic were almost comical. Usually, a case presentation was made, and Dr. Sabiston would then spend the remainder of the time asking us questions about the case and the surgical principles involved.

Occasionally, however, after returning from surgical conferences, the residents would be asked to present short summaries of what they had learned at the conferences. It was the job of the chief residents to speak beforehand with each junior resident and tell them which lectures they would be asked to discuss.

Near the end of my junior resident year, I had the opportunity to attend a surgical conference at The Homestead in Hot Springs, Virginia. Now, it should be pointed out that I was less than one month away from becoming a resident in orthopaedic surgery, and my interest in general surgical problems was by then, admittedly, waning. I found the Homestead to be a beautiful place with many temptations and, in the company of my fellow residents, Mike McNamara and Sam Currin, was tempted by most of them, usually capping off the evening with some lively darts battles at the Sam Snead Tavern in the small village of Hot Springs. To us as surgical students, these darts contests were also physiological experiments in seeing how well we could toss the little suckers while simultaneously quaffing a few cold ones.

My attendance at the surgical lectures that week was less then exemplary, as you might imagine from the above. But, when I returned to Duke, I was expected to present at "Man Rounds" a short summary of one of the lectures I had heard. My chief resident was Dr. Bill Holman, now an esteemed cardiac surgeon. He was a good man and had been my chief resident earlier in the year when I rotated on cardiothoracic surgery. We got on well, but when we discussed which lectures I would present, he became more and more frustrated. The conversation went something like this:

"How about discussing this one on platelet-derived growth factors in wound healing?" asked Holman.

"Well, uhm, Bill, I didn't get a chance to hear that one."

"OK, what about this lecture on Goretex grafts in abdominal aortic aneurysms?"

"Uhm, yeah—that was a good one, ... I think, but I can't remember too much about it."

"I see. What about this paper from the Mayo on laparoscopic cholecystectomy?"

"Gee, Bill, I think I was kinda sick that morning. Some virus I picked up, maybe."

Bill was quickly becoming exasperated and he knew my virus was probably due to the dreaded Molson aureus. Finally, he asked the obvious question. "Well, did you go to any lecture you think you can talk intelligently about?" I did have an answer for this. I agreed to discuss the lecture concerning "that Boston surgical dude with the cartoon."

"That Boston surgical dude with the cartoon" was Ernest Amory Codman, and thus did I first come to know him. I discussed the lecture that had been presented at The Homestead in which I learned about Codman and his emphasis on outcomes and when I first heard about the meeting at the Boston Medical Library at which he unveiled his famed cartoon of the ostrich kicking out the Golden Eggs.

Now I know him well. I met him while dissecting out some shoulder, noting that what he first pointed out ninety years ago is exactly correct. I met him while a resident on the orthopaedic oncology service, learning of Codman's Tumor and Triangle. I met him while studying shoulder surgery, hearing of Codman's Paradox and Codman's sign. And I have encountered him frequently while attempting to design a database to track outcome studies of shoulder problems.

To me, my interest in Codman's life seems an obvious one because of the many similarities with my own. I must reveal them to you here, but Codman would approve, for he stated in his book, *The Shoulder*, that he felt an author should reveal something about himself in the preface to his books. It is noteworthy that many surgeons feel the most valuable portion of the book is the preface, which has little to do with the shoulder.

When I first started delving into Codman's life, I was struck by the analogies to my own. We grew up within ten miles of one another. He attended prep school in a neighboring town only five miles from my high school. His primary interests were shoulder surgery, bone sarcoma, and outcome studies. My practice is primarily that of a shoulder specialist in orthopaedics, but as a resident, my secondary interest was bone tumors and sarcoma. As a Fellow in shoulder surgery, I became very interested in tracking the outcomes of shoulder surgery. Codman married a woman named Katherine Bowditch, whose family's name graced my high school's track and football stadium. Finally, Codman settled in retirement and died in a development named Ponkapoag, south of Boston, where in my premedical career as a professional golfer, at Ponkapoag Golf Course, I would win more tournaments than at any other course.

There have been no previous book-length biographies of this fascinating Boston surgeon. With my own interest in writing, my interest in Codman, and the almost eerie parallels that kept evolving, I thought it natural to write the first. My writing assistant, Jane White Bason, as always, was instrumental in helping produce and edit the manuscript. My medical assistant, Kim Tuck, was helpful with everything, as she always is, despite, during some of the early days of the research, her questions about why I was getting all these calls about this Dr. Codman fellow.

Many other people have lent their help. Nobody can fully understand Codman without spending time at the Rare Book Room of the Boston Medical Library at the Countway Library of Medicine in the Harvard Medical School. There one can find Codman's Papers in eleven large boxes of folders and clippings. My time there was fun and enlightening and I would like to thank the librarians at the Rare Book Room for their support, especially Lucretia McClure, Madeleine W. Mullin, Corinne Blakeslee, and Richard J. Wolfe.

Many other people helped along the way. Edmund Kenealy, reference librarian at the Canton Public Library in Canton, Massachusetts, helped me find information on Codman's retirement home. I owe a huge debt to Warren B. Ervine of Halifax, Nova Scotia, who helped track down information about Codman's medical relief efforts after the Halifax Explosion. Jane Bihldorff, John Hemenway, and Gerard McEleney were very helpful in tracing Codman's retirement home in the Ponkapong region. Monique Rasetti and Anthony J. deV. Hill of Saint Mark's School provided me with information concerning his years at this esteemed prep school, as did Nick Noble, historian at The Fay School. Laura Shedore at the Joint Commission for Accreditation of Healthcare organizations, Wendy Thomas at the Schlesinger Library of Radcliffe College, and Brian Sullivan of Harvard Archives also provided assistance. Steven Borack of Randolph, Massachusetts, helped with many of the photographs including herein.

Physicians who provided assistance include Drs. Julia Crim, Clyde Helms, Lanny Johnson, Nancy Major, T. J. "Jock" Murray, Douglas Reintgen, Marcia Scott, Hilliard Siegler, Daniel Sexton, and Donald Sweet. Finally, notes from a few doctors who had trained under Codman were quite useful, notably, Dr. Carter Rowe, Dr. Francis D. Moore, Dr. Edward B. Twitchell, and Dr. William Quimby. During the last stages of my research, Dr. Charles A. Rockwood kindly sent me a copy of a very rare book on Codman and also lent his support. Dr. Kevin McGuire provided me a copy of his Princeton honors thesis on Codman, which was very helpful. I thank them all.

Three doctors deserve a special word of thanks. I owe a large debt to Dr. David Sabiston, who wrote a foreword to the book, and who will, for the last time, find out the truth about that Monday conference at which I discussed the Codman paper. Dr. Sabiston helped me become a surgeon in more ways than one, for which I am eternally grateful. Dr. James Urbaniak, Chief of Orthopaedics at Duke University Medical Center, likewise provided me with the opportunity that allowed me to establish my current career, and I thank him for that opportunity and for all that he has taught me, both in and out of the operating room. Dr. Clement Sledge, who has taken up Dr. Codman's cause as a current orthopaedic expert on outcomes, was kind enough to review the manuscript and provide a foreword as well.

I offer special appreciation to Drs. Duncan Neuhauser and Susan Reverby, both medical historians who had previously written well-known journal articles concerning Codman, and Mr. Michael Millenson, who supported the project in his "dark" days. All were excited by this project and read drafts of the manuscript for me. Their comments, criticism, support, and assistance were invaluable, and I thank them all.

Special thanks are due to Lewis Reines and Richard Lampert of W. B. Saunders for agreeing to take on the task of publishing this biography. To them, and John Feagin, M.D., who first put me in touch with Saunders, I offer my appreciation.

I owe a lot to my family. Karen has suffered many nights while I banged away on the computer or was at the library, writing about or researching that eccentric and irascible old Boston surgeon, but she has accepted my own eccentricity and irascibility, for which I love her. Our three dogs, Kamper Mallon, Kelly Mallon, and Mickey Mantle Mallon, have cheerfully stood by, wishing I would take them for another walk, or throw them their tennis ball for a few more hours, but they have usually asked no greater privilege than to sit at my feet while I worked and wrote. My father, John Mallon, and sister, Jessie M. Spence, have lent their love and moral support, as always.

In addition, I would like to thank the four men I consider to be my orthopaedic mentors, to whom I dedicate this volume, and who helped with this book by their examples as orthopaedic surgeons, as doctors, and as men. There is much talk in the 1990s of the quality of medical care and the quality and caring nature of doctors. If you ever find yourself in the hands of Drs. Frank Bassett, Tom Dimmig, John Harrelson, or Rich Hawkins, sit back and relax, and rest, assured you will receive superb treatment and receive it with compassion. I can only aspire to their level.

And finally, this one's for my Mom and her many nights at Howard Johnson's. She is at least now resting more comfortably.

Bill Mallon, M.D.
Durham, NC
September 1998

PREFACE TO THE NEW EDITION

Not too much different to add from 1998. Codman still remains little known to the medical world although he deserves so much more. Hopefully making the biography accessible digitally will allow this to happen.

Since the first edition Frank Bassett, one of the orthopaedists to whom it was dedicated, has passed on and my wife and I still miss hearing all his stories. Our dogs at the time—Kamper, Kelly, and Mickey Mantle—are also now up in doggie heaven, replaced by five equally wonderful pooches.

Finally, my Dad passed away shortly after the original book was published. He's now resting more comfortably with my Mom, to whom the original edition was dedicated. This one is still for her, and for my Dad.

Bill Mallon, M.D.
Durham, NC
June 2012

PROLOGUE
WHO HE WAS

Through the woodland, through the valley, comes a horseman wild and free.
Tilting at the windmills passing, who can the brave young horseman be?
He is wild but he is mellow; he is strong but he is weak;
He is cruel but he is gentle; he is wise but he is meek.

Gordon Lightfoot, *Don Quixote* [1969]

Ernest Amory Codman tilted at windmills much of his life, and he longed to be wild and free among the woodlands. He was at times wild and mellow, strong and weak, and cruel and gentle. He was very wise, though he was never accused of being meek. But who was he?

Codman was a surgeon whose life spanned the end of the 19th and the beginning of the 20th century. He was a pioneer in several fields of medicine, notably the study of the shoulder and bone sarcomas. To many physicians, he is remembered only for this. But to Codman, neither field was what truly motivated him. Codman wanted to be a pioneer, but his goal was far greater; he wished to reform medicine and how it was practiced in the 20th century. His primary interest in medicine was what he called the End Result Idea. A simple idea, really, it consisted only of the notion that doctors should follow all their patients long enough to tell if the results of their treatment worked. But in Codman's era, it was completely revolutionary, and not at all well accepted among his peers. From his first mention of it around 1905, much of his life would be spent attempting to convince the medical world of the importance of the End Result Idea—to little avail. It was the windmill at which he tilted, but never managed to fell.

Two things best define the essence of Ernest Amory Codman. One was a simple notebook, with cardboard covers, which was filled with the notes he made over more than 45 years of hunting in the woods. The other was a meeting that he chaired at the Boston Medical Library on 6 January 1915. Though his life and personality were complex, one can gain a basic understanding of Codman by studying these two primary events in his life.

The first entry in Codman's hunting notebook was dated 1889. For the next 48 years, with only a few gaps during the 1910s, he documented the record of his hunting forays. He included everything concerning those days in the woods. For each day that he hunted, he recorded assiduously the day, the friends with whom he hunted, and the place that they hunted. He listed the name of the dog who accompanied him, and when he brought along a new dog, that dog's name, breed, and how he was obtained were usually described. He recorded the number and type of birds killed, and the number of shells used for the day's catch. The weather was often recorded, and the method of transport to the site is occasionally noted.

The journal is methodical, complete, and precise, with almost 200 pages filled with Codman's notations. At the end of each season of hunting, there was often a short note concerning his efforts for the year. Notably, he discussed whether he had had a good year or not, and *how it could have been improved.*

In short, it is an almost fanatical description of the hobby of a lifetime. But when examined more closely, it is an impressive effort in which Codman sought, not only to record what he had done, *but how he could have done it better.* The notebook is a demonstration of Codman applying the End Results Idea to his hobby and leisure time. The End Result Idea would become his life's work, and professionally it would cost him dearly. But to see this man apply the same system to his hunting gives us clues as to what it meant to him, and also to what he meant to it.

Surely, Codman must have known that what he would do that January night could be the end of his professional career, but it was of no concern to him. As Codman faced the gathering crowd at the Boston Medical Library, chairing the meeting he had planned and designed, all the fury of his passion for the End Result System had to be churning within him. He was never known for his tact. But now, in front of the elite of the medical society of Boston and neighboring towns who had gathered for this meeting of the Surgical Section of the Suffolk District Medical Society, his inner fury would come unbridled.

The people gathered there were not only the elite of the medical profession, but included several hospital trustees and administrators, efficiency experts, and notably, the Mayor of Boston, James Curley. They had come for "A Meeting for the Discussion of Hospital Efficiency." In front of this esteemed audience, Codman, who knew little of the word compromise, would effectively watch his promising, young surgical career immolate. He cared not a whit.

It was the End Result Idea that mattered to him, and only the End Result Idea. It was then, and would remain forever the Holy Grail of his life. He himself described his quest as Quixotic, and throughout his life, he would tilt at windmills frequently. On that night in Boston, all that mattered to him was his presentation of the End Result Idea to the medical elite of Massachusetts, and his method of presentation was chosen specifically for its dramatic and shocking effect.

At the end of the meeting, Codman rose to speak. First, he criticized several of the earlier speakers, showing less than a modicum of grace. Then, he gave his own presentation. It included the unveiling of a large cartoon,[1] which he had had drawn by an artist friend. In the center of

---

1 The cartoon still exists today. Originally drawn by Philip D. Hale, an artist friend of Codman's, it is kept at the Boston Medical Library Rare Book Room at the Countway Medical Library of the Harvard Medical School. The cartoon is in three panels and must be pieced together. Often described by other writers as 8' in length, it is a little smaller, measuring 3' x 6' in size when fully assembled. It is drawn on bland, light brown wrapping paper, reminiscent of a shopping bag. It will never be mistaken for great art.

the cartoon stood an ostrich with its head buried in the sand. Behind the ostrich stood the Trustees of the Massachusetts General Hospital, who sat idly by while this ostrich kicked out its Golden Eggs to the professors and surgeons of the hospital. The Golden Eggs represented the rich fees collected by the Harvard doctors, as the Trustees watched mindlessly, not caring at all that the ostrich kept its head in the sand, and never looked at the results of its efforts, thereby not implementing Codman's beloved End Result System. He described the cartoon and its implications in detail, leaving out nothing, and openly criticized everyone involved with the current system of medical education and its lack of follow-up. He offended virtually everybody in the room.

Many of the doctors in attendance got up and left in a huff. A few days later, the *Boston Post* ran a large story about the meeting under the headline, "Cartoon by Physician Causes Stir." Codman was asked to resign from his position as chairman of the Surgical Section of the Suffolk District Medical Society. Over the next few months, he received hundreds of letters. Many of them were of a similar vein, effectively asking, "We don't really disagree with your ideas, but did you have to present them in such an embarrassing manner?"

After that night, his life would never be the same. Before that winter's night, he had been thought of as among the best and the brightest. Graduate of a leading prep school, Harvard College, and Harvard Medical School, he was immediately appointed as an assistant surgeon at the renowned Massachusetts General Hospital. His best friend was Harvey Cushing, known as the first great neurosurgeon, with whom he had attended medical school, and who said of Codman that he had always bested him [Cushing] in their contests for medical knowledge. By 1915, Codman had published copiously in the medical journals, and was already an expert on anesthesiology, radiology, and abdominal surgery (notably of duodenal ulcers). He was the first surgeon to become interested in the problems of the shoulder, and is today considered *the* great pioneer of shoulder surgery. He had it all.

But burdened forever after by the reprobation of his peers, he would never become much of a financial success as a practicing surgeon, and his career after 1915 tumbled. In the last decade of his life, he was almost a pauper, even given to fighting the banks to avoid repossession of his house. In spite of these difficulties, however, he continued his Quixotic quest to the end,[2] never flagging in his efforts to reform the medical system of the early 20th century. He never did.

Now, 80 years later, Codman is seen not as a heretic, but a pioneer who was far ahead of his time. His place in history has become as he predicted, "But if the prophet is confident of the value of his service, he may keep his equanimity in spite of the jeers of his contemporaries. Although the End Result Idea may not achieve its entire fulfillment for several generations, I hope to be as content when dying as any soldier on the battle field, who, although he may have fought for quite the wrong side, feels the glow of patriotism, or as many an old fashioned baron, breathing his last in his four-poster, convinced that he has left his children protected from a wicked world. Honors, except those I have thrust upon myself, are conspicuously absent on my chart, but I am able to enjoy the hypothesis that I may receive some from a more receptive generation."[3]

Codman finished medical school in 1895, and was thus a surgeon of the 90's; but the question must be asked—of which century? Perhaps, of which millennium? To fully understand him, it is necessary to look further, deep into the man who pushed back the envelope of medical knowledge in many ways, perhaps on as many sides as any other doctor of the 20th century, but one who remained unheralded and unappreciated for most of his lifetime.

---

[2]Codman described his own work as Quixotic, using it in the Preface to his book on the shoulder on both pp. xxxii and xxxvii.

[3]Preface, p. xxxviii. All future footnote references to "Preface" refer to the Preface to *The Shoulder: Rupture of the Supraspinatus Tendon and Other Lesions In or About the Subacromial Bursa*, by E. A. Codman, M.D.; published in 1934 by Thomas Todd Printers of Boston.

CHAPTER 1
A BRAHMIN BEGINNING

He comes of the Brahmin caste of New England.
This is the harmless, inoffensive, untitled aristocracy.

Oliver Wendell Holmes, *The Brahmin Caste of New England*, [1860]

Ernest Amory Codman has been described as being of Brahmin descent or, more properly, a Boston Brahmin.[4] While certainly correct, it is hardly complimentary. Brahmin is a slightly pejorative description of the older, conservative, socially exclusive families of New England, who were often noted to be culturally and aristocratically pretentious. The term is derived as a humorous reference to the Brahmins, the highest caste of the Hindu society.

The Brahmins produced many distinguished writers in the 19th century, including Oliver Wendell Holmes, Henry Wadsworth Longfellow, and James Russell Lowell, and they helped shape literary and cultural opinions and tastes in that era. They made themselves the arbiters of literary taste and established Boston as the literary capital of America in the 1800s. They were very conservative, and advocated what has been described as a genteel rational humanism, "quite out of step with their brilliant contemporaries."[5]

4Reverby S. Stealing the golden eggs: Ernest Amory Codman and the science and management of medicine. *Bulletin of the History of Medicine*, 55: 1981, p. 156.

5*Encyclopedia Brittanica*, MICROPÆDIA, Volume II, (London: 15th edition, 1978), pg. 226.

In his book, *The Rascal King*, Jack Beatty described the Brahmins and their influence in *fin de siècle* Boston, "Boston was home to the most influential upper class in American history, the Brahmins of Beacon Hill and the Back Bay. These 'sifted few,' in Oliver Wendell Holmes's phrase, had power over city and state out of all proportion to their numbers. Long after they ceased to count politically, they weighed on the psyche of aspirant groups, making the hope of rising seem futile and intimidating the rare instances of immigrant wealth with the scepter of good taste. They controlled the citadels of culture—to the Irish, as Upton Sinclair wrote in his novel *Boston*, 'A far-off mysterious thing, but awe-inspiring, like the power of a voodoo magician.' They manned the redoubts of finance."[6]

Ernest Amory Codman's family was of a decided Brahmin bent. His earliest known ancestor on his father's side was Robert Codman, who emigrated over from England following many of the early Pilgrims, settling in Charlestown, Massachusetts. Robert Codman (1637-1678) received a grant of land in Salem, Massachusetts in 1637 and established the Codman line in Colonial America. From Robert Codman, the line of descent went through his son, Stephen Codman (1650-1706), and his wife, Elizabeth Randall; to John Codman (1)[7] (1696-1735) and Parnell Foster; John Codman (2) (1719-1792) and Abigail (Soley) Asbury; and then to John Codman (3) and Margaret Russell and eventually to John Codman (4) and Mary Wheelwright.

John Codman (3) (1755-1808) was Ernest Amory Codman's great grandfather and was a prosperous Boston merchant. His son, John Codman (4) was E. A. Codman's paternal grandfather, and became a well-known theologian, who served as the pastor of the Second Parish in Dorchester, Massachusetts, from 1808 until his death. He was described as a very conservative, orthodox minister who upheld his

---

6Beatty, *The Rascal King*, p. 10.

7There are six (6) "John Codmans" in E. A. Codman's ancestry. It is not possible to distinguish them from one another easily and I have chosen simply numbering them. Unfortunately, middle names for this group of John Codmans have not survived in most cases. Several of them had to have middle names, however, even when not listed, as Amory Codman's brother, John Codman, definitely had no middle name and is listed in his Harvard records simply as John Codman, Jr. This actually must be an error, as his father was not a John Codman, and he should correctly be termed John Codman, II, since the name skipped a generation, but it implies that several of the other John Codmans had more complete names not known to us.

principles against some of the newer Unitarians and other religious revolutionaries of the era. [8]

It has been said that Ernest Amory Codman inherited his vigorous mind and unconventional methods from his grandfather, John Codman (4), whose conservative nature and adamantine tendencies were described thusly, "... when this Congregational minister became aware that his flock was likely to be contaminated by the teachings of his brother preachers, he refused to allow any other than his own discourses in his church in Dorchester. A hostile element placed another minister in the pulpit and protected him there by a guard. But John Codman climbed up the steps as high as he could, addressed the congregation and walked out with a large majority of those in the church. The opposition soon gave in."[9]

John Codman (4), the minister, had two male children, John Codman (5) and William Coombs Codman. John Codman (5) (1814-1900) was Ernest Amory Codman's uncle and his most famous ancestor.

John Codman (5) was born in Dorchester, where his theologian father lived. John and William were exposed not only to the teachings of their father but the teachings of many clergymen as well. Their home was a favorite gathering place for clergymen on their travels through Boston and many evenings were spent with the children receiving extensive theological education as their father and his friends argued doctrinal questions from dinner until bedtime while they indulged freely of the Codman family's supply of rum and smoking tobacco.

However, John Codman (5) was more entranced by his maternal grandfather, Henry Wheelwright, who was a Newburyport (Massachusetts) sea captain. His interest in seafaring stories told to him by grandfather Wheelwright eventually led to his first career, that of a sea captain. John Codman (5) briefly attended Amherst College, but withdrew to go to sea in a clipper ship. His nautical career lasted until the end of the Civil War. He made numerous trips to China and the East Indies and during the Crimean War, commanded the *William*

8Homans, pg. 296.

9*Ibid.*

Penn, which carried troops from Constantinople (Istanbul) to the Crimean region. During the Civil War, Captain Codman was the captain of the *Quaker City* which was used to transport stores and supplies to South Carolina.

After giving up his life at sea, John Codman (5) settled near Boston and became a writer, borrowing heavily from his wartime and seagoing adventures. He was also an enthusiastic horseman who occasionally traveled from Boston to New York on horseback and briefly owned a ranch in Idaho. His books included *Sailors' Life and Sailors' Yarns* (1847), *Ten Months in Brazil* (1867), *The Roundtrip* (1879—"describing a tour of the western states"), *Winter Sketches From the Saddle* (1888), and *An American Transport in the Crimean War* (1896).

John Codman's (5) brother, William Coombs Codman (1821-1903), lived a slightly more pedestrian life. He began his business career engaged as an importer in the East India trade. When he was 37 years old, he married a younger woman, the former Elizabeth Hurd, who was then 22. Their marriage would produce four children. The Codmans settled in Boston, eventually living at 23 West Cedar Street in Boston from the 1860s until their deaths. He survived Elizabeth Hurd (1836-1896) by seven years.

The first of William and Elizabeth Codman's children was Anna Gertrude Codman, who was born on 1 May 1859. Few details are known of her life although notes in the Codman Archives make it obvious that she was not a normal child. There are no precise descriptions of the nature of her physical or mental disabilities, but she was institutionalized from a young age.[10] There are numerous letters to and from Ernest Amory Codman which discuss Anna and her problems. He was left as her overseer although it does not appear that he visited her often after she was institutionalized.

Despite the distance of separation and her disability, Ernest Amory Codman took great care of his sister. A 1903 letter which he received from the Hotel Chasen in St. Louis, notes, "I made a good long call on Annie at the Grafton in Washington and we also saw Miss Von

---

10In the Codman Archives, there are several letters from Anna Codman to Amory Codman but, unfortunately, her handwriting is virtually unintelligible.

Nordeck and Miss Putnam. I think we were with Annie almost an hour. She seems serene and at peace with the world, and it is a great pleasure to me to carry away such a memory of her. You must feel great satisfaction, after all your years of anxiety, and brotherly care, to have such a fortunate outcome."[11] Anna Codman died in 1937 leaving only a few small personal possessions that were noted to have a total value at her death of $107.50. [12]

The next Codman child was William Coombs Codman, Jr. who was born on 6 August 1860. He was Ernest Amory Codman's older brother and would not survive him, dying in 1938, two years before Amory. With another brother, John, he would inherit his father's real estate and insurance business, which the father had entered after giving up the East India Trade. Their brokerage firm, Codman & Codman, was based at 40 Kilby Street in Boston, but they were in business together for only a few years. John Codman, Jr. was born on 16 January 1863, and was the first member of his family to finish college, graduating from Harvard in 1885. Unfortunately, John Codman died fairly young, on 31 August 1897, after having suffered for many years with a congenital heart ailment.

Ernest Amory Codman was William and Elizabeth Codman's last child. (Figure 1) Born on 30 December 1869, he would eventually become the most famous and most successful member of the family, but with a success that would never be measured in financial terms. He spent his early years living with his family at 23 West Cedar Street, until he entered boarding school. [13]

11CA 7/139. All future footnote references to "CA #/#" refer to holdings of the Codman Archives found in the Rare Book Room of the Countway Medical Library at Harvard Medical School in Boston. The numbers refer to the box and folder numbers. Thus, this reference is to "Codman Archives, Box 7, Folder 139."

12CA 7/139.

13The house at 23 West Cedar Street, an old Boston brownstone, was built in 1836, and still exists to this day, with the exterior of the building apparently being little changed from the late 19th century, although plumbing and electricity has been added. It was one of a pair of mirror image houses, the other now being 25 West Cedar Street. The Codman's old house at 23 West Cedar Street was later converted into apartment buildings, but has since been re-converted into a single family dwelling. Almost no structural changes to 25 West Cedar Street have been made since its construction in 1836.

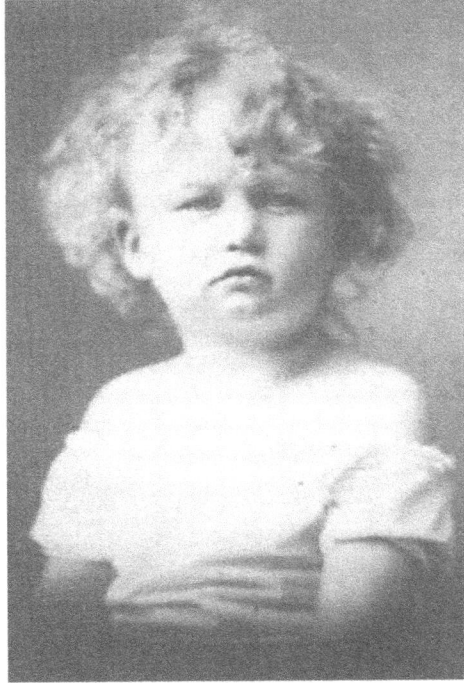

Figure 1—"Baby Codman with eyes so blue, crown with curls like glory."
The first known photograph of E. Amory Codman. (Courtesy Francis A.
Countway Library of Medicine, Rare Books and Special Collections
Department)

Many of his most important letters, papers and books were written under the name E. A. Codman, and one often sees the name Ernest A. Codman used to describe him by writers of the later 20th century. However, he almost never used the name Ernest, being known to his family and to his friends in his early life as Amory, although strangely, it was pronounced "Emery."[14] In his later life he was usually called "Cod" by his closest friends.[15]

14Twitchell EB. Personal correspondence.

15Quinby WC. "Recollections of Grouse Hunting with Amory Codman," in *Codman, A Study in Hospital Efficiency*, pg. 1 (Oakbrook Terrace, Illinois, Joint Commission and Accreditation of Health Organizations, 1996)

The first recorded mention of Amory Codman as a child is in a poem, written by a family friend, Miss Bailey, when he was only three years old:

Baby Codman with eyes so blue, crown with curls like glory,
Cheeks of the fair azalea's hue—
Thus I commence my story.

Baby Codman is so pretty, and also very fair;
He ne'er is a child who is fretty,
Showing a good mother's care.

In slumber sweet unconscious sprite!
Bright angels guard thee from all harms;
I think of thee a vision bright,
But not without alarm. [16]

How prophetic that last stanza would prove to be.

Codman's upbringing was definitely that of the elite, cultured class—the Brahmins. By all accounts, his was a happy childhood, although he did not spend much of it at home, which was a relatively normal occurrence for children from his class in that era. His early years, in fact, gave no hint whatsoever that young Codman would become, to the medical world, a heretic and iconoclast.

16CA 10/199.

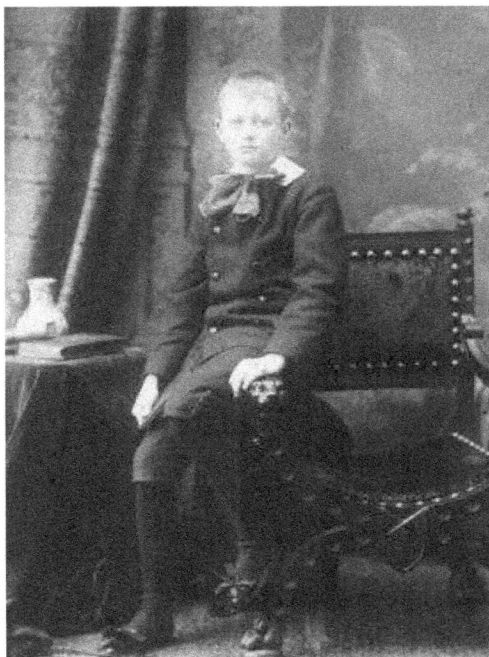

Figure 2—Codman during his days as a student at The Fay School in Southborough, Massachusetts. (Courtesy Francis A. Countway Library of Medicine, Rare Books and Special Collections Department)

After finishing the 2nd grade, Codman spent ten years in school in Southborough, Massachusetts, a Boston suburb about 25 miles west of Boston. From the 3rd grade through the 6th he attended The Fay School, a private boarding school, and from then until high school graduation, he went to Saint Mark's School in Southborough. (Figure 2) The two schools were located within a mile of one another and were ideal training grounds for a life in medicine and science in the late 19th century.

Saint Mark's School (Figure 3A) was founded by Joseph Burnett, a doctor who never practiced, but worked as a chemist and apothecary. The chemical company he founded eventually provided much of the ether which was used for early anesthetics. Joseph Burnett settled in Southborough, where he used his chemical fortune to settle in as a gentleman farmer, and he became the largest employer in the town. All of his family had had a rich educational background, especially scientific, and Burnett wished to carry on that tradition with his several sons. His oldest son attended St. Paul's Academy in Concord, New Hampshire, but the headmaster there suggested that Burnett should start his own independent boarding school for the rest of his sons. This led to Saint Mark's, which opened in 1865 (Figure 3B-C), attended in the early years mostly by Burnett's sons and their friends.

Joseph Burnett's sister, Eliza Bell Burnett Fay, wished to be a Chinese missionary, but her brother needed a "feeder" school for Saint Mark's and asked her to open a small boarding school for the elementary grades. Originally called Mrs. Fay's School, it opened in 1866, and was also populated early on by Burnett cousins, friends, and many of the Southborough neighborhood children.

Both schools emphasized science from the very beginning. By the 1880s, Saint Mark's established itself among the top tier of New England prep schools. In that time, almost 100% of the Saint Mark's' graduates attended either Harvard or Yale, with an occasional student going to another well-known institution, such as Dartmouth, Amherst, or West Point. It would have been difficult in 1880 to find better preparatory schools for a young man who wished to pursue a career in the sciences or medicine.[17]

During Codman's years at Saint Mark's School, his hobbies were those which would remain with him his whole life, hunting, fishing and trapping. He also showed some interest in both baseball and football, and despite some knee problems, he played on the Saint Mark's baseball team during his sophomore year.[18] It is during his years at Saint Mark's that we first come to know something of Amory Codman, as the Codman Archives contain numerous letters to and from his parents and his brothers and sister.

The first known description of Codman as a student came from the headmaster at Saint Mark's School, William Peck on 20 September 1881. He noted, "Amory is doing well, I never saw so great a change in

---

17My sources for background information on the history of The Fay School and Saint Mark's School are Mr. Nick Noble, historian of both schools, and a teacher at The Fay School (and formerly Saint Mark's), and the current headmaster of Saint Mark's School, Mr. Anthony J. deV. Hill.

18*Ibid.*

any boy. Your visit has wrought wonders in the boy; he is at his best, and we enjoy his good behavior and so does he."[19]

Once he began school, Codman lived with his family and his parents for only a few months of each year. But this was typical of the Boston Brahmins, who often sent their children away to boarding schools. There is no indication that he felt unloved or neglected. An example is the first recorded note to his mother, written in February 1883 in the form of a Valentine poem.

This Valentine I send to one, who's just "fair, fat and forty".
She is not a little nun so very high and haughty.
She is just as sweet as sweet can be though loved by none so well as me.
Her hair is brown, her eyes are blue, she is just the daisy I bet you.
You ask, "Who is this little dame of whom you so highly raise the flame,"
Then I shall vow she is no other than my sweet dear darling Mother.[20]

However, he was not above admonishing her occasionally, as he did in a letter of April 1886, "I was surprised to find a mistake in your English in your last letter-you used 'between all those' instead of 'among'."[21]

Amory Codman's love for the outdoors, and hunting and fishing, first began to surface in 1883, when he was 14. He was apparently promised a gun by his older brother, John, and asked about this several times during letters home, including one in which he emphatically asked, "Has John picked out my gun yet???"[22]

During his time at Saint Mark's, Codman wrote fairly typical letters back to his parents, often related to his hobby involving the out-of-doors. In July 1883 he wrote to his parents asking for money for some slugs and darts for his air pistol. In July 1884 he asked his father for eight dollars for money to take "stuffing" (taxidermy) lessons which he had arranged to take from a man in nearby Sterling, Massachusetts.

19CA 7/141.

20CA 7/128.

21CA 7/131.

22CA 7/129.

Of course, like many children away at school, the occasional letter to his parents concerning his grades was necessary. Although Codman later became an esteemed doctor, he was far from one of the outstanding pupils at Saint Mark's early in his career.

> **Southborough, 1883**
> **Dear Father:**
> I received your letter reproving me for my bad scholarship and I had a talking to from Mr. P. My average last month was only .7 lower than the month before when I stood second in my class. Last month there were seven fellows below me and only five above. I will try to do much better this month. I like this school very much and hope to graduate from it.
> **In great haste,**
> **E. Amory Codman**[23]

Codman occasionally combined the two most common topics of correspondence from schoolchildren to their parents at home by discussing both his need of money and his problems with his grades. In a letter dated 18 January 1885 he prepared his father for the worst in a letter:

> **Dear Father:**
> On my next report you will probably see 0 for decorum. It is not for anything so very bad. It was only a prank such as I do very often and happened to be caught. I am to be punished pretty severely for it. I am need of money and a fiver would be very acceptable. Trying to do better I remain,
> **Your affectionate son,**
> **E. A. Codman**[24]

---

[23]CA 7/131.

[24]CA 7/128.

Amory Codman also began to have some occasional physical problems while in school, one of which, a problem with his left knee, would bother him much of his life. He mentioned it several times in his letters home.

> July 1885:
> **My dear Father:**
> **I am having quite a nice time up here and have some very fair fishing. I am giving my leg a good rest and it is very much better.**[25]

He then went on to ask his father for further money.

> February 19, 1886
> **My dear Father:**
> **I am very sorry to be obliged to tell you that my knee is a good deal worse. Please don't tell Mamma, however, she might be worried and it is no worse than it has been before.**[26]
> April 18, 1887
> **My dearest brother:**
> **My knee did not think I had better go to church so I do the next best thing and write to you. Jack has got home and I think looks much better.**[27]

The last letter above also mentioned the health problems of his brother, John, for the first time in the archival record.

Amory Codman was the son of very Puritanical parents and descended from very conservative religious families. However, he himself was never highly religious. He was raised an Episcopalian but, after his school days, he never practiced formal religion to any degree. Even during that time it was obvious he was having questions

---

25CA 7/130.

26CA 7/131.

27CA 7/132.

concerning his own faith and beliefs as noted in two letters he sent to his mother from Saint Mark's.

> **January 11, 1885**
> **Dear Mother:**
> I went to the Holy Communion on last Sunday as you wished, and I think it did me some good. Just before I left, Papa said to me that he wished me to go at least once a fortnight—but I did not promise.[28]
> **21 March 1886**
> **My dear Mother:**
> I am afraid I cannot come down to see you this week. I cannot think of any rational excuse. I went to Communion this morning. Have you the remotest idea where you are going next summer?[29]

Though the mentions of faith and religion in the Codman Archives are brief, it is certainly in character with Amory Codman. He would later profess to be an atheist.

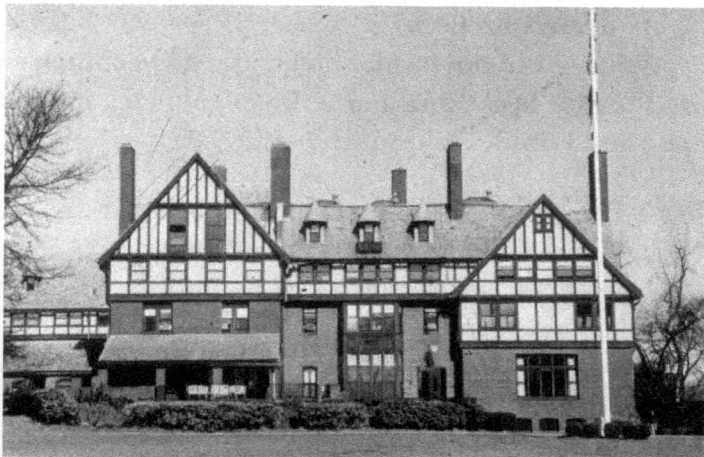

28CA 7/130.

29CA 7/131.

Figure 3A—Saint Mark's School, where Codman attended high school, as it looks today. (Courtesy Saint Mark's School, Southborough, Massachusetts)

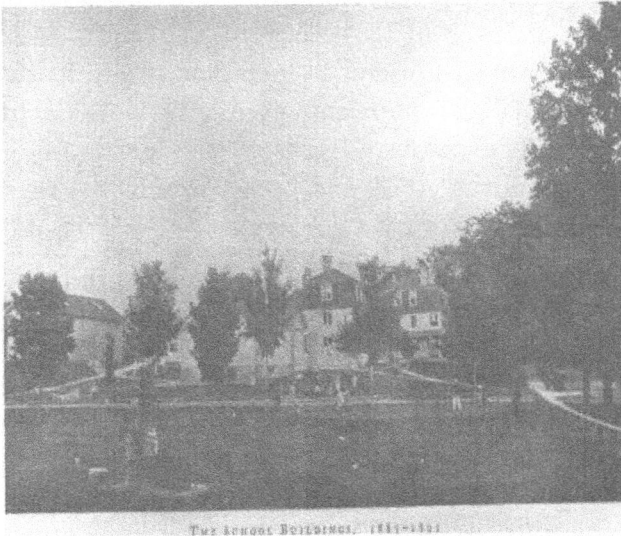

THE SCHOOL BUILDINGS. 1865-1891

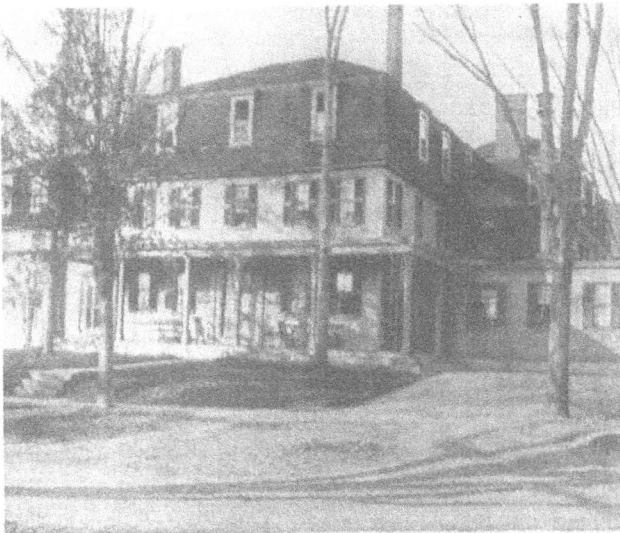

THE OLD SCHOOL BUILDING. ABOUT 1887

Figure 3B-C—Two views of Saint Mark's School in the era in which Codman attended school there. (Courtesy Saint Mark's School, Southborough, Massachusetts)

Codman's early performance as a student at Saint Mark's was only average although he improved significantly during his stay there, eventually reaching the top of his form, which was then Saint Mark's terminology for a class.[30] In 1881-82, in the first form (seventh grade), he was ranked 18th of 58 students in the school. Saint Mark's graded at that time on a 0 to 10 scale, although giving the marks to the tenth of a point, so effectively it was similar to later standard grading of 0 to 100. Marks were given out monthly and were based on a series of tests and classroom recitations. Codman survived only on his ability in class recitation—his test grades were initially very poor.

Codman's grades in the fall of 1882, starting second form (eighth grade), ranged from a 4.0 for decorum to a 10.0 for neatness. His best subjects at that time were science, for which he received a grade of 9.3 in November. In 1883-84, in the third form (ninth grade), he was noted to have actually gone backwards somewhat, ranking now 39th in a class of 60, with relatively low grades. However, Amory Codman's last three years at Saint Mark's were decidedly better academically. In his sophomore year he ranked 14th in the school and second in the fourth form (tenth grade).

In the spring of his sophomore year, despite his knee problems, he did play baseball, although he appeared in only two varsity games. Perhaps his sophomore athletic feats inspired him, for in the fall of 1885, then a junior (fifth former), he was a rusher (lineman) on the football team and also played in the annual school tennis tournament, partnering another student described in the Saint Mark's Archives only as Barnes. They won one match, and were eliminated in the second round.

And Codman continued to improve academically during his junior year. He was now sixth in the school and second in the form, although he led the form in November. In the spring of his junior year, Amory received a 5.0 for decorum in April. Was he punished for this? We

---

[30]All of the following data on Codman's grades can be found in the Archives at Saint Mark's Academy. They were unearthed for me via the daunting work of Mr. Nick Noble, historian at The Fay School (where Codman attended school from the 3rd through the 6th grade), and former archivist at Saint Mark's. All of Codman's grades can be found. I have not included them in their entirety, as it seems a bit pedantic, but will leave a copy of them to the Codman Archives at the Countway Library, for the use of future Codman biographers.

cannot tell precisely, but he was not at school in May 1886, returning in June, and Noble speculates that it may have been a punishment for something he did in April. Was it possibly early signs of Codman angering the establishment?[31]

By his senior year, Codman was the top student at Saint Mark's, but the year is a bit of a puzzle. He ranked first in the school in December (9.02) and first in the form for the year, and he received the highest honor given a graduating Saint Mark's student, The Founders' Medal, signifying him as the best student in the sixth form (senior class). But he inexplicably missed three of the 10 months of the school year. He did not start school in September, although the reason is not given to us. And he was not there in April or May of 1887, although he returned for June, in time to receive marks above 9.0 on all his final exams.

It is not exactly certain why Codman missed April and May of his senior year, but his letters do tell us that he was travelling. During those months, Amory and his brother, Jack, took a trip together to North Carolina. They arrived in Asheville, North Carolina on 10 April 1887 and Amory wrote identical letters that day to his mother and father. He noted that Jack had gone away for a trip on horseback for a few days and would be back on Thursday. Several other letters from this trip are written from Hot Springs, a town very near the western border of North Carolina. Thermal springs had been discovered in Hot Springs in 1778, and it had been a health resort since the early 1800s.

Amory had several problems during this trip with his knee, described it limiting his activities several times, and also noted that it had swelled up on him frequently. In addition, he also mentioned Jack's health problems in his correspondence. From the letters it is apparent that Jack, who would die young, was already somewhat ill. Most likely, the trip to the spas of Hot Springs and Asheville were to help Jack's health, and maybe even Amory's. Or perhaps they simply wished to spend some time together, knowing Jack's condition to be tenuous, and his time short.

---

31 Noble N. Personal correspondence, 9 February 1997.

Codman returned in early June, in time to graduate from Saint Mark's at the top of the class. His headmaster sent the following letter to Amory's parents:

> July 13, 1887,
> My dear Mr. Codman,
> Ernest leaves Saint Mark's with an excellent record for behavior and scholarship. He takes with him my best wishes for future success.
> Virtually yours,
> William E. Peck[32]

Noble, who has studied many Saint Mark's student records from that era, has summarized his findings of Codman's years in Southborough, "Very bright, fastidious to the point of obsessiveness (neat, punctual, precise), independent, something of a loner, not a joiner, marches to his own drummer (hence erratic conformity and behavior), congenial and popular despite (or perhaps because) of this. Perhaps some of his decorum difficulties stem from constant questioning and challenging ... not uncommon in a mind like Codman's. But frustrating as hell for the typical teacher of the 1880s. A bit mischievous, and not reluctant to accept a challenge (this might also account for his popularity)."[33]

All this foreshadows his later life. Fastidious—the record keeper, the hunting diary, the End Result Idea; marches to his own drummer— he would later demonstrate this in spades; constant questioning and challenging—again presaging his work on End Results, and much of his other medical work; mischievous and not reluctant to accept a challenge—with the End Result Idea, he would never back down; and finally, congenial and popular.

But however difficult he may have been for the teachers at Saint Mark's, the school had prepared him well for the next part of his life. Codman took the natural next step for a Saint Mark's graduate by proceeding on to Harvard College. It was a step he took easily and what

---

32*Ibid.*

33Noble. *Op. Cit.*

should have been Codman's assumed ascendancy to the top of the medical world was well on its way.

CHAPTER 2

HARVARD SCHOOLDAYS

You can always tell a Harvard man, but you can't tell him much.

Attributed to James Barnes [1866-1936]

In October 1887 Amory Codman began his college career at Harvard in Cambridge, Massachusetts. The eight years he would spend in college and medical school at Harvard were apparently happy ones, "I was a conventional enough Boston-Harvard boy, with relatives and acquaintances among the well-to-do ... "[34] In his own description of his college days at Harvard, Codman noted that he had a successful first two years and in the third year began his travels to Europe.

Codman traveled a great deal during his college and medical school years. He spent the summer break after his freshman year in college in Vermont and New Hampshire where he stayed very active, and further cultivated his love of the outdoors. In a letter to his father, dated 20 July 1888, he wrote:

> **Dear Father:**
> I have arrived here in Brattleboro after having passed through a great deal of good times with just enough of hardship to make it sweeter. I leave here tomorrow and Monday I am going to Princeton for a

---

34Preface, p. viii.

week. While in Connecticut we ran the 15 Mile Falls, an almost unheard of exploit for canoes. We got through somehow with six or eight tip overs—once in the very worst place. This time my foot caught in this fall and I was dragged along down the falls under water.[35]

In the summer before his senior year he spent time in New Hampshire, Western Massachusetts, and on Cape Cod.

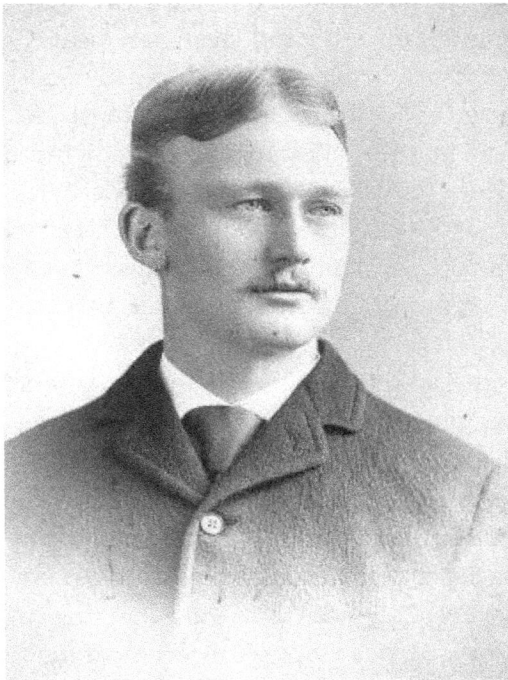

Figure 4—Amory Codman's Harvard College graduation photograph. (Courtesy Francis A. Countway Library of Medicine, Rare Books and Special Collections Department)

Unfortunately, little is known about his years at Harvard College as an undergraduate. The *Harvard Annual Report for 1886-1890*, however, lists the following classes as the most popular among

35CA 7/132.

Harvard students, in this order: 1) Latin, 2) Greek, 3) Latin Composition, 4) Greek Composition, 5) Solid Geometry, 6) French, and 7) Logarithms and Trigonometry. Given the era, his pre-medical bent, and the fact that he had studied them at Saint Mark's, it is almost certain that Codman studied both Latin and Greek. Further clues concerning his knowledge of these languages were given in his papers, when he frequently interspersed his writing with Latin and Greek phrases.[36]

Codman's freshman class consisted of 295 male students, but of that number, only 145 finished all four years, with many students in the Class of '91 being added after the freshman year. On 18 June 1891, Codman graduated *cum laude* from Harvard College having been accepted to Harvard Medical School. (Figure 4) He was one of 288 graduating seniors in 1891. Why he chose medicine as a career is not mentioned precisely in his books and journal articles, the writings of Harvey Cushing, or his papers. Nor does his ancestry help us, as there are no other doctors in his family tree. Perhaps his years at Saint Mark's School, with its strong emphasis on science inspired him to pursue medicine.

At this time the structure of medicine in America was changing rapidly, with specialization becoming more common among doctors. In addition, hospitals such as the Massachusetts General, were becoming of increasing importance to American medicine. Previously, hospital privileges were not deemed necessary to a physician's practice of medicine. However, with clinical medicine becoming increasingly dependent on the basic sciences, this was changing rapidly at the turn of the century. Harvard was among the foremost medical schools (as it remains to this day) in the United States, with its emphasis on clinical practice and a close affiliation with several Boston hospitals, including the Massachusetts General Hospital.[37]

At that time Harvard Medical School was located at the corner of Boylston and Exeter Streets in Boston, and Codman began his studies

---

36Unfortunately neither the Harvard Archives, Countway Medical Library, nor the Codman Archives provides us with any significant description of Codman's undergraduate years.

37Reverby, p. 157, quoting from her own source, S Reverby, "The search for the hospital yardstick: nursing and the rationalization of hospital work," in *Health Care in America: Essays in Social History*, ed. by Susan Reverby and David Rosner (Philadelphia: Temple University Press, 1979), pp. 206-225.

there in September 1891. In medical school Codman continued his successful academic career, earning a Ballard Scholarship and a George Cheyne Shattuck Scholarship. When he began medical school, he moved into his brother John's home, renting a room at 104 Mount Vernon Street. He would live there until 1904, after John's death and even after his own marriage. As a medical student, Amory also met the man who later became his best friend, Harvey Williams Cushing, who would become America's first well-known neurosurgeon. Cushing lived at 32 West Cedar Street during medical school, just down the road from Codman's birthplace, and diagonally across the corner from 104 Mount Vernon.

As with his undergraduate days, Codman's exact course of study in medical school has not survived, but he almost certainly took the standard courses required of all first- and second-year medical students. The standard first-year curriculum in 1891-92 consisted of anatomy, physiology, and medical chemistry. The standard second-year curriculum for 1892-93 consisted of advanced anatomy, pathologic anatomy, and therapeutics.

Near the end of their first-year in medical school, on 3 April 1892 to be precise, Codman and Cushing were both elected to the prestigious Boylston Medical Society.[38] They worked together as prosectors in the lab of Dr. Maurice [Howe] Richardson (1867-1912), of which Cushing noted, "Dr. Richardson's demonstrations have begun and are good fun though they have not given us much dissecting to do as yet."[39]

In John Fulton's excellent biography of Cushing, the friendship between Codman and Cushing is discussed frequently. Cushing obviously admired Codman greatly, as we can deduce from the following: "Went to Nahant with Codmans [for several days]. Rather cold for first few days but got warm enough by the fifth [June]. Got our meals for two days, then to club. I could not study well—was grouchy because Codman learns so much faster than I that I came back after six days—not a very pleasant guest."[40] And further: "I am now writing you

---

38Fulton J, *Harvey Cushing: A Biography*, (Springfield, IL: C. C. Thomas, 1946), p. 60.

39Fulton, p. 68.

40Fulton, p. 76.

while Codman sits here grinding over my Surgery notes and swearing at my writing. I wish I had his fourteen hours a day energy and enthusiasm. I get 'woozy' after about three."[41]

Codman and Cushing's time together did not consist only of academics and studying medicine. There are many passages in Cushing's writings about walking across bridges while looking at beautiful sunsets, walking out to the park and observing the first robin of spring, and going to pop concerts. Their friendship would continue throughout their lives.

During his third-year of medical school, beginning in December 1893, Codman took advantage of the opportunity to travel and study in Europe and Egypt. He commented on this in his Preface[42] to *The Shoulder*: "In the third winter I had the opportunity to travel in Europe and Egypt with a friend, on the understanding that I could spend as much time as I wished at the Clinics in various cities we visited, London, Paris, Berlin, Vienna, Cairo and others. This experience and some study on the way enabled me to pass my third year examinations and get my degree on my return."[43]

Codman wrote his parents several letters concerning those travels during his third year in medical school, including some from Berlin, London, Rome, and Cairo. There was little of note in the letters although he did mention that his knee was swelling up and bothering him again.

The European trip was very important to Codman's future career. While in Vienna, Codman studied with Professor [Eduard] Albert (1841-1900), who was the chief of the clinic at which Codman visited. This is probably what prompted his original interest in shoulder surgery and he described it in the Preface, "It was in Vienna that my attention was first attracted to the subdeltoid bursa, because it was mentioned in a little book by [Professor] E[duard] Albert, *Diagnöstik der Chirugischer Krankheiten* (Alfred Holder, Wien, 1893). I had never heard this bursa spoken of at home by my teachers, nor do I think it

---

41Fulton, p. 87.

42All future references to "the Preface (capitalized)" are to the Preface to Codman's last book, *The Shoulder*, pp. v-xl.

43Preface, p. vii.

was mentioned in American medical literature at that time. Soon after my return I served two years as surgical intern at the Massachusetts General Hospital in Boston, and during this period, sometimes made diagnoses of subdeltoid bursitis, which were ignored by my seniors."[44]

Codman completed his medical school studies after only three years, in 1894, although he would not graduate officially until 1895, with his entering class. He served what would have been his last year of medical school as an intern at the Massachusetts General Hospital. That year he was a house officer (resident) on the East Surgical Service, along with George L[awrence] Barney (1868-1898), Richard E[dward] Edes (1867-1901), and Frederick W[arren] Pearl (né 1868).[45] It was an important year in Codman's life, and also for the history of anaesthesia. During this year, Codman and Cushing worked together on what they called "ether charts." These were the first instance of monitoring a patient's anaesthetic course during a surgical procedure.

Several years later Codman remembered their development of the anesthesia charts in a letter to Cushing:

> **February 9, 1920**
> **Dear Harvey,**
> **Having nothing better to do lately I have been trying to put my effects into order again after the volcanic dislocation caused by the war and incidentally the renting of our house.**
> **Katie, after my departure, dumped all the accumulation of years into one pile. So during this [survey] weeks I have had old diaries, letters and unpublished attempts at "papers", mercilessly put them in the wastebasket. There are many things which remind me of you and show the stimulus you were to me. I am sorry that age now prevents me from reacting to your enthusiasm, and that I have ceased to cultivate**

44Preface, p. viii.

45Washburn FA, *The Massachusetts General Hospital: Its Development, 1900-1935*. Boston: Houghton-Mifflin, 1939, p. 617.

my mind enough to follow your soaring in pituitary function.

One of the things I cannot bear to dump in the wastebasket is a collection of ether charts which we made thirty years ago! In connection therewith I find a long <u>unpublished</u> paper on "etherization" in which I described <u>vividly</u> the process as we then knew it. I must say I never read anything better on the subject. I recall the reasons for not publishing it was, that I took it to "Coll Warren", who regarded it as too frank for the good of the hospital for it described in detail the case which I lost in the O.R. because I was paying attention to some tomfoolery which <u>you</u> (who had come in the theater) were entertaining us with, while the poor devil was inhaling vomitus! and also spoke of the case which stopped breathing under ether and interested you in brain surgery. So I send you these charts to destroy with some solemnity for you and I are the only persons that give a— — — — —for them. Do they give this ether per hour now?

Sincerely,

E. A. Codman[46]

It seems to us now the two cases Codman mentioned were devastating medical complications, and to Cushing it seemed that way as well. But anesthesia in 1895 was a poorly developed science and it was not uncommon for people to die during relatively simple operations. Part of the problem was that their condition could not be followed closely, as the monitors and machines which today accurately trace the patients' vital signs did not exist when Cushing and Codman were in medical school. And even if they did exist, prior to 1895 the patients' condition was simply not recorded while under ether (anesthesia). The development of the anesthesia record gave doctors a method to record their monitoring of the patient. Though this seems

---

46Beecher HK. The first anesthesia records (Codman, Cushing). *Surg Gyn Obst*, 71: 689-693, 1940, also contained in the Anaesthesia Charts contained in the Codman Archives.

basic to us at the end of the 20th century, it was anything but 100 years ago.

After receiving Codman's letter in 1920, Cushing wrote the next day to the superintendent of the Massachusetts General Hospital, Dr. Frederic A. Washburn, concerning the anesthesia charts:

> 10 February 1920
> My Dear Dr. Washburn:
> I have just received the accompanying note from Codman with these old ether charts of the year 1895. So far as I am aware they represent the first attempt made anywhere to keep charts during anaesthesia, and the story is as follows:
> When Dr. Codman and I, having entered the hospital together, were "Junior House Pupils" I believe was the official term, or "House Pups", the unofficial one, we gave the anaesthesia, as is the custom I believe now, twenty-five years later.
> I hesitate to recall what an awful business it was and how many fatalities there were.
> My first giving of an anaesthetic was when, a third-year student, I was called from the seats and sent in a little side room with a patient and an orderly and told to put the patient to sleep, for Dr. ... was to operate for the class. I knew nothing about the patient whatsoever, merely that a nurse came in and gave the patient a hypodermic injection. I proceeded as best I could under the orderly's directions, and in view of the repeated urgent calls for the patient from the amphitheater it seemed to me an interminable time for the old man, who kept gagging, to go to sleep. We finally wheeled him in. I can vividly recall, even now, just how he looked and the feel of his bedraggled whiskers. The operation was started and at this juncture there was a sudden great gush of fluid from the patient's mouth, most of which was inhaled, and he died.

I stood aside, burning with chagrin and remorse. No one paid the slightest attention to me, though I supposed that I had killed the patient. The operation was completed in spite of the episode, as a demonstration to the class. I slunk out of the hospital, walked the streets of North Boston the rest of the afternoon, and in the evening went to the surgeon's house to ask if there was any possible way I could atone for the calamity to the man's family before I left the Medical School and went into some other business.

To my perfect amazement I was told it was nothing at all, that I had nothing to do with the man's death, that he had a strangulated hernia and had been vomiting all night anyway, and that sort of thing happened frequently and I had better forget about it and go on with the Medical School. I went on with the Medical School but I have never forgotten about it.

Now, to come back to these ether charts, Codman and I resolved that we would improve our technique of giving ether, which in those days in the large majority of cases meant crowding the patient into the second stage of anaesthesia as quickly as possible, and for the most part we used old sea sponges.

In order to make a game of this task before us we made a wager of a dinner as to who would learn to give the best anaesthesia. We determined to let the test of satisfactory anaesthesia rest with the patient's behavior in the ward, and though I have forgotten just what was our skill of marking the cases, a perfect anaesthesia was supposed to be one in which the patient was sufficiently conscious to respond when left on the ward with the nurse and did not subsequently vomit. You will recall in those days we had no ether recovery room for general use, except for the Saturday clinics.

I think we both became very much more skillful on our jobs than otherwise would have become, owing to this competition, but it was particularly due, I think, to the detailed attention which we had to put upon the patient by the careful recording of the pulse rate throughout the operation.

...

I have been moved to write all of this because of the memories which have crowded in owing to a sight of these old charts, and, simple as they are, you will see that Codman and I each got up our own type of chart. I am sorry the final score is not given, nor do I remember who had to pay for the dinner. I am quite sure, however, that I did, for Codman usually managed to beat me in most things.

...

We are still, some of us, only too careless in its use, and some studies as Dr. Cutler's and Dr. Morton made during their term of residency at the M.G.H. pointing out the frequency of post-anaesthesia pulmonary complications, are but a further step in the direction of improving our technique in its administration. I still feel that one of the most important elements in the giving of an anaesthetic is to have the anaesthetist keep during its administration a detailed chart of pulse, respiration, and blood pressure. At the time of his notable address some years ago on Ether Day, Dr. Keen, who took up this subject, intimated that too elaborate a record of this kind might take the administrator's mind from his primary job. I feel most emphatically this keeps his mind <u>on</u> his job.

Please put this in a corner of the Treadwell Library, where someday some young fellow may brush the dust from it and say who were these fellows anyway and what is this "ether" they are talking about? "Do

you mean people used to be put to sleep by the inhalation of drugs in the 19th century?"
Very sincerely yours,
Harvey Cushing[47]

Again, Cushing's admiration of Codman is evident from the line in the above letter, "I am quite sure, however, that I did, for Codman usually managed to beat me in most things."[48]

Codman's contribution to the development of the anesthesia record, or ether charts, is probably his first foray into the End Result Idea. Essentially, the End Result Idea is nothing but closely monitoring the patient to determine outcomes. The anesthesia record was initially developed not for this end, but as a way of improving the delivery of anesthesia, and to improve the safety of surgery for the patient. However, it is Codman's first known effort at better monitoring of medical interventions, and, as he would say later in his life, using it as a method to improve medical care.

In 1939, Dr. Henry K[nowles] Beecher (1904-1976) of the Massachusetts General Hospital researched Cushing and Codman's early anesthesia records and unearthed the above two letters. He corresponded with Codman on the topic who, characteristically, gave the credit elsewhere, to Dr. Francis B. Harrington, who was to become his surgical mentor. Codman wrote,

I have not seen the exhibit [the anesthesia records] in the Treadwell Library but I shall take an early opportunity to look at it, and have no doubt that I will not have any objection to its publication.

I do not wish to take any credit for starting the charts because of my recollection the keeping of these charts was suggested by my chief, Dr. F. B. Harrington. I, of course, did the work but it was Dr. Harrington who thought that such a study would be valuable. If I recollect correctly, Doctor Cushing took up the work

---

47*Ibid.*, pp. 689, 691-693.

48CA 5/109.

after I had finished my work as etherizer for I am quite sure that Doctor Cushing got his appointment about eight months later than I did, although we were in the same class in medical school.[49]

A week later Codman wrote another letter to Dr. Beecher:

I have been to the Treadwell and seen the charts. Dr. Cushing has a way of making things interesting and dramatic even at the expense of a little inaccuracy. I recall nothing about the dinner he speaks of, or of our determination to improve the techniques of anæsthesia, but we were anxious to train ourselves to be good etherizers!

I took the opportunity to find the dates of our appointments as H.O.'s. As I thought, I preceded him about 8 months and am quite sure that I had already begun the use of charts at the suggestion of Dr. Harrington before H.C. appeared on the scene at all![50]

Beecher concludes his article by summarizing that the first anesthesia records were kept at the suggestion of Dr. Harrington, first by Amory Codman and later by Harvey Cushing. They are an important milestone in the history of anesthesiology and their use early in the 20th century was probably responsible for saving the lives of many patients undergoing surgery. They are Codman's first major contribution to improving the quality of medical care.

Amory Codman graduated officially from Harvard Medical School on 26 June 1895, after serving his surgical internship. There are vague references by Cushing that Codman was either at the top or near the top of his class, although again, as with his college records, details are lacking. Already he had made a landmark contribution to one field of medicine, anesthesiology, and he was given an appointment as an Assistant Surgeon to Out-Patients at the Massachusetts General

---

49Beecher, p. 693.

50*Ibid.*

Hospital. His life would be forever inextricably intertwined with the Massachusetts General Hospital, though the relationship would not always be a friendly one. Codman's pugnacity and obstinacy, which we have had not yet seen demonstrated overtly in his life, would be the cause of that.

CHAPTER 3
FIRST DECADE OF PRACTICE

Things are always at their best in their beginning (Les choses valent toujours mieux dans leur source).

Blaise Pascal, *Lettres Provinciales*, No. 2, [1656-57]

After graduating from Harvard Medical School, Codman began the practice of medicine. Today, after finishing medical school all doctors are required to serve an internship and virtually all doctors then finish a residency in some area of specialization. In 1895 it was common for medical school graduates to go directly into the practice of medicine, after finishing a one-year internship. Codman served his internship this during his last year in medical school, and began the practice of medicine in the summer of 1895.

Codman's initial position in practice was as an Assistant in Anatomy at the Harvard Medical School. In addition, however, he did take on a type of residency position, or what was then called an apprenticeship, to the Chief of the Surgical Service at the Massachusetts General Hospital, Dr. Francis Bishop Harrington (1854-1914), as Assistant Surgeon to Out-Patients, while, "… still continuing to work in the Surgical Outpatient Department of the M.G.H. and to assist the late Dr. F. B. Harrington in the practice of surgery."[51]

---

51 Preface, p. ix.

Frank Harrington was one of the most revered surgeons in Boston in that era, and served as a mentor to Codman. Harrington had graduated from Tufts in 1877, and received his M.D. degree from Harvard in 1881. From 1911-14 he was the Chief of the East Surgical Service at the Massachusetts General Hospital. It was written of him, "Honest and straightforward, he was friendly and sympathetic. His patients were devoted to him. The world was poorer when he died. Drs. E. A. Codman and Lincoln Davis (né 1872) were his pupils."[52] Harrington obviously had a great influence on Codman, as he thanked him often in his early medical papers.

From 1896 to 1899 Codman worked diligently in the anatomy department, mainly dissecting the shoulder and exploring the joints and bursae of the shoulder. He had become interested in the subacromial bursa during his medical school trip to Vienna when he read about it in the aforementioned book by Albert, *Diagnöstik der Chirugischer Krankheiten.*

At almost the same time as Codman began his practice, in December 1895, the German Wilhelm Conrad Röntgen (1845-1923) discovered X-rays. Röntgen's discovery was a landmark in the history of medicine, although it was somewhat serendipitous. Röntgen used what was known as a Crookes tube which was a vacuum tube named for Professor, Sir William Crookes (1832-1919) of England. In many laboratories throughout the world, scientists had been studying the effects of electrical current in a Crookes vacuum tube. On the day of Röntgen's initial discovery, a piece of barium-platinum-cyanide paper was lying on the laboratory floor near a Crookes tube and the paper became luminous when an electric current was passed through the tube. Röntgen immediately realized that some form of radiation had been generated from the tube and was being projected beyond the glass walls of the tube. He then carried out a carefully designed set of experiments which first elucidated the salient features of X-radiation.[53]

Codman was fascinated by the new X-ray device and immediately began to explore its ability to aid in the study of anatomy and to help

---

52Washburn FA, p. 74.

53As of this writing, the centennial of the discovery of X-rays and Röntgen's first paper on that subject has only recently been celebrated.

understand more about disease processes. He combined his anatomic dissections with X-ray studies of bones and joints. For his X-ray studies, Codman sought the help of Professor William Trowbridge (1843-1923) of Harvard and also Professor Elihu Thomson (1853-1937) of the General Electric Company in Lynn, Massachusetts. Trowbridge and Thomson taught him the basics of working the Crookes tube and creating X-radiation, and Codman began his clinical work with X-rays in 1896.

Based on a comment made by Codman in May 1940, as recorded by Fulton in his biography of Cushing, it is not certain if the Massachusetts General Hospital had a Crookes tube or any other device capable of generating X-radiation in 1895: "Thomson (Elihu) invented the double focus tube for alternating current at almost the same time in this country. My recollection is that Dr. [John Collins] Warren brought the tube home at my request because I had read of it in the *Lancet* or *B.M.J.* [*Boston Medical and Surgical Journal*] .... I don't think that I have ever written anything on the early X-ray days except what is in the preface to my book, *The Shoulder*."[54]

Apparently Codman collaborated with Harvey Cushing once again in his early work with X-rays. Cushing, himself, noted, "No X-ray photos had been taken at the Johns Hopkins Hospital when I came down in the fall of 1896. Codman and I had been fooling with some exposures at the Mass. Genl. using an old static machine, and he continued for about ten years more until it obviously affected his physical condition."[55] Despite Cushing's comment concerning Codman's health, there are no further notes in the Codman Archives concerning his physical condition during this era, except for a brief mention in the Preface that, in 1897, he had had the lateral meniscus of the left knee removed, which was the knee that had bothered him all of his years at Saint Mark's and at Harvard.

Codman also worked on X-rays with Walter Bradford Cannon (1871-1945), a Harvard physiologist, who pioneered X-ray studies of the alimentary tract. In an article written in 1990, Neuhauser noted that,

---

54Fulton, p. 115.

55*Ibid.*

"On December 29, 'the first demonstration of movement of the alimentary canal by means of x-ray in the conscious animal' was presented by Codman and W[alter] B[radford] Cannon to participants of the annual meeting of the American Physiological Society. They created a sensation when they were the first to use Roentgen's x-rays for physiological purposes."[56]

In another recent article, Dr. Francis Moore mentioned Cannon's own description of his early collaboration with Codman:

> Almost fifty years later, Dr. Cannon wrote to Dr. John Fulton at Yale, (under date of April 16, 1942) some details of this early experience with the new rays, "The early apparatus used in Boston came altogether from Swett and Lewis of Bromfield Street. It was their tubes which we used in the early work by Dr. Codman and by me. They were trifling affairs compared to the modern tubes and fairly soon became useless because of a hole burned through the very thin anode. I was not at any time associated with Walter Dodd. Dr. Amory Codman, however, brought a tube, a large secondary coil and an interrupter to the Medical School early in December, 1896. The apparatus was set up in the small prosectors' room in the anatomy department of the Medical School at the corner of Boylston and Exeter Streets. It was thought best to try first a small dog as a subject and I was commissioned to get a card of globular pearl buttons for the dog to swallow. Dr. Dwight, professor of anatomy, and Dr. Bowditch, Dr. Codman and I were the only witnesses. We placed a fluorescent screen over the dog's esophagus and with the greenish light on the tube shining below we watched it glow on the fluorescent surface. Everyone was keyed up with tense excitement. It was my function to place the pearl button as far back

---

56Neuhauser D. Ernest Amory Codman, M.D., and end results of medical care. *Int J Tech Assessment Health Care*, 6: 307-325, 1990, p. 308.

as possible in the dog's throat so he would swallow it. Nothing was seen! As the intensity of our interest increased, someone exploded "Button, button who's got the button!" Then we all broke out in a sort of hysterical laughter.[57]

Thus, while working as an Assistant in Anatomy, and Assistant to Dr. Harrington as essentially a surgical resident, Codman continued his work with X-rays and became one of the nation's first skiagraphers, now called radiologists.[58] After two years of these radiographic studies, Codman published his first paper in the medical literature entitled, "Experiments on the Application of the Roentgen Rays to the Study of Anatomy."[59] (He had earlier had five letters published as "Correspondence" in the *Boston Medical and Surgical Journal*—see Codman's *curriculum vitæ* in the appendices for these references)

The article was published in the *Journal of Experimental Medicine* in March 1898, and was the result of his two years of anatomic studies of normal joints in various positions. Concurrent with this he produced a huge album of normal anatomic X-rays of each joint of the body in varying positions—flexion, extension, and various positions of deviation and rotation. Codman later commented, "It was a tremendous piece of work, and for me at that time, a very expensive one. Recently, in poking around the Museum, I came across this album covered with dust. It probably had not been open since left there … Furthermore the fact that my atlas of the normal joints was not used by my colleagues, was a good lesson to my personal sensitiveness and taught me, to some extent, to postpone hope of recognition of labor."[60] It was not the last time that Codman would find little recognition for

---

57Moore, p. 17.

58Skiagraphy is the original name for radiology in this country and a skiagram is the original name used in the early literature for X-rays. *Skia-* is a Greek root meaning shadow, hence the obvious use of the name for X-rays.

59*J Exp Med*, 3(3): 383-391, 1898.

60Preface, p. x.

his work, and presaged the reception his End Result Idea would receive from the Boston medical community.

Codman's first paper on X-rays and the study of anatomy was, like much of his future work, quite prescient, anticipating much of what we know about the normal function of joints today. By measuring the joints near the extremes of flexion and extension, and using fluoroscopy to watch those movements, he was the first to really study the biomechanics of the movements of joints. Some of the radiographs that are reproduced in this article show the wrist in positions of neutral, radial and ulnar deviation, and his comments on them anticipate our studies of today, describing the motions of the wrist at both the radiocarpal joint and the midcarpal joint in various types of motion. These motions of the skeleton had not been seen previously or studied in living subjects. Codman immediately realized the clinical importance of X-rays to medicine and the importance of being able to recognize normal X-rays, "For this reason it is important to have a knowledge of the normal X-ray anatomy of the bones, for the X-ray picture differs from the photograph of the bare bones and from the frozen section, as it shows outline, internal structure and differences in density."[61]

Of significant importance in this article, however, was the amount and type of radiation that was necessary to take these radiographs in 1898. Codman noted that the skiagraphs in the article were taken from cadavers by using a focus tube stimulated with a 7-inch spark induction coil with a current of about 15 amperes and a pressure of four volts in the primary coil. In addition, the body parts were exposed at a distance of about 12 inches [30.5 cm.] for three to five minutes. Modern radiographic technique uses milliamperes and kilovolts and the body parts are usually exposed at about 40 inches [101.6 cm.] for milliseconds. Codman's atlas has hundreds of radiographs, all taken with these high radiation doses, and it is almost certain that he took little or no precautions to protect himself from radiation exposure. The resultant enormous amount of radiation generated by these machines

---

[61]*J Exp Med*, p. 383.

supports Cushing's earlier postulate that it was affecting Codman's physical condition.

In the summer of 1899, Codman added another title to his job duties. He was given the official position as the first skiagrapher (radiologist) to the Boston Children's Hospital. It was on a part-time basis and he continued to do anatomic dissections, as well as assist in surgery.

Codman obviously enjoyed the early work he did with X-ray machines, even if it may have eventually been at the expense of his own health. He stated in the preface to his book that:

> It would be impossible to give the reader an idea of the thrilling experience of those of us who did the early X-ray work. We each made weekly discoveries, only to find that our fellow workers in the same city and all other cities had made the same ones at the same time. Announcements of new uses of the X-ray, which are now familiar came with every issue of the Medical Journals. Each of us had the self-importance to think that we were the first to show fractures of various types, diagnose bone tumors, to locate foreign bodies and new parts of the anatomy. I remember that an early contribution of mine in the Boston Medical and Surgical Journal was to show that the X-ray was likely to help us in studying the epiphyseal lines! My plate, which was made with a tube which did not focus, after an exposure of over fifteen minutes, showed the epiphyses in the arm of a dead baby. Yet what I wrote was then unknown to the great majority of readers. We almost forgot that it was all because of Röntgen had noticed something which many others might have observed.[62]

Codman then ended this long comment on his early experience with X-rays by philosophizing a bit, as he often did, "Probably other

---

62Preface, p. x.

things of great importance are showing themselves to us daily, and we look but we do not see." .[63] Was Codman possibly referring here to the fact that other doctors never recognized his X-ray studies? As these comments were made later in his life, perhaps it was a reflection on how his End Result Idea had never received the recognition for which he was hoping?

Codman reflected further on his early days in the X-ray research, "There were many amusing, exciting and tragic episodes in those days, for we all had burns and some of us gave them. Many of my old friends are now dead from X-ray cancer. It was fortunate for me that my interest in surgery was greater than in Röntgen's discovery."[64] But it is not certain that Codman survived his early research around the huge radiation fields of early X-ray machines with no cost to his own health. As noted, Cushing thought that it had affected Codman's physical condition, and it has been postulated that Codman sterilized himself because of his work around X-rays as he and his wife never had children.[65] Codman eventually died from malignant melanoma, a skin cancer with known association with radiation exposure. However, it is not known to be associated with exposure to X-radiation, but these studies have all been done with modern doses, which are minimal in comparison to that which Codman received during his research.

Codman's early work on X-rays at the Massachusetts General Hospital was performed in the laboratory of Professor Henry Bowditch. During his time working with Bowditch, Codman took X-rays of numerous body parts of the people working in the laboratory. One X-ray of Bowditch's forearm revealed a bullet near the ulna which he had received during the Civil War while leading a charge at New Hope Church on 27 November 1863.

Codman was gone from Boston for at least eight or nine months during the late 1890s on two trips out West. The first trip was made in late 1898 and early 1899 along with his brother, William, to whom he

63Preface, p. x.

64Preface, p. xi.

65Neuhauser D. "Introduction: Ernest Amory Codman and the end results of medical care." In: *Codman: A Study in Hospital Efficiency. As Demonstrated by the Case Report of the First Five Years of a Private Hospital*, Oakbrook Terrace, IL: Joint Commission on Accreditation of Healthcare Organizations, 1996. pp. 10-11.

referred several times in his letters home as "Buffalo Bill." During most of this trip they stayed near Sheridan, Wyoming at the Sheridan Inn. However, in September 1898 a letter to his father noted they were departing for two weeks of bear hunting in the mountains at a place called Black's Canyon on the Crow Reservation in Montana.

After a few years in practice, Codman was becoming well-known as a surgeon in the Boston area. On 5 November 1898 he received a letter from W[illiam] Cameron Forbes (né 1870), a wealthy Boston banker who knew Codman from their days together at Harvard. Forbes invited Codman to serve as personal physician to him and his brother, Waldo E. Forbes, while they traveled in the West. The trip was made in the summer of 1899 and Codman was paid $10,000 by Forbes, an enormous sum for the time. To the Forbes family, it was money well spent, as evidenced by the many letters in the Codman Archives from the Forbes to Codman.

One of these letters was from Cameron Forbes' mother, Edith Forbes, thanking Codman for saving her son's life. While in Montana on the trip out West, Cameron Forbes' horse reared back and threw him to the ground, where he landed on his head. The incident made the newspapers out West and noted that Codman was fortunately at Cameron Forbes's side to provide the proper treatment to help him recover.[66]

During these early years of his practice, Codman fell in love and married. Coincidentally his research work had some relation to this. While working in Bowditch's lab, he met one of the professor's nieces, Katherine Putnam Bowditch, known as Katy.[67] They became engaged in November 1898 and were married on 16 November 1899. (Figure 5) Neuhauser noted, "Although Codman kept a detailed diary of this year, November 1899 was left blank, a rare lapse into Boston reticence by this outspoken man."[68] A few years after their marriage, Katherine and

---

66CA 7/145.

67Her name is spelled variably in this book as "Katy" and "Katie." Katherine Codman usually signed her letters with her full first name, Katherine, but on the rare occasion she used her nickname, she spelled it Katy. Amory Codman always spelled her name Katie in his letters, and his friends, notably Harvey Cushing and Edward Martin, invariably used this spelling. I have preserved the original spellings in the letters, but use Katherine's preferred "Katy" when not quoting a source.

68Neuhauser, p. 9. Neuhauser is referring to the hunting and fishing diary that Codman kept throughout his

Amory Codman moved into a home at 227 Beacon Street in Boston, a home in which they would live throughout the rest of both their lives.

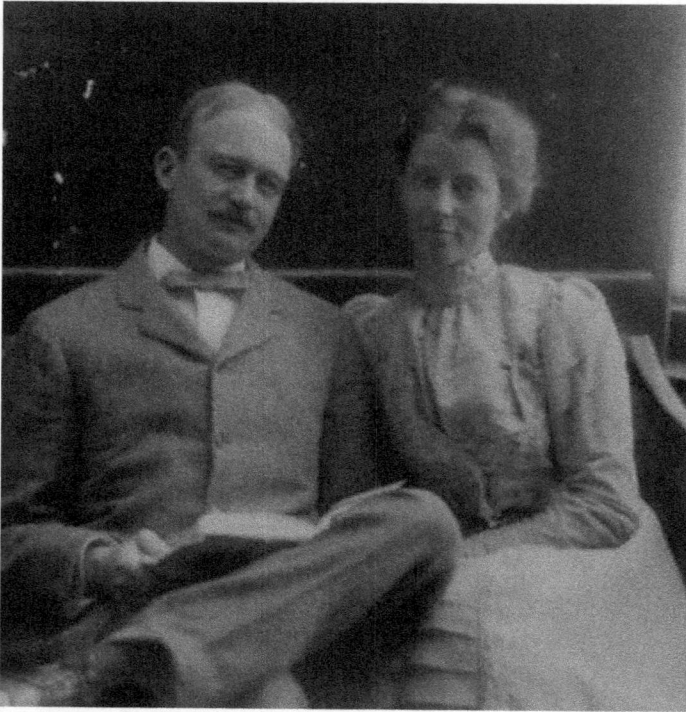

Figure 5—Amory Codman and his bride, Katherine Bowditch Codman, shortly after their marriage. (Courtesy Francis A. Countway Library of Medicine, Rare Books and Special Collections Department)

Codman enjoyed travel and the outdoors and the trip out West with the Forbes was something he probably would have enjoyed doing, even if he had not been paid a huge amount of money for it. Despite his busy schedule at the Massachusetts General Hospital and the Boston Children's Hospital, he continued traveling during these early years of his practice. In the detailed chart of his life in the Preface[69] he described several trips that he made between 1896 and 1899. One of them was the trip out West with the Forbes. However, he visited the

---

life and which is kept in the Codman Archives.

69Preface, p. vi.

Canadian Maritime Provinces frequently, having first travelled to Nova Scotia in 1891, and he later visited New Brunswick in 1896.

In 1897 Codman again traveled to New Brunswick and Nova Scotia with his close friend, Samuel Barlow. In a letter to his father from the Queen Hotel in Yarmouth, Nova Scotia, he described Barlow as "very amusing and entertaining" and the people as "very hospitable, especially Charles Robbins, who was a descendant of Chandler Robbins who came over on the Mayflower." In several letters home he noted that he and Barlow shot together frequently and that the shooting was "fair."[70]

Upon Codman's return to Boston and Mass General he continued his research and published many papers on X-rays. His use of X-rays may have been responsible for leading him to his study of orthopaedics, as evidenced by his third published paper (1900) in the *Boston Medical and Surgical Journal*[71] which was entitled, "A Study of the X-ray Plates of One Hundred and Forty Cases of Fracture of the Lower End of the Radius." Prior to its publication, Codman read this paper before the Boston Society for Medical Improvement on 19 March 1900. This paper is noteworthy because it presents Codman's study of what was known then and is known today as a Colles' fracture. Although this fracture had been described in the 18th century by Abraham Colles, his diagnosis was made on clinical evaluation and eventually autopsy studies. Codman was the first person to study the fracture with radiographs and also to develop a classification of Colles' fractures, one of the most common fractures treated by orthopaedists.

Today, there are several classifications of fractures of the distal end of the radius that are used by orthopaedists. Codman;s classification separated this fracture into ten classes, as follows:

Class I: Fracture through the base of the styloid process of the radius.

70CA 7/136.

71BMSJ, 143 (13): 305-308. All future footnote references to "BMSJ" refer to the *Boston Medical and Surgical Journal*, the journal in which Codman published the bulk of his medical literature. In 1929, this journal changed its name and became the *New England Journal of Medicine*.

Class II: Fracture of the inner angle of the lower end of the radius.[72]

Class III: Transverse fractures at or a little above the epiphyseal line (in adults) without displacement.

Class IV: The distal fragment is comminuted, either as a simple T-fracture or into several smaller pieces.[73]

Class V: Separation of the epiphysis of the lower end of the radius.[74]

Class VI: Separation of the epiphysis of the lower end of the radius with chip off the posterior surface of the diaphysis.[75]

Class VII: Impaction of lower fragment into the shaft.

Class VIII: This is the typical Colles' fracture and may itself be divided into two forms: that with marked radial displacement of the fragment and that which the posterior deformity is more decided.

Class IX: Stellate fracture of the lower end of the radius with longitudinal fissures extending into the shaft.

Class X: Reverse Colles' fracture, that is, anterior displacement of the lower fragment.[76]

As he often did, Codman anticipated much of modern orthopaedics in studying of this very common problem. In fact, this remarkable article on distal radius fractures describes precisely almost all of the types of distal radius fractures that we know well today, over 90 years later.

In 1902 Codman published two papers in the *Philadelphia Medical Journal* that were essentially a two-part series, in which both articles were entitled, "A Study of the Cases of Accidental X-ray Burns Hitherto

---

72This fracture would be classified by orthopaedists today as having what is known as a die-punch fragment.

73This fracture would probably correspond to the fracture that is described by a classification we use today from Dr. Charles Melone. In this classification he describes two-, three-, and four-part fractures of the distal radius and this would certainly be a four-part fracture.

74This would correspond to what is known today as a Salter-Harris type I fracture.

75This would correspond to what is known today as a Salter-Harris type II fracture.

76This is usually termed a Smith's fracture today, although the drawing Codman has in the article may actually make it what is now termed a volar Barton's fracture.

Recorded."[77] The articles described in detail all the X-ray burns that he was able to find in the literature. He observed that the incidence of X-ray burns was decreasing with time, finding that 55 cases were reported in 1896, 12 in 1897, 6 in 1898, 9 in 1899, 3 in 1900 and only 1 in 1901. The doctors of this era were obviously learning the dangers of X-rays and using them more safely, partly through better techniques and partly through better equipment.

Codman classified X-ray burns into five types: 1) what he called skiagrapher's dermatitis; 2) a milder case of a transient erythema followed by an exfoliation of superficial epidermis; 3) cases of the second degree with formation of blisters following the erythema; 4) more severe cases in which the burn would extend to the deeper layers of the skin and subcutaneous tissues; and 5) a fifth case in which he noted there was some internal lesion attributed to the X-ray. Analyzing his descriptions, the first two burns were probably different stages of what are now known as first-degree burns, while the third and fourth lesions were second- and third-degree burns. Codman concluded in this paper that, "The important factors which contribute to the production of X-ray burns are: the intensity of the current used to stimulate the tubes; the quality of the tubes, the distance and time of the exposure; and the idiosyncrasy of the patient."[78]

Codman was becoming a recognized expert on X-rays based on his publications and the anatomic atlas he provided to the Massachusetts General Hospital (MGH). As an example that many of the problems attendant to the practice of medicine today also existed in that era, he was even asked to serve as an expert witness in at least one medical malpractice cases. In a letter dated 6 February 1905, W. A. Cleland, a lawyer from Portland, Oregon, asked Codman to testify on behalf of his doctor/client who was being sued by one of the doctor's patients because of X-ray burns. Codman refused to testify.[79]

Codman published one other excellent paper on X-rays in his early career. This was entitled, "The Open Use of X-ray in Surgery," and

---

77*Phil Med J*, <u>10</u>: 438-442, 499-503.

78*Phil Med J*, <u>10</u>: 503.

79CA 5/95.

appeared in the *Johns Hopkins Hospital Bulletin* in May 1903.[80] His candor showed up dramatically in this article and also showed early signs of his philosophy of being honest and forthright in publishing his outcomes. He stated, "We use the X-ray as a routine method in fractures. I am personally thankful that my house officer experience was in the days before the X-ray ... You have read, as I have, certain rosy articles on the use of the X-ray and their more terrible forms of malignant disease, of the disappearance of sarcoma and cancer, but all I can tell you is that at the Massachusetts Hospital we do not get such good results and I in my private practice do not get such results."

Codman would continue to be recognized as one of the world's top experts on X-rays. In 1905 he submitted a paper, "The Use of the X-ray for Diagnosis of Bone Diseases." hoping to win the Gross Prize, which was given every five years by a committee of doctors in Philadelphia for the best medical paper. The paper did not win the award and Codman commented on this in the Preface:

> **The prize for that year was awarded for an essay on ligation of the carotids and cases of malignant disease of the face! The author claims that thus starving the growth of the tumors by stopping their blood supply was of great help in controlling the disease. The method is now seldom if ever used, yet today, practically everything my paper contained is common knowledge among röntgenologists. It is hardly possible to realize now, that at that time (1905), busy surgeons had no idea of the practical value of the X-ray and the diagnosis of bone disease and that the pictures which I presented to this committee were to them unintelligible![81]**

However, Codman did not discard the paper that he had submitted for the Gross Prize. One of the committee members was a Philadelphia surgeon named William W[illiams] Keen (1837-1932). Keen wrote a

---

80*Johns Hopkins Hosp Bull*, 14(146): 120-124.

81Preface, p. xi.

textbook on surgery, *Surgery: Its Principles and Practices*, which was one of the leading surgical texts of its time, and he asked Codman to write a chapter on the use of X-ray in surgery for the book. Although Keen's committee had not awarded Codman the Gross Prize in 1905, in 1911 he accepted the paper almost exactly as Codman had written it, for use as a chapter in his textbook.[82]

Between 1900 and 1905 Codman was very busy in his own private practice of surgery. In 1900 he was promoted from Assistant Surgeon to Surgeon to Out-Patients at the Massachusetts General Hospital and he was also an Assistant in Clinical Operative Surgery at the Harvard Medical School. This was in addition to his continued duties as the Skiagrapher at the Boston Children's Hospital, although he no longer worked in Bowditch's lab as an Assistant in Anatomy.

In his early career, Codman wrote eclectically on various subjects in surgery, reflecting his practice as a general surgeon but with an emphasis that was developing, and would continue to grow, in orthopaedic surgery. In 1905 he published an article in *the Boston Medical and Surgical Journal* on rhinoplasty as a plastic procedure for "rodent ulcer of the face," i.e., an ulcer caused by a rat gnawing on the victim's face.[83] That same year he described the results of nontraumatic surgery of the brain and spinal cord, or one of the earliest forms of neurosurgery, at the Massachusetts General Hospital.[84] Codman described very poor results from early neurosurgery in that era, which would not be unexpected in the first decade of the 20th century. In Cushing's biography, Fulton writes, "During the first years his (Cushing) mortality rates from [neurosurgical] operations were high, so high, indeed, that he was many times discouraged and on more than one occasion the questions was raised whether he was justified in proceeding."[85] Codman, however, continued his emphasis on orthopaedic injuries with an article in 1903, (which may have been

---

82*Ibid.*

83BMSJ, 152(10): 275-278, 1905.

84BMSJ, 153(3): 74-76, 1905.

85Fulton, p. 268.

based on his own personal problems) entitled, "The Formation of Loose Cartilages in the Knee Joint."[86]

During this time he wrote prolifically in medical journals, publishing 19 papers, most of them in the highly prestigious *Boston Medical and Surgical Journal*.[87] Codman published papers on many different subjects, including several on orthopaedics that were aided by his use of X-rays. In 1904 he published the first description of a bone cyst in the fingers, "Report of a Case of Bone Cyst of a Digital Phalanx."[88]

Codman wrote a series of four articles between 1902 and 1904 that began to take him away from the practice of radiology, and gave the first inklings of his interest in both shoulder surgery and outcome studies. One was a very interesting article published in the *Boston Medical and Surgical Journal* in 1904: "Some Points on the Diagnosis and Treatment of Certain Neglected Minor Surgical Lesions."[89] In this article he discussed scaphoid fractures, giving the first X-ray description of this fracture, and a problem on which he would publish more extensively one year later. In addition, he noted that, reflecting the medical practice of the times, differential diagnosis of this lesion must include tuberculosis of the wrist joint, adding, "I have never known syphilis to affect the wrist joint except in one case of Charcot's disease."[90]

The seminal portion of this paper, however, was Codman's first description in print of the subacromial bursa and painful shoulder problems. He described what we now would term a "painful arc syndrome" and "impingement sign." He ended the paper by discussing fractures of the calcaneus, describing what is so common today, which is the long-term disability relating to this fracture, "I have never seen one of these cases as a late result, who did not complain of

---

86BMSJ, 149(16): 427-428, 1903.

87The *Boston Medical and Surgical Journal* was the top medical journal of the time and it is actually still considered so, although now under its current name of *The New England Journal of Medicine*.

88BMSJ, 150(8): 211-212, 1904.

89BMSJ, 150(14): 371-374, 1904.

90BMSJ, 150(14): 372, 1904.

some soreness in his foot on unusual exertions, such as extreme flexion of the ankle, walking on rough ground, long standing, etc."[91] It was further evidence of Codman's developing interest in orthopaedics.

However, his major publication on orthopaedic problems during this time came one year later when he and Henry Melville Chase (né 1874) published two extremely long articles in the *Annals of Surgery*, entitled, "The Diagnosis and Treatment of Fractures of the Carpal Scaphoid and Dislocation of the Semilunar Bone."[92] Codman and Chase described in detail 30 cases of scaphoid fractures and produced multiple X-rays that were reprinted. Again demonstrating that Codman seemed more a surgeon of our era than his, these articles again anticipated much of what we know about these difficult fractures today.

In 1905, nonunion of the scaphoid was controversial, as it remains to this day. Codman explained, "Professor Dwight, looking at the subject from a developmental and anatomical point of view, explains these lesions as instances of bipartite centers of ossification which never unite by true bony union, and thus are easily separated by violence."[93] Codman demurred however, "Yet I still believe that, putting aside extraordinary cases of injury, the normal scaphoid is never broken, and that the separation into two parts, which undoubtedly occurs, is the result of violence acting on a bone composed of two pieces united merely by cartilage." Codman was describing what we recognize as a common problem today, in which a fibrous nonunion of the scaphoid occurs and eventually becomes symptomatic when the fibrous nonunion is disrupted. In concluding this article, Codman and Chase noted that sprains of the wrist were often due to injuries of the carpal scaphoid. They recommended excision of the proximal half of a fractured scaphoid if it had proceeded to nonunion, and they also noted that the occurrence of a bipartite scaphoid was very rare in comparison with a fracture. Though their work was new and

---

91BSMJ, 150(14): 374, 1904.

92*Ann Surg*, 41(3): 321-362, March 1905; and *Ann Surg*, 41(6): 863-902, June 1905.

93*Ann Surg*, 41(3): 323, March 1905.

important, it could not have been done without their X-ray studies, for which Codman was largely responsible.

Codman first works on outcome studies were published in 1902 and twice in 1904 in three remarkable articles simply summarizing the results of Dr. Harrington's practice for several months. These articles were, "A Resume of the Results of Dr. [F. B.] Harrington's Service From June to October 1, 1900, As Seen in the Following June or Later,"[94] "Remarks on the Resume of Dr. F. B. Harrington's Service for the Year 1902,"[95] and "Results of Dr. F. B. Harrington's Service 1 June to 1 October 1900."[96] These were Codman's first papers on the End Result Idea. It is unlikely that these articles would be published today, as they do not deal with any specific problem but simply list all the cases that Dr. Harrington treated for several months and their outcomes—no conclusions are reached. In the 1902 article, Codman reviewed all the cases which did not come out perfectly under the subtitle, "Remarks on the Cases in Which the Results Were Not Perfect." Today this section would likely engender a rash of malpractice lawsuits.

He anticipated his later comments on and study of the End Result Idea in his closing paragraph of the article, "Remarks on the Resume of Dr. F. B. Harrington's Service for the Year 1902,"

> **If some arrangement could be made by which the house officer should see these late results, it would be very instructive for them, for I feel sure that the house officer in graduating from this institution gets a very much more favorable idea of the results of surgical operations than he is really justified in having.**[97]

The stage was set. Finished with his first decade of medical practice by 1905, Codman was becoming a prominent surgeon in the Boston area. His background was perfect—his Brahmin upbringing, an exclusive prep school with a strong scientific background, Harvard

94BMSJ, 146(20): 515-517, 1902.

95BMSJ, 153(3): 74-75, 1904.

96BMSJ, 150(23): 618-622, 1904.

97BMSJ, 153(3): 75, 1904.

College, Harvard Medical School, the Mass General. He had already been a pioneer in two fields of medicine, anesthesiology and radiology, but more importantly, his interest had been piqued in orthopaedics, in the shoulder, and the study of End Results and outcomes. At this time there seemed to be no limits to the heights his career would reach.

CHAPTER 4

EARLY INTEREST IN THE SHOULDER

There is nothing more difficult to take in hand, more perilous to conduct, or more uncertain in its success, than to take the lead in the introduction of a new order of things.

Niccolò Machiavelli, *The Prince*, [1532]

Codman's powers of observation and clinical judgment had to be remarkable. He began his clinical practice at the dawn of the X-ray era, and he never had the advantage of the advanced medical tests so well known to modern orthopaedic surgeons. Yet, what he eventually learned about the shoulder would stand up well and likely surpass the knowledge of most orthopedic surgeons of the 1990s.

As mentioned in Chapter Two, Codman stated that he first became interested in the shoulder, especially the subacromial bursa, while a Harvard medical student traveling in Europe, and studying at the clinic of Professor Eduard Albert in Vienna. His first paper on shoulder problems appeared in the *Boston Medical and Surgical Journal* in April 1904.[98] The article began with a discussion of scaphoid fractures and ended with a discussion of fractures of the os calcis. But there is one page (373) that was devoted entirely to the shoulder and contains the first mention in the English literature of what is often called "impingement syndrome." Codman noted, "We all know how often

---

98BMSJ, 150(14): 371-374, 7 April 1904.

the shoulder remains crippled for life and the patient complains he is unable to get his hand to the back of his head. This term, peri-arthritis, is a sort of surgical wastebasket in which we throw our diagnostic failures."[99] Demonstrating his superb powers of observation and presaging our current knowledge of this clinical entity, he described what are known today as the "painful arc syndromes" and the "impingement sign".

> **In raising the arm over the head, the first third of the motion may be accomplished by the rolling of the head of the humerus and the glenoid cavity but to move beyond this if the scapula be fixed, the great tuberosity and capsule of the joint must also roll under the acromion process. This would bring into play the two surfaces of the acromial bursa which, if inflamed, gives great pain and causes the muscles about the joint to fix the humerus at this point, and the remaining arc of motion is carried by the movements of the scapula on the thorax.[100]**

Codman read this article at the meeting of the Worcester District Medical Society on 9 March 1904. The paper came to the attention of Dr. George [Washington] Crile (1864-1943) of Cleveland who invited Codman to visit that city and present the paper before their Society, which he eventually did, on 16 March 1906. During that presentation, Codman learned that he had not been the first to describe the clinical entity of subacromial bursitis, or impingement syndrome.

> **During the discussion Dr. Carl Hamann of Cleveland mentioned a paper by Küster published in 1902. I had, at that time, never seen this article and, though I am frequently quoted as having been the first to describe subdeltoid bursitis, this paper shows clearly that I was not. After seeing Küster's paper I**

99*Ibid*, p. 373.

100*Ibid*.

> **adopted his name of subacromial bursitis as better than the term subdeltoid.**[101]

The controversy over the name of this clinical problem still exists to this day. The most common term for it is "impingement syndrome," as the rotator cuff is felt by some surgeons to become impinged mechanically under the acromial process of the scapula, as Codman described above. Other terms for it, which are virtually synonymous, however, are "subacromial bursitis," "rotator cuff tendinitis," and in Europe, "painful arc syndrome."

In two great bursts of effort Codman eventually published 19 articles in the medical literature on the shoulder. Between 1904 and 1912, 13 shoulder articles appeared under his name, and between 1926 and 1937 his final six papers on the subject, as well as his shoulder book, were published. The intervening 14 years saw him publish nothing on the shoulder—he was concentrating on End Results during that time.

His first paper devoted solely to the shoulder was published in the *Boston Medical and Surgical Journal* in 1906, and was entitled, "On Stiff and Painful Shoulders. The Anatomy of the Subdeltoid or Subacromial Bursa and Its Clinical Importance. Subdeltoid Bursitis."[102] This paper was essentially a summary of Codman's discussion of the subject in Cleveland, and it was his most complete single paper on the subject during his early work.

The paper began with the description of the anatomy of the subacromial bursa and the rotator cuff. He then described the pathology of the region, commenting that the three causes of subacromial bursal inflammation were trauma, inflammation, and sepsis, but he included several subcategories of each type. Codman then described the four basic types of sub-acromial bursitis with respect to the causation. He described Type I as acute or recent cases; Type II would now be termed adhesive capsulitis; Type III was chronic subacromial bursitis; and Type IV was a complete rotator cuff tear. He

---

101Preface, p. viii.

102BMSJ, 154(22): 613-620, 31 May 1906. The exact same article also appeared in *The Ohio State Medical Journal* in August 1906.

then described the treatment of these four types suggesting that both manipulation under anesthesia[103], and the use of his own abduction splint were very helpful in treating these problems. During the discussion of treatment of the adhesive cases, he made the now well-known anatomic point, "Complete abduction (elevation) of the humerus necessitates external rotation,"[104] and later in the same article, he stated that this biomechanical description was original with him. Codman noted that the use of his abduction splint shortened the period of rehabilitation by preventing adhesions from forming and allowed the patient to begin early motion exercises.

In 1908 Codman published an even more exhaustive treatment of subacromial bursitis, with a seven-part series that appeared from October to December of that year in the *Boston Medical and Surgical Journal*, with all seven articles bearing the same title, "Bursitis Subacromialis, or Peri-Arthritis of the Shoulder Joint (Subdeltoid Bursitis)."[105] His opening statement in the first part of the series is a fact known by all modern orthopaedists but which was first described by Codman in 1908. "It is the writer's experience that more patients seek hospital treatment for lesions involving the subacromial bursa than for all other lesions of the shoulder joint, including tuberculosis and fractures, added together."[106] This seven-part series then described in detail the various classifications discussed in his 1906 paper. In addition, he gave detailed case studies on all 75 cases that he had been able to treat to that time.

The anatomy section of the first paper provided biomechanical descriptions of the motions of the humerus with numerous illustrations. In this section, Codman used the word "impingement" for the first time in reference to this clinical problem. He also touched on bicipital tendinitis, having commented, "I am inclined to think that lesions of the serous sheath about the biceps tendon are rare, but it is possible that in some cases I had confused them with subdeltoid

---

103Although he describes this as manipulation under ether.

104*Ibid*, p. 617.

105BMSJ, 159(17-23): 533-537; 576-582; 615-616; 644-648; 677-681; 723-726; 756-759.

106BMSJ, 159(17): 533.

bursitis."[107] This confusion in the clinical diagnosis of these similar problems exists to this day.

Codman based most of his anatomy description on dissections he had performed himself, and he described his findings in detail. One particularly cogent point that he made concerned the shoulder capsule, "Another anatomical factor of great importance is: that the ligamentous capsule of the shoulder-joint is not a very significant structure in that the real capsule of the joint is a muscular one formed by the subscapularis, the supra- and infra-spinatus and teres minor. These muscles have tendinous expansions at their insertions, but the muscular bellies completely surround the joint."[108] Though today we understand that the shoulder capsule is actually a dynamic one, maintained mostly by the tendons of the rotator cuff, Codman's description of this was the first in the medical literature.

In the second part of the series, published 29 October 1908, Codman discussed the pathology, symptoms and diagnosis of subacromial bursitis. He described three types of the problem, as mentioned in his earlier paper, this time omitting the Type IV or rotator cuff tear. He also discussed a clinical sign which is often now called the "painful arc" but was then known as Dawbarn's Sign. However, this point of physical examination has, with only slight modifications, also been termed Codman's Sign.[109] Codman noted, "In a small portion of the cases (those in which no adhesion had as yet taken place and in which the spasm can be overcome), this tender point, being on the base of the bursa, will disappear beneath the acromion when the arm is abducted. When it occurs this sign is almost pathognomonic."[110] He also described a clinical finding, abnormal scapulo-humeral rhythm, which many modern shoulder surgeons use frequently in their clinical descriptions of shoulder problems: "The scapula does not accompany

---

107*Ibid.*, p. 537.

108*Ibid.*

109See a more detailed description of this in Appendix II.

110BMSJ, 159(18): 577.

the motions of the humerus, but, as said above, the relative motions may be jerky and uneven."[111]

In this paper, Codman then listed the differential diagnoses of subacromial bursitis, which reflected the era in which he practised. Among these he listed tuberculosis, fractures of the tuberosity and of the anatomical and surgical neck of the humerus, deep axillary abscess, muscular rheumatism, chronic rheumatic conditions, acromioclavicular arthritis, circumflex (axillary nerve) paralysis, inflammation of the sheath of the biceps tendon, and brachial neuritis (plexitis). Note the diagnoses—several of these are almost never used today. A surgeon of the 1990s would rarely even consider tuberculosis or axillary abscess in the differential diagnosis of shoulder pain.

Interestingly, Codman later criticized the article in which [Robert Hugh MacKay] Dawbarn (né 1860) described his sign, sending a letter to the *Boston Medical and Surgical Journal*. Dawbarn stated that his sign was pathognomonic of sub-acromial bursitis, whereas Codman stated that all cases of sub-acromial bursitis will have Dawbarn's sign, but that not all patients with Dawbarn's sign will have sub-acromial bursitis. He further stated that Dawbarn misunderstood pathognomonic but Codman had it backwards. In this matter, it appears that Codman was wrong and Dawbarn correct.[112]

Part three of the series discussed the prognosis of sub-acromial bursitis and began the discussion of its treatment. Of interest in this paper was Codman's description of the prognosis in Type II lesions, or what is now termed adhesive capsulitis. He stated, precisely as is often done today, "It is fairly safe to say that even without treatment the disability seldom lasts over two years."[113] He continued his discussion of treatment in the fourth part of the series. He listed three treatments for the Type II lesion, or adhesive capsulitis: gradual stretching, rupture under an anesthetic, and division, or lysis of adhesions. These are exactly the three options that are still offered to patients, now usually termed physical therapy, manipulation under anesthesia, and surgical lysis of adhesions, now most often done arthroscopically.

111*Ibid.* p. 578.

112BMSJ, 154(26): 750, 28 June 1906.
113BMSJ, 159(19) 615, 5 November 1908.

Should we have expected anything less from this brilliant student of the shoulder?

The remainder of part four, and sections of part five-seven contain case reports of 26 cases treated by Codman between 1906 and 1908. In the seventh and last part of the series, Codman summarized his findings on this topic:

Summary:

1. The subacromial bursa and supraspinatus muscle are of essential value in abduction of the arm.
2. Lesions of the subacromial bursa and of the tendon of the supraspinatus are the common causes of stiff and painful shoulders.
3. Many cases which pass into diagnoses of contusion of the shoulder, neuritis, peri-arthritis, circumflex paralysis and muscular rheumatism are in reality due to lesions of these structures.
4. The final prognoses of these cases is good, but when pain is severe, and disability is great, relief may be obtained by a simple operation of little danger.[114]

In May 1911 Codman published a landmark article in the medical literature when he gave the first known description, in English, of repair of a rotator cuff tear[115] entitled, "Complete Rupture of the Supraspinatus Tendon. Operative Treatment With Report of Two Successful Cases." In the article, Codman remarked, "I have had two cases of complete rupture of the supraspinatus tendon on which I have operated, and in both of which I was able not only to demonstrate the existence of the anatomical lesion in conjunction with the above symptoms, but succeeded by suturing the tendon to the tuberosity and bringing about complete restoration of the function of abduction."[116]

114BMSJ, 159(23): 759, 3 December 1908.

115BMSJ, 164(20): 708-710, 18 May 1911.

116*Ibid.*, p. 708.

His first rotator cuff repair was performed on a 52-year-old woman (J.A.) on 11 March 1909. He was not able to effect what we would now term a "watertight repair," and he described the procedure as follows, "By holding the bursa wide open, pulling down on the arm and raising the elbow from the table, the retracted end of the supraspinatus could be seen. This was caught with a tenaculum and pulled down enough to suture with four heavy silk threads to the remaining portion still attached to the tuberosity. This could not be done exactly but was done nearly enough so that it seemed possible for repair to take place along the silk sutures. A little gap was also left on each side which was not covered with tendon substances. It was in a sense a *suture à distance*."[117]

Three months after the surgery, Codman described the patient as having good use of her arm and able to do her own work, able to button the back of her dress, style her own hair, and abduct her arm to 135 degrees. He later demonstrated her shoulder function to the Interurban Orthopedic Club in Boston on 25 March 1911 (a two-year follow-up), and commented in the paper, "The arm is perfectly well and the function is perfect. The only abnormal sign is the deltoid is unusually prominent due to the presence of joint fluid in the bursa."[118]

Codman's second rotator cuff repair was performed on a 40-year-old man (D.R.) on 10 January 1911. The patient again did well, although Codman was still unable to achieve complete repair, "With some difficulty the supraspinatus tendon was caught with a tenaculum, freed and pulled forward. It was then sutured '*à distance*' to the tuberosity with heavy silk prepared with paraffine after the manner of Lange. As in the previous case, the retracted tendon could not be entirely united, but enough strands of silk were put in to make it possible for the function of the tendon to be replaced."[119] This was obviously a very large, or massive, rotator cuff tear as Codman also

---

117*Ibid.* p. 708.

118*Ibid.* p. 709. We would now consider the joint fluid in the bursa and the swelling of the shoulder to be signs that the rotator cuff repair had failed. However, with such excellent shoulder function that would be of little clinical importance.

119*Ibid.*, p. 709

noted that at first the supraspinatus had retracted so far that he could not see it.[120]

On 25 March 1911 Codman presented this patient to the Interurban Orthopedic Club and wrote, "Patient is working everyday—can chop wood and do other chores without pain. He can easily place his hand on top of his head or behind his back. Full abduction of the humerus on the scapula is, however, weak, and although he can elevate his arm, he cannot hold it in an abducted position against the downward pull of even moderate force. This strength in the arm in other respects is excellent and the patient is well satisfied. The function of the supraspinatus is fully as good as it was in Case 1, at the same length of time after the operation."[121]

In the same paper, Codman described one other case in which he had made a clinical diagnosis of a rotator cuff tear, but the patient would not submit to surgery. Codman noted that four years after the injury, the patient was still doing very poorly with very limited motion and great weakness in the shoulder.

Codman ended the paper with the rather prescient sentence, "Twice I have seen a longitudinal split between the tendon of subscapularis and that of the supraspinatus."[122] We would now describe this as a rotator interval lesion, although it would not be described as such with any frequency until the 1980s.

Later in 1911, Codman followed this landmark paper by publishing an interesting article in the *Boston Medical and Surgical Journal*.[123] In this article he responded to another article that reviewed one of his earlier shoulder papers. In April 1911 Dr. T[homas] Turner Thomas (né 1866) published an article entitled, "Stiff and Painful Shoulders, With Loss of Power in the Upper Extremity," in the *American Journal of the Medical Sciences*. Codman discussed Thomas's paper as follows, "In this article Dr. Thomas devoted most of his attention to discussing a paper of mine published in the *Boston Medical and Surgical Journal* in 1906, Vol. cxliv,

120*Ibid.*

121*Ibid.*

122*Ibid.* p. 710.

123BMSJ, <u>165(4)</u>: 115-120, 20 July 1911.

p. 613. Dr. Thomas had evidently not seen the much more extensive paper of mine on the same subject which appeared in the *Boston Medical and Surgical Journal* for Oct., 22-29, Nov. 5, 12, 19, 26 and Dec. 3, 1908."[124] Codman continued to discuss Thomas' paper quite honestly. He went page-by-page through the paper in which he both agreed and disagreed with certain of Thomas's comments, and gave the reasons why in every case. It was a clear and lucid analysis of the shoulder by the man who already knew it better than any other surgeon.

In 1912 Codman published another paper on shoulder problems, one which would again bring him eponymic fame. The paper was entitled, "Abduction of the Shoulder. An Interesting Observation in Connection With Subacromial Bursitis and Rupture of the Tendon and Supraspinatus."[125] In this paper he described a clinical finding that allows pain-free motion of the shoulder, even among patients with rotator cuff pathology. This finding was responsible for a series of exercises now known as pendulum exercises, or often termed Codman's Exercises.

Codman described this phenomenon, "When a person stands with the knees straight and the fingertips close to the floor, the humerus is abducted on the scapula by gravity alone without muscular effort."[126] He continued further, "In treatment, too, this observation can be utilized by beginning the mobilization of very acute cases and postoperative cases by simply having them lean the body forward with the arm hanging instead of making an attempt at abduction against gravity in the usual way."[127] He also recommended use of this exercise for all patients with rotator cuff problems, "Finally let me say this, that, simple as to which this point I call attention is, its proper appreciation by the medical profession will materially help to relieve the suffering and hasten the recovery of *all* stiff and painful shoulders. Obvious and trivial as it may seem, I am sure that from now on it will prove of assistance in *every* shoulder case and should become of daily use in

---

124*Ibid*. p. 115

125BMSJ, 166(24): 890-891, 13 June 1912.

126*Ibid*. p. 890.

127Ibid. p. 891.

every hospital clinic."[128] Though many of his ideas to reform medical care would meet with little acceptance, this idea has been embraced by modern shoulder surgeons and physical therapists. Codman's Exercises remain a staple of many shoulder therapy programs to this day.

With the publication of his 1912 paper, Codman's intense interest in the shoulder, and his flurry of articles on the rotator cuff, was now over, at least temporarily. He then turned his attention to other matters, specifically the End Result Idea. He would not publish another paper on the shoulder until 1926, and that one was in an obscure journal, *The Industrial Doctor*. One year later, he had another article published in the *Boston Medical and Surgical Journal*, this one entitled, "Obscure Lesions of the Shoulder; Rupture of the Supraspinatus Tendon."[129] By 1927, the rotator cuff tear was still considered an unusual entity and not a common problem. In fact, Codman wrote in this paper that he had operated on only 20 to 30 cases of complete rupture of the supraspinatus tendon, and this was 18 years after he had performed his first repair.

However, although never published, Codman compiled a complete description of his early work on the rotator cuff. This work listed and described, in detail, the 89 cases of rotator cuff tears and subacromial bursitis for which he treated his patients between 1902 and March 1914. Left as a manuscript, which can now be found in the Codman Archives, it is entitled: "Abstracts And References To Hospital Records Of The Cases Hitherto Operated On By Dr. Codman For Lesions About The Shoulder Joint. Bibliography." He stated that, "It is on these cases only that he can rely as evidence for any general statements which he has made in his publications as to points in the clinical pathology or results of operative treatment, by which he claims to have added to the general knowledge of the subject."[130] He closed by stating, "This list is offered to the surgical staff of Massachusetts Hospital as a Standard in shoulder surgery, with the hopes of the staff may assign this class of

---

128*Ibid.*

129BMSJ, 196(10): 381-387, 10 March 1927.

130CA 5/98.

surgery to someone of their number and order that he may raise the Standard but further contributions to the knowledge of the subject has demonstrated by improved results of the patients."[131] It was evidence of his desire to improve the Standard of medicine in general, and again foreshadowed his coming work on End Results.

Codman would begin work on his shoulder book in 1927, and publish it in 1934. In the last decade of his life, he would publish four more papers on rupture of the supraspinatus tendon. But for now, the shoulder would have to wait. He would turn away from its study and pursue his Quixotic quest of the End Result Idea. His early interest in studying the End Results of a surgical service was soon to become the obsession of his life. And he still had further work yet to do in other areas of medicine.

131CA 5/98.

CHAPTER 5
PERIPHERAL INTERESTS IN MEDICINE

I am the teacher of athletes. He that by me spreads a wider breast than my own only proves the width of my own.

Walt Whitman, *Leaves of Grass* [1855]

Despite his pioneering work on the shoulder in the first decade of the century, Codman was still considered merely one of the lower level surgeons at the Massachusetts General Hospital. At the beginning of the 20th century, like many hospitals in the United States, Mass General worked on a strict seniority system. Promotion could only occur if a senior surgeon left the hospital or died. No matter his publications, no matter his technical skill as a surgeon, there was no chance for Codman to improve his status among the surgeons except through attrition of the senior staff. Quality counted for nothing. This certainly rankled him, and may have been the stimulus which eventually led to his work on the End Result Idea.

In that era the younger and lower level surgeons did most of the night emergencies at the MGH, and on one Christmas night (1901), Codman made a preoperative diagnosis of a perforated duodenal ulcer and successfully operated on the patient. It was the first case thus diagnosed and operated upon at the Massachusetts General Hospital and stimulated his interest in this problem, then thought to be very unusual.

As it was uncommon for surgeons to specialize solely in orthopaedics at that time, Codman continued practicing as a general surgeon. His papers and research during the 1900s reflect his generalization, as he began to write several medical articles on the topic of duodenal ulcers. In addition to these, several of his other papers published in the literature concentrated on abdominal lesions. He did not stop there, publishing on urologic problems, gynecologic problems, and cases which would now be dealt with by plastic surgeons. His interests seemed to encompass all of medicine within their purview.

An example of the lack scientific knowledge that permeated medicine in those days can be gleaned from an unusual paper that Codman published in 1906 dealing with a case report of a 16-year-old girl who developed spontaneous gangrene of her index finger. Despite serial deletion of the tip of the finger the gangrene continued to spread up the finger and to her hand. The wound refused to heal and, after disarticulation at the metacarpophalangeal joint, he then embarked on a radical treatment of the nerves of the arm, which would today be considered malpractice. He noted, "At this time I saw the patient again in the Out-patient Department and made an incision under cocaine, about halfway up the arm and *excised two or more inches of the radial nerve*,[132] starting at the point where it emerges from the fascia; at the same time I excised and curetted out the gangrenous area."[133] Codman discussed the case with several prominent surgeons including George Crile of Cleveland and his good friend, Harvey Cushing. They agreed it was not a problem of Raynaud's phenomenon and suggested that stretching of the brachial plexus might be of help. He further embarked on treatment of the peripheral nerves of her arm to heal her lesion, "On May 15th the patient was again admitted to the hospital, and on May 16th I gave her ether, *dissected out the median nerve in the middle of the forearm and stretched it as much as I dared to do without breaking it.*"[134] Despite this treatment, which would never be recommended today

---

132 The italics are mine.

133 The italics are mine.

134 The italics are mine.

because the excision or stretching of the nerves would cause significant loss of motor function, Codman noted that she went on to heal the lesion.

The 13 February 1908 edition of the *Boston Medical and Surgical Journal* contained two non-orthopaedic articles by Codman. The first was a case report describing the successful removal of a bullet from the brain, while the second was his first of numerous articles on duodenal ulcers. In this first paper on duodenal ulcers, Codman reported on six cases of acute perforation of the ulcers, beginning with the one noted above when he was taking night call. He also gave credit for much of his experience to his mentor, Francis Harrington.

After this paper, the duodenal ulcer would be Codman's main interest for the next several years. He had somewhat abandoned his research on the shoulder, though this would not last, and his medical interests remained widespread. In the April 1908 issue of the *Boston Medical and Surgical Journal* he published a review of all the cases of intussusception which had occurred at the Massachusetts General Hospital. He described 27 cases, 11 in infants under one year of age, of whom only two survived.[135] It was another early example of Codman publishing the End Results of the treatment of a single disease.

Later that same April Codman published another paper on the duodenum this one entitled, "Chronic Obstruction of the Duodenum By the Root of the Mesentery."[136] The paper began with the descriptions of the anatomy and embryology of the duodenum. He went on to describe the pathology of the obstruction of the duodenum by the root of the mesentery, relating it back to an anatomic etiology. It was a superb example of relating patho-physiologic entities back to their anatomic causes.

In May 1908 Codman published a report of a case of an intravesicular cyst of the ureter. He discussed both cystoscopy of the bladder and of the base of the ureter, as well as having performed a suprapubic cystostomy.[137] Both of these are now mainstays of modern

---

135BMSJ, 158(16): 439-446, 2 April 1908.

136BMSJ, 158(16): 503-510, 16 April 1908.

137BMSJ, 158(22): 828-831, 28 May 1908.

urology, but in 1905 they were rarely done, and they were unusual enough to warrant a case report in a major medical journal.

In February 1909, Codman published one of his rare papers which dealt with an orthopaedic problem outside the shoulder. It was also one of his few papers that did not appear in the *Boston Medical and Surgical Journal* or *Surgical Gynecology & Obstetrics*. The title of this paper was, "Bone Transference: Report of a Case of Operation After the Method of Huntington."[138] The case was one of a patient with long-standing osteomyelitis of the tibia. Codman stated that it had been described that complete resection of the diseased portion of the shaft would allow periosteal regeneration, but he was concerned in this case, that the diseased bone entailed such a large segment of the tibia that periosteal regeneration would not allow it to heal fully.

A 1905 paper in *Annals of Surgery* by Dr. Thomas Huntington had reported a similar case in which the shaft of the fibula was transferred to take the place of the tibia after the diseased segment had been resected.[139] Codman performed the same operation on 26 October 1905, after receiving permission to do so by Dr. Harrington, his chief of service. At the time, Codman noted that he thought the only option was amputation. Using his X-ray experience, he followed up on the patient with serial radiographs, both before transference of the fibula and one year and three years after.

He described the final follow-up thusly, "The functional value of the leg, without support, was nevertheless practically normal in less than a year. It is now normal except for a slight limp caused by the shortening (1 inch) and some stiffness of the ankle. It seems perfectly strong, although patient is wisely somewhat careful subjecting it to severe strains."[140] Codman, however, emphasized his now developing devotion to reporting all outcomes including the unsuccessful ones, although, in this case, he had been successful. He noted at the end of the article, "It seems to me that it is important to report these cases *whether they are successful or not* (italics mine), because in the next

---

138*Ann Surg*, 49(6): 820-823, February 1909.

139*Ann Surg*, 41: 249, 1905.

140*Ann Surg*, 69(6): 823, February 1909.

decade subperiosteal resection is likely to be a common operation and is likely to fail in a considerable percentage of cases."[141] The italicized segment shows that, to Codman, the End Result and its use to report outcomes, even poor one, was the most best method to improve medical care.

Codman then turned his attention almost entirely to the duodenum and duodenal ulcers. Between 1908 and 1911 Codman would publish nine seminal papers on duodenal ulcers. In this country, along with the Mayo brothers, he would become one of the experts on the topic. In the *Boston Medical and Surgical Journal* he published two sets of serial articles. The first set was a three-part series that appeared in September 1909, entitled, "The Importance of Distinguishing Simple Round Ulcers of the Duodenum From Those Ulcers Which Involve the Pyloris Or Above It."[142] In November and December of that same year he published a four-part series entitled, "The Diagnosis of Ulcer of the Duodenum."[143]

In the first series of articles he noted that most surgeons of his era thought duodenal ulcer to be a rare disease. He commented that, according to current teaching, gastric ulcers outnumbered duodenal ulcers by 12:1, but his clinical suspicion was that the ratio was closer to 2:1. He described the symptoms of both the chronic ulcer as well as acute perforation of the chronic ulcer. In his descriptions of how duodenal ulcers may cause death, his colorful phrasing shone through, "These insignificant ulcers may prove fatal in three different ways: (1) by perforation, (2) by hemorrhage and (3) by starvation due to stricture of the pyloris. But if they do not cause death, they may heal in time; we do not know how long this takes because in cases with a long chronic history there are always periods of comparative freedom. In such cases we do not know whether this is the same skunk under the barn all the time or another one."[144] In this series he also quoted freely from a well-

---

141*Ibid.*

142BMSJ, 161(10-12): 313-318, 351-355, and 359-403. September 1909.

143BMSJ, 161(22-25): 767-774, 816-822, 853-857 and 887-891, November and December 1909.

144BMSJ, 161(10): 316, 2 September 1909.

known British surgeon of the time, Lord Berkeley Moynihan (1865-1936). He would later come to know Moynihan well as his patient.

In the second article in the four-part series entitled, "The Diagnosis of Ulcer of the Duodenum," Codman had changed his emphasis on the importance of duodenal ulcer. Although it was only a few months later, he stressed its frequency as a clinical diagnosis even more. In the opening paragraph, he described its occurrence, "It is at least twice as common as gastric ulcer, and nearly as common as acute appendicitis."[145] In this series, he helped students of that time learn to distinguish between gastric ulcers and duodenal ulcers by describing the differences in the symptoms.

When a young or middle-aged man complains of a severe though bearable pain when the stomach is just becoming empty a couple hours after his last meal, and if at times he is subject to relatively acute attacks with continuous pain, epigastric tenderness and vomiting, you may suspect duodenal ulcer.[146]

Codman described the three important differential diagnoses in this case as: (1) gastric ulcer, (2) gallstones, and (3) acute appendicitis. Further emphasizing his use of the End Result Idea, the last three parts of this series were entirely filled with case reports in which he described all 50 cases of duodenal ulcer that he had treated between August 1903 and June 1909.

In July 1911 Codman published one more paper on duodenal ulcers, that in the *Boston Medical and Surgical Journal*. It was entitled, "Progress and Surgery, Duodenal Ulcer,"[147] and was essentially a review, or current concepts, article in which Codman discussed a committee investigation by a commission appointed by the United States Government to investigate the treatment of duodenal ulcers. He referenced several articles and a book by Lord Moynihan and began this article by noting that the recent writings of Moynihan and the

---

145BMSJ, 161(22): 767, 25 November 1909.

146*Ibid.*, p. 768.

147BMSJ, 165(2): 54-59, 13 July 1911.

Mayos had aroused an intense interest in the diagnosis and the value of operative treatment in duodenal ulcer. Codman was too modest— his own work was also important in this regard.

Codman published nothing further in the medical literature on duodenal ulcers although he had become one of the world's foremost on the subject. However, although he did not publish more on duodenal ulcers in medical journals, he did not stop studying them. The Codman Archives contain a manuscript he wrote, dated 24 April 1914, in which he listed and described, in detail, the 89 cases of duodenal ulcer that he had treated between 25 December 1901 (mentioned above) and 16 March 1914. Codman's manuscript was entitled "Abstracts and End Result Reports in Reference to the Hospital Records of the Cases Hitherto Operated on by E. A. Codman for Lesions of the Stomach and Duodenum." He also noted the manuscript was to be presented as a standard to the surgical staff of the Massachusetts General Hospital, similar to the manuscript that he had provided of his own study of rotator cuff tears and subacromial bursitis.[148] (See Chapter Four)

Note that this manuscript report left to the Mass General contains the words "End Results" in the title. It should be noted that, at this time, it was unheard of for surgeons to publish large series of results such as this. Most of the articles in medical journals at that time consisted of either case reports or a small series of cases that they had treated on a single problem. There was rarely any lengthy follow-up mentioned, and often only good results would be described, omitting the poor ones—unfortunately, this bias continues somewhat to the modern medical era. For Codman, all his medical interests seemed only a means to his goal of proving to the world the utility of the End Result Idea as a way to improve the quality of medical care.

Codman was a teacher. His role as a surgeon at MGH, a renowned academic institution, required that he teach medical students and lower-level house officers and surgeons. He also used his interest in duodenal ulcers, and other abdominal problems, to teach other doctors. In 1913 Codman gave a course on the diagnosis of abdominal diseases

---

148CA 5/106.

and many of the doctors who attended the course were very impressed by Codman's ability as a teacher. All of them said they would return if he gave another such course and numerous letters attesting to this fact can be found in the Codman Archives.[149]

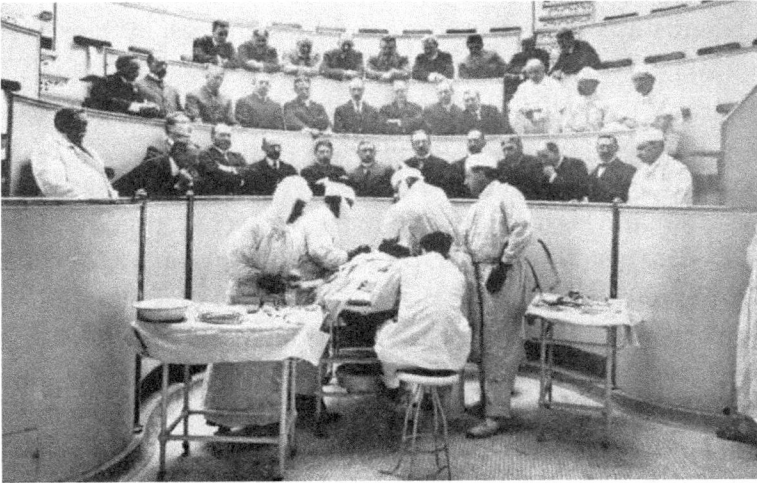

Figure 6—Amory Codman operating in the Bigelow Amphitheatre at the Massachusetts General Hospital, during the 1908 Meeting of the Society of Clinical Surgery. Codman is the tall figure to the right of the operating table, wearing the mask, his back turned towards us, and his left arm over the patient. (Courtesy Benham Press, Indianapolis, Indiana)

With his pioneering papers on the shoulder and duodenal ulcer, Codman was developing a national reputation as a surgeon, even if the advancement he sought at the MGH would never be dependent on that distinction. His developing reputation is probably best exemplified by the letter he received from Dr. James Mumford of Boston dated 17 July 1903 informing him of his election to the newly formed American Society of Clinical Surgery, later the Society of Clinical Surgery. (Figure 6) Composed only of the elite American surgeons of the era, membership in this Society established that Codman was highly considered by his peers, as there were only 32 founding members.[150]

149CA 3/57.

150Shumacker HB Jr. *History of The Society of Clinical Surgery*. Indianapolis: Benham Press, 1977.

In 1910 the Society of Clinical Surgery met in England and Codman spent at least three months there with his wife, staying after the meeting ended in early July. It was to be one of the most important trips of his life, for on this trip his End Result Idea would find a receptive ear in Dr. Edward Martin of Philadelphia. Martin and Codman formed a close friendship on this trip that would last the rest of their lives. (See Chapter Six)

On this trip Codman also met the renowned British surgeon, Berkeley, Lord Moynihan, 1st Baron of Leeds (1865-1936), whose work had greatly influenced him. Born Berkeley George Andrew Moynihan, Lord Moynihan was one of the most respected British physicians during Codman's lifetime. A professor of surgery and consulting surgeon at the University of Leeds, he was knighted in 1912 and became a baron in 1929. During his career he received over 15 honorary degrees from several different nations. Among his publications were included *Abdominal Operations* (4th ed., 1925) and *Duodenal Ulcers* (2nd ed., 1912), and he considered among the world's top experts on the problem which both interested and afflicted Codman, duodenal ulcer.

Codman had suffered with abdominal pain for years that he had suspected was a duodenal ulcer. In August 1910, Moynihan operated on him, almost certainly at the Leeds Council Infirmary, performing a gastric jejunostomy which brought Codman some relief from his chronic abdominal problems.[151] No doubt Codman was grateful.

Codman returned to the United States in September 1910. He continued to work as an assistant surgeon at the Massachusetts General Hospital. With his developing reputation he was also doing better now financially, increasing his annual salary from $3,000 in 1907 to $7,500 in 1911. This reputation was primarily based on his work on the shoulder and abdominal diseases. Recognition came from several sources, but probably none meant more than that which he received from his closest friend, and renowned surgeon, Harvey Cushing. Cushing wrote to him on 5 November 1910:

151Of note, Codman had previously undergone abdominal surgery. In the preface to his book he notes that in 1907 he underwent an abdominal exploration. Nothing in the Codman Archives or in his preface described further the details or results of that surgery.

Dear Amory:
I have just read these two papers on duodenal ulcer. They are the best things ever written. Wish I was capable of anything half as well done.
Affectionately,
H.C.[152]

Harvey Cushing and Amory Codman continued their close friendship which they developed in medical school. Cushing was a powerful ally for Codman to have in the medical community. Considered the father of modern neurosurgery, Cushing graduated from Harvard Medical School, with Codman, in 1895. He then spent five years as an assistant surgeon, effectively a resident, at The John Hopkins Hospital in Baltimore, and then joined the staff there in 1902, after spending two years studying in Europe under Theodor Kocher.

After several years at Johns Hopkins (1902-1910), returned to Harvard, remaining there until 1932, at which time he joined the faculty at Yale. He is remembered for his many pioneering surgical procedures on the brain and spinal cord, especially on neurologic tumors. In his laboratory his physiology research made important discoveries concerning the function of the pituitary gland. Cushing was also a renowned teacher, establishing the Hunterian Laboratory of Experimental Medicine at Johns Hopkins (1905) and the Laboratory of Surgical Research at Harvard. In addition to his clinical work, he wrote a Pulitzer Prize-winning biography of Sir William Osler in 1925.

On 17 May 1910, Cushing was appointed to the Senior Chair of Surgery at the Harvard Medical School and as Chief of Staff of the Peter Bent Brigham Hospital, which was being built adjacent to Harvard Medical School. Of interest, the architects of the Brigham were the firm of Codman & Despradelle. Codman, in this case, was Richard Codman, Amory's cousin, and a well-known Boston architect.[153] Codman wrote Cushing after the appointment: "I was delighted with your little note. Not only pleased for you, for Boston, and the Harvard Medical School,

---

152CA 2/24.

153Despradelle was Constant Désiré Despradelle, a Boston-based French architect.

but inwardly tickled with my own good judgment in picking out the man for this job nearly twenty years ago when I first saw you..."[154]

Cushing wrote back to Codman on 3 January 1911:

> **I have been going over the MGH 'publications' and rereading your duodenal papers. They are simply 'bang up'!—by far the best things that have been written, and written—what's more—in by far the most effective, readable and telling way. You're a wonder as I have always secretly thought. The only reason they didn't make you the prospective surgeon to Brigham was that it would have looked like a family affair— architect et al. I wish they would do it now and let me back out. You only have an occasional bellyache while I have perpetual cold feet. Then I have got the dickens of a lot to do here and my head buzzes with hemianopsias, carbohydrate assimilation limits, plasma in which things grow, dyspituitarism, and pinealismus, not to speak of Willy, Mary, Betsy and Henry.**
>
> **Yours admiringly, with love and Happy New Years to you and Katie**
>
> **Harvey Cushing[155]**

Over the next decade, Codman concentrated his time and his research on the End Result Idea and began to publish primarily on that topic. However, he never abandoned his interest in the abdomen and general surgical problems and his reputation as an expert in this realm was secure. In June 1911 Dr. S[amuel] W. Goddard wrote a paper before the Massachusetts Medical Society on "Surgical Treatment of Pyloric Stenosis, With Report of Cases." When published in the *Boston Medical and Surgical Journal*,[156] it also contained a long discussion in which Codman, by then acknowledged as an expert on abdominal

---

154Fulton, pp. 339-340.

155*Ibid*. p. 317

156BMSJ, 165(13): 479-483, 28 September 1911.

problems, was asked to give his comments and lead the discussion between several other well-known surgeons.

In 1912 Codman combined his interest in abdominal problems with his earlier research on X-rays in the paper "Diagnosis of Disease of the Stomach and Intestines by the X-Ray." [157] This paper described what we know today as a barium swallow. Codman described it as a "bismuth meal" that was swallowed and then traced serially down the alimentary canal by the use of fluoroscopy.

In 1913 Codman used his interest in End Results to summarize his work on abdominal problems. He published, "Observations on a Series of Ninety-Eight Consecutive Operations for Chronic Appendicitis." In this paper Codman made the rather blunt statement, which would be considered heretical today, "I believe that any surgeon who is willing to follow the facts to their logical conclusion will say, if he is not too much afraid of ridicule, that routine appendectomy is logical and reasonable for every child."[158]

He ended this paper with a call for other people to follow his lead and report large series of cases such as this one, presaging his End Result work.

Although this paper is brief and perhaps offers no new points of interest, I hope you will agree that the method which it illustrates is an important one. Great hospitals like the Massachusetts General Hospital have a duty to perform to medical and surgical science. Their clinical material should not be used haphazard to perfect the skill of a few favorite operators without scientific study of the cases. By grouping cases into series large enough to favor comparative study and by observing definite previously-determined points a rational and clinical science can be established. By putting the results on record the patient will not only be protected, but each operator will have the strongest incentive to excel in all the details of diagnosis and

---

157BMSJ, 166(5): 155-159, 1 February 1912.

158Ibid. p. 495

technique which count toward a successful result. This method will put an end to the old experimental surgery for each operator took a try at each new operation and reported only the good results.[159]

Codman published his last few papers on abdominal problems between 1918 and 1920. The first appeared in the *Transactions of the American Surgical Association* and was entitled, "The Treatment of Malignant Peritonitis of Ovarian Origin."[160] This paper was of particular interest for a comment he made early on in the text, "My hobby for looking up end results has led me to some pleasant surprises in this type of case ..."[161] By 1918, after the events of the previous few years, there were few doctors in Boston that would have termed Codman's obsession with End Results, "a hobby."

In 1920 Codman ended his published literature on abdominal problems with a two-part series in the *Boston Medical and Surgical Journal* on intestinal obstruction, again using this disease process to illustrate the use of the End Result Idea. He described his own experience treating 40 patients, of which he noted, to his great surprise, that the last 27 cases had all fully recovered, an exceptional surgical result for that era.

These last two papers of Codman's on abdominal diseases were written summaries of a talk he gave before the Springfield (MA) Academy of Medicine on 11 November 1919. The opening paragraph describes quite well where his emphasis lay by this time:

I feel it a great honor to be asked a second time to speak before this Academy, and only regret that I could not have been here on the first occasion. Besides the honor of being asked to address you, I find myself indebted to you for other things. In the first place, any medical society which asks me to address it, thereby puts itself, in a measure, on record as approving of the

---

159*Ibid.* p. 498.

160*Trans Amer Surg Assoc*, 36: 483-494, 1918.

161*Ibid.* pp. 483-484.

movement towards hospital standardization, even though, as in the present instance my subject is a surgical one.[162]

By 1920, however, Codman was not known as an abdominal surgeon, nor was he known primarily as a shoulder surgeon. He was considered a man obsessed, obsessed by his own desire to reform medical science by looking at the End Results of all medical and surgical treatments.

162BMSJ, 182(17): 420, 22 April 1920.

CHAPTER 6
THE GENESIS OF THE END RESULT IDEA

When you can measure what you are speaking about, and express it in numbers, you know something about it; but when you cannot measure it, when you cannot express it in numbers, your knowledge is of a meager and unsatisfactory kind: It may be the beginning of knowledge, but you have scarcely, in your thoughts, advanced to the stage of science.

William Thomson, the Lord Kelvin, *Popular Lectures and Addresses* [1891-1894]

A monomaniac has been defined as a person with a mental derangement restricted to one idea or group of ideas. [163] By the 1910s Codman was definitely monomaniacally obsessed with the End Result Idea but was he mentally deranged? Delusional? Crazy? Though some surgeons and doctors contemporary with him might have thought so, the quote that probably best describes him comes from the end of a popular movie of the 1970s, "He wasn't a loonie. He was the sanest man I ever knew in my life … He wasn't a lunatic. He was a hero."[164] He almost had to be, to endure what the End Result Idea would do to him. In a recent paper on Codman, Donabedian states that

---

163*Webster's Third New International Dictionary*, 17th edition, Volume II (Chicago: G & C Merriam Co., 1976), p. 1463.

164Ted Spindler (played by Wilford Brimley) commenting on the character of Jack Godell (played by Jack Lemmon) in "The China Syndrome", ©Columbia Pictures Industry, Inc., 1979.

the obsession, "… led him to disgrace, notoriety, isolation, and near financial ruin."[165]

Was Codman the first to write about outcome studies—did he invent the idea? Not exactly, but he was the first doctor to embrace the idea. The true pioneer of outcome studies was a nurse, and quite a famous one at that. Florence Nightingale (1820-1910) first achieved fame during the Crimean War in the 1850s, when she volunteered to tend to soldiers at the front. She was appalled at the unsanitary conditions she found there and the extremely high mortality rates in the military hospitals. Nightingale eventually wrote a paper on her plans to solve this problem, *A Proposal for Improved Statistics of Surgical Operations*. This paper urged hospitals and doctors to report the outcomes of their care in a standardized manner.[166] But no doctor prior to Codman followed Nightingale's lead, and the years between Codman and Nightingale are a void in this important area of medicine. And there is no evidence that he actually followed her lead; Codman never mentions Florence Nightingale in any of his writings.

As 1910 approached, Codman was writing more and more about the End Results of medical outcomes (Figure 7). Though most of his writing at this time usually discussed shoulders and abdominal problems, he usually made some references to the importance of studying the outcomes of medical interventions. His first real attempt at analyzing End Results in the literature occurred as early as 1902 when he published the results of the service of his surgical mentor, Francis Harrington, in the *Boston Medical and Surgical Journal*.[167] (See Chapter Three) He followed this several years later in 1904 with a follow-up review on Dr. Harrington's service.[168]

165Donabedian A. The end results of health care: Ernest Codman's contribution to quality assessment and beyond. *Milbank Quarterly*, 67(2): 234-235, 1989.

166Millenson ML. *Demanding Medical Excellence: Doctors and Accountability in the Information Age*, p. 141.

167BMSJ, 146 (2): 515-517, 15 May 1902

168BMSJ, 151 (3): 74-75, 21 July 1904.

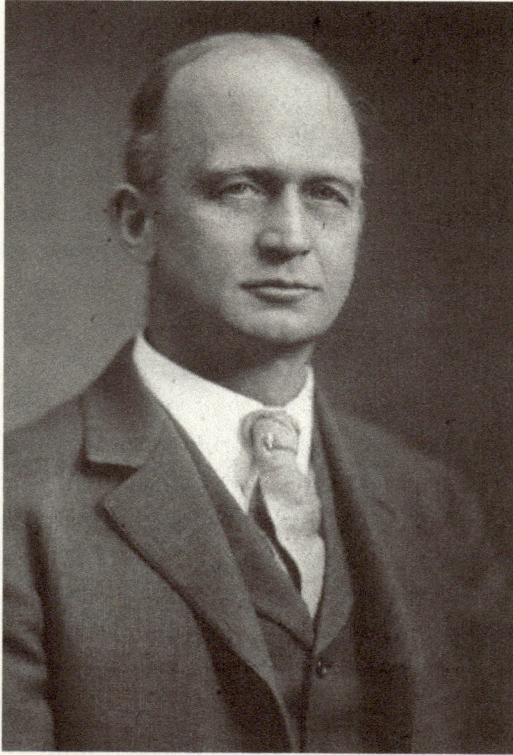

Figure 7—Amory Codman at the height of his surgical career, near the time of the opening of the Codman Hospital in 1911. (Courtesy Francis A. Countway Library of Medicine, Rare Books and Special Collections Department)

Codman never tells us exactly why he became interested in the End Result Idea, but there are clues available. McGuire has discussed the influences on Codman extensively in his thesis on Codman and the End Result Idea,[169] and feels that there were many influences. There are actually four major reasons that influenced Codman to begin espousing the End Result Idea, which we will examine each in detail. The first was a personal, and somewhat selfish one—he wanted to be promoted at the Massachusetts General Hospital. It is almost certain that the idea began with this in mind. The second reason, emphasized by McGuire, relates to the era of medicine in which he practised, termed the

---

[169]McGuire KJ. "The End Result System: Ernest Amory Codman and the Origins of Accountability in American Medicine, 1910-1934." B.A. Thesis, Princeton University, 1993. Much of what follows is based, to a large degree, on Dr. McGuire's study of this relationship.

Progressive Era of Medicine. McGuire noted that the era encouraged and promoted medical reform via entrance standards and organizational consolidation.[170] But here we will emphasize the reform of medical education. Thirdly, a major influence on Codman and all of medicine in this era, was work done in the area of scientific management, especially that by Frederick W. Taylor. Finally, between 1900 and 1915, when Codman did most of his work on End Results, doctors, and especially surgeons, were beginning to organize into groups on a national basis. This organizational movement, mentioned by McGuire as part of the Progressive Era, allowed doctors to meet at least yearly, and compare notes, theories, techniques, and methods, and possibly begin to standardize the practice of medicine. It furthered the education of the doctors after their medical training had ended, and prior to this time, that rarely occurred.

Self-Promotion

Codman began his career as a young junior surgeon on the staff of the Massachusetts General Hospital. As a junior surgeon, Codman's chances for promotion depended, not on the quality of his work, but only on time and the attrition of the senior staff above him. And Codman at least had a chance for promotion. His Brahmin background, his scientific pre-medical education, his training at Harvard and the MGH, all provided him with the opportunity to be promoted, which would have been denied to someone of lesser schooling and background.

Codman was obviously cocky, thinking a great deal of his own abilities—his letters reflect this. Perhaps the End Result Idea began only as a selfish attempt by him to help his own chances for promotion? However altruistic he may have been, he certainly had selfish motives early in his career, when he fought the seniority system at the Massachusetts General Hospital. Codman wanted to be promoted above surgeons he considered his inferior, even if they were senior to him, and he used End Results to come up with statistics which would

---

170*Ibid.*, pp. 27-28.

enable him to prove his own superiority—and possibly support his own promotion.

At any rate, he quickly saw the utility of the idea as a method to better the quality of a medical staff, by promoting only the best surgeons and physicians, rather than those who had been around for the longest time. He realized that this was a way to study the best methods of medical practice. And eventually, selfishness played little role. In fact, as Donabedian notes above, the idea almost destroyed him in the end. If he were not trying to improve medical care in general, surely he would have abandoned the idea when it turned against his original selfish goals.

Reform of Medical Education

At the beginning of the 20th century it was realized that medical education was far from ideal, and the quality of medical care was less than it should be. The training of doctors was haphazard and minimal at many schools. Medical school education was all book learning, given as two series of lectures over 20 weeks of each year for two years. Doctors who attended a third year of medical school could graduate *cum laude*.[171] The medical reforms of the Progressive Era received their greatest boost from the work of Abraham Flexner (1866-1959), whose work was instrumental in improving the quality of medical education.. Flexner was hired by the Carnegie Foundation to produce a report on medical education and the report was frequently scathing.[172] Many hospitals and medical schools were forced to close because of the revelations in Flexner's report.

In 1909, there were 155 medical schools in the United States and Canada and Flexner visited all of them. At each school, he examined five factors: 1) entrance requirements, 2) size and training of the faculty, 3) endowment support of the school, 4) quality and adequacy of the laboratories, and 5) relationships between medical schools and

---

171Davis L. *Fellowship of Surgeons: A History of the American College of Surgeons*. Springfield, IL: C. C. Thomas, 1960, p. 9.

172Neuhauser, p. 321.

hospitals. He eventually produced a report[173] that made seven major recommendations for the reform of medical education.

Flexner first two points were to reduce the number of poorly trained physicians and to reduce the number of medical schools, specifically from 155 to 31. He further contended that pre-medical education required a minimum of two years of college with a strong scientific background. In 1909, only 16 of the 155 medical schools required their entering medical students to have more than two years of college and only about 50 required education beyond high school. There was no emphasis at all on pre-medical education emphasizing the sciences. Flexner's fourth conclusion was the most controversial one. He emphasized that medical practice and scientific investigation should be done concurrently, stating that investigation and practice were "one in spirit, method, and object."[174] He combined this idea with his fifth suggestion—medical school faculty members should engage in research. He stated, "... only research will keep the teachers in condition."[175] Sixth, Flexner stated that medical schools should operate in association with hospitals. As incredible as it may seem to us in the 1990s, it was possible in 1900 for a medical student to graduate as a doctor without actually seeing or caring for patients, but only studying medicine from a textbook. Finally, Flexner recommended that the states should increase their regulation of medical licensure.

And what became of Flexner's recommendations from this report? Most of them were followed closely, and the report definitely reformed medical education in North America. The number of medical schools never approached 31, but the number decreased from 155 in 1909 to 76 in 1930. Improvements in pre-medical education were slower in coming, as Flexner noted in 1925 that only "a few medical schools required three or more years of college preparation."[176] His next two precepts—combining clinical practice and investigation, and requiring

---

173Flexner A. *Medical Education in the United States and Canada: Report to the Carnegie Foundation for the Advancement of Teaching.* New York: Merrymount Press, 1910.

174*Ibid.,* p. 56.

175*Ibid.*

176Hudson RP, "Abraham Flexner in Historical Perspective," p. 9. In: *Beyond Flexner: Medical Education in the Twentieth Century*, eds. B Barzansky, N Gevitz. New York: Greenwood Press, 1992.

faculty members to do research—were, for the most part, followed by most medical schools. Flexner's sixth recommendation, combining medical education with hospitals was eventually followed almost completely, and led to the development of "teaching hospitals" over the next 20 years. Flexner's final recommendation re state licensure was actually already underway, to a degree, but his report emphasized its importance.[177]

Not unexpectedly, the Harvard Medical School and the Massachusetts General Hospital (MGH) fared well by Flexner's analysis, though not in every respect. In particular, Flexner did not like the seniority system used by the MGH and at most other hospitals. Neuhauser has noted that this system was coming into disfavor in this era, primarily due to Flexner, "This seniority system at the MGH was Flexner's major criticism of the Harvard Medical School in his famous report."[178] This was support for Codman's criticism of the system, and eventually Codman and the Flexner report served as the impetus for reforming the system at the MGH.

Frederick Taylor and Taylorism

Although improving medical education was important, Codman thought this was not enough. He still felt it was necessary to study End Results and compare the results, to evaluate the quality of care. And Codman based this idea, not necessarily on anything he learned from within the medical world, but on another significant influence outside of the world of medicine, a movement called "Taylorism." Taylorism was the theory of scientific management espoused and promoted by Frederick W[inslow] Taylor (1856-1915) in the first decade of the 20th century.[179] Taylorism was essentially a movement in manufacturing, studying ways in which workers could perform their tasks more efficiently in order to increase production. The workers were monitored and watched closely, often under the eyes of a supervisor

---

177Most of my background on the Flexner report comes from Hudson's chapter (see previous footnote), and the Flexner report itself.

178Neuhauser D. Ernest Amory Codman, M.D. and end results of medical care. *Int J Tech Assess Health Care*, 6: 321, 1990.

179Taylor FW. *Principles of Scientific Management*. New York: W. W. Norton, 1911.

with a stopwatch that recorded their every movement. Taylorism was not popular among the workers, but management loved it.[180]

Codman embraced Taylorism and hoped to apply its principles to medicine and surgery. Presenting before a meeting of the Taylor Society, Codman related the two ideas of End Results and Taylorism. I quote from McGuire, who cited the published version of Codman's talk:

> Codman asked his audience to consider a hypothetical problem of soda fountain staffing. Codman described two positions: one a small store where the trade was not large, but steady and easy to handle; the other was a railroad station which on hot days made enough money to last the entire year. Codman asked rhetorically, what sort of boys would you want for each position? He answered that for the small store you would want a careful, meticulous boy who would "wash out the glasses, careful, thorough ... who would take care not to break any glasses and spill soda over the counter and so forth." At the railroad station, on the other hand, you would want a boy who was "naturally quick and dextrous and flew fast in one direction and then in another, and was perhaps a little careless about dropping a glass now and then or spilling a soda or handing it to you without wiping it thoroughly," for your profit depended on quantity. The point was that, in his opinion, hospital physicians conducted themselves too much like the second boy, instead of combining the positive attributes and avoiding the drawbacks of both. ... What Codman sought in a hospital surgeon was a "combination of that quick, dextrous boy, and the boy who is very careful and cleans the glasses thoroughly ... You want one so careful that he can deal with broken glasses" for in a hospital, each "glass" dropped or cracked

---

180McGuire discusses Taylorism and its effects on Codman's thinking on pp. 31-35 of his thesis.

> meant disability or death. In summary, Codman
> sought an "efficient" surgeon.[181]

Codman was not alone in supporting Taylor's theories as a means to better the practice of medicine. Other doctors, notably Robert Dickinson, and an industrial engineer named Frank Gilbreth, also embraced the idea and attempted to apply it the medicine. Dickinson, Gilbreth, and Codman were the "great triumvirate" of medical reform by one writer. [182] We'll hear much more about Dickinson and Gilbreth later.

The Organization of Surgeons

The political structure by which doctors and surgeons organized at the turn of the century was far different from what we know today. Whereas, today, there are multiple organizations and societies of doctors, it was only in the era from 1900 to 1915 that physicians were first starting to form such groups. Prior to this time, the only national association of surgeons was the American Surgical Association, formed in 1887 by Samuel Gross. With this trend towards organization, certain physicians came to positions of political power as leaders of these groups. There are three doctors who were especially influential in the formation of surgical societies, and who directly influence our story — Harvey Cushing, Edward Martin, and Franklin Martin. And Codman was fortunate that the first two were his close friends. We discussed Cushing and his career in Chapter Five.

Dr. Edward Martin (1859-1938) of Philadelphia was a gynecologic surgeon. He graduated from Swarthmore in 1878 and received his medical degree from the University of Pennsylvania in 1883 before interning at University Hospital in Philadelphia. From 1902 until his death in 1938 he was Clinical Professor of Surgery at the Women's Medical College of Pennsylvania. He joined the faculty at the University of Pennsylvania in 1903 as a professor of surgery and, in

---

181McGuire. pp. 33-34.

182Wrege CD, "The efficient management of hospitals," p. 117, quoting Gilbreth from RL Dickinson's paper, "Standardization of surgery: an attack on the problem," *JAMA*, 63(5): 763-765, 29 August 1914.

1910, was made John Rhea Barton Professor of Surgery. Edward Martin became a founding member of the Society of Clinical Surgery in 1903, and served as president of the Clinical Congress of Surgeons of North America in 1911 and 1912. In 1912 he presided over a meeting in Philadelphia at which the American College of Surgeons was formed on paper. He would eventually be a member of the Board of Regents, Board of Governors, and several other important committees of the American College of Surgeons. For his work in the organization of surgery in this country, as well as for his clinical acumen and surgical skills, Martin was awarded honorary degrees from several institutions: the University of Pennsylvania (1919), Swarthmore College (1920), and Temple University (1935).

Dr. Franklin Martin (1857-1935) of Chicago was also a gynecologic surgeon, but was not related to Edward Martin. Franklin Martin graduated from the Chicago Medical College (later Northwestern) in 1880, and opened his practice shortly thereafter. He served on the staff and faculty at the Polyclinic Hospital Medical School and the Women's Hospital in Chicago. He is best known for starting the respected surgical journal, *Surgery, Gynecology & Obstetrics*, in 1905, and he served as its managing editor until 1935. He was also the doctor behind the series of meetings known as the Clinical Congress(es) of Surgeons of North America, and he and Edward Martin were the primary impetus behind the formation of the American College of Surgeons. Unlike Cushing and Edward Martin, Franklin Martin and Codman did not get along well at all.

In 1900, Cushing was attending the 13th International Medical Congress in Paris, when he sat down to talk with two other distinguished American surgeons, Albert [John] Ochsner (1885-1925) and William Mayo. Both Ochsner and Mayo would later help form two of the best known medical institutions in American, the Ochsner Clinic in New Orleans and the Mayo Clinic in Rochester, Minnesota (formed with his brother, Charles Mayo). The three were quite weary of hearing endless papers presented at the Paris meeting, and proposed a new society which would meet and watch surgery performed at large surgical amphitheatres in the major cities of the United States and abroad.

92 / Bill Mallon, M.D.

This idea became the American Society of Clinical Surgery, with the name later changed to the Society of Clinical Surgery, the name by which it exists to this day. It was formed at a meeting in New York at the home of George Brewer on 11 July 1903. The founding members were Dr. George [Emerson] Brewer of New York (1861-1939), Dr. Charles [Harrison] Frazier of Philadelphia (1870-1936), Dr. George [Washington] Crile of Cleveland (1864-1943), Dr. John [Cummings] Munro of Boston (1858-1910), Dr. James [Gregory] Mumford (1863-1914) and Codman's close friend, Dr. Harvey Cushing. The members present at that meeting elected Codman as one of the 32 founding members of this early surgical society, and he received a letter from the first Secretary of the organization, James Mumford, documenting that fact. Brewer was elected as the first President and served in that capacity through 1905. The first meeting was held in Philadelphia and Baltimore on 13-14 November 1903, with the 21 attendees watching surgery in Baltimore at Johns Hopkins on the first day, traveling overnight to Philadelphia and observing surgery there. Codman attended the meeting.

Over the next few years the Society of Clinical Surgery grew in importance and esteem. Meetings were held in New York, Cleveland, Buffalo, Boston, Chicago, and the Mayo Clinic. Codman organized the meeting in Boston on 21-22 April 1905, and demonstrated surgery before the group at the meeting in Boston in 1908.. The group also decided to travel overseas and this first occurred in 1910 when the Society met in England.

The members of the Society left New York on 22 June 1910 by ship, arriving in Liverpool for the start of the meeting on 28 June. Over the next ten days, the American group observed surgery in London, Oxford, Middlesex, Edinburgh, and ended up in Leeds. Amory and Katy Codman attended the meeting, which ended on 7 July.[183] But the Codmans stayed in London for a holiday and also to allow Amory to have his aforementioned surgery by Lord Moynihan. After his recovery, Amory Codman was also able to do some hunting in Scotland in September. The meeting in London was quite important to Codman,

[183]All of this background on the Society of Clinical Surgery is derived from Shumacker's book on the history of the Society.

because of several talks he had with Edward Martin. We'll return to that in a moment.

Franklin Martin was never elected as a member of the Society of Clinical Surgery, for reasons not known. But he had similar desires to bring surgeons together to observe prominent surgeons in action, but his ideas were far more grandiose. He proposed a huge "Congress" of surgeons to come together and spend almost two weeks watching the top surgeons of the major cities in America. The idea came to fruition and in 1910 approximately 1,500 surgeons spent almost two weeks in Chicago (7-19 November 1910). A second meeting of the organization occurred in Philadelphia in 1911, also in November. The third meeting was held in New York in November 1912, and at that meeting, Franklin Martin and Edward Martin sat down together and formulated the first plans for the American College of Surgeons. In May 1913, Edward Martin was chairman of the meeting in Washington, D.C. at which the American College of Surgeons was formally recognized.

With this background—the reform of medical education, the scientific management of industry, and the organization of surgeons—the stage was set for Codman to promote and attempt to establish the End Result Idea.

The End Result Idea

What, exactly, was the End Result Idea? What did Codman mean by it? Here I must digress for a moment. We have used the terms "End Result Idea" and "End Result System" almost interchangeably. But other phrases have appeared with similar meanings—"Efficiency," "Standardization of Hospitals," and "Outcome Studies." The terms are not all strictly synonymous, but they are similar. The "End Result Idea" was Codman's term as defined above—basically all patients should be followed long enough to determine the outcome of medical care. The "End Results System" was another "Codmanism" which was the method by which he implemented the End Result Idea. It entailed keeping cards on each patient—more on the cards later. (Figure 8) "Efficiency" was a generic term used in that era to describe how well hospitals and doctors functioned. It loosely meant the quality of care. "Standardization of Hospitals" referred to requiring hospitals to meet some minimal standards of quality of care. It did not require hospitals to study outcomes, although Codman recommended it. "Outcome Studies" is the modern term, which is essentially identical with Codman's End Result Idea.

Fortunately, Codman has defined the End Result Idea for us many times in many articles and written publications. Codman called it, "The common sense notion that *every* hospital should follow *every* patient it treats, long enough to determine whether or not the treatment has been successful, and then to inquire, 'If not, why not?' with a view to preventing similar failures in the future."[184] However, he gave a longer, more complete definition as follows:

The End Result System

We have advocated a simple system of hospital organization first recommended by the Committee on Standardization of Hospitals of the Clinical Congress of Surgeons.

In brief, it is this:

That the Trustees of Hospitals should see to it that an effort is made to follow up each patient they treat, long enough to determine whether the treatment given has permanently relieved the condition or symptoms complained of.

That they should give the members of the Staff credit for taking the responsibility of successful treatment and promote them accordingly. Likewise they should see that all cases in which the treatment is found to have been unsuccessful or unsatisfactory are carefully analyzed, in order to fix the responsibility for failure on:

1. The physician or surgeon responsible for the treatment.

2. The organization carrying out the detail of the treatment.

184Preface, p. xii.

3. The disease or condition of the patient.

4. The personal or social conditions preventing the cooperation of the patient.[185]

Note the emphasis at the beginning of the fourth paragraph above: "That they should give the members of the Staff credit for taking the responsibility of successful treatment and promote them accordingly."

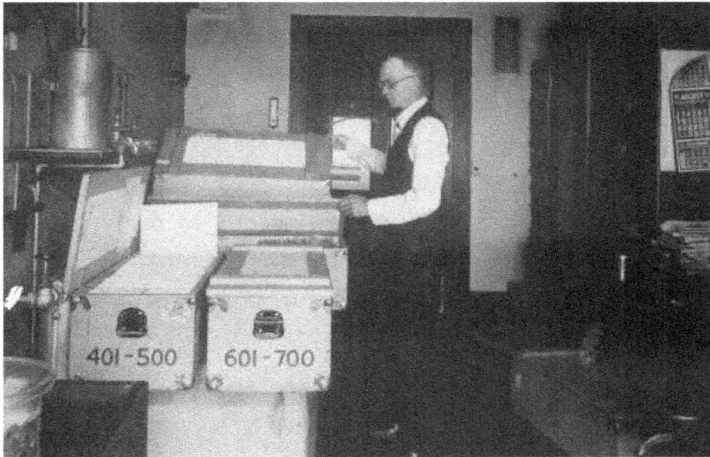

Figure 8—Codman working with his End Result Cards in their elaborate filing system. (Courtesy Francis A. Countway Library of Medicine, Rare Books and Special Collections Department)

Was it important to use the End Result Idea in 1910? Or in 1999? In 1910, Codman was probably the only doctor who thought so, though over the next few years he would receive the support of a few prominent doctors. But today his ideas are considered as necessary and important—by doctors, by patients, by lawyers, and even more, by insurance companies—even if the medical world of the near-21st century still does not strictly follow his system. As he always did, Codman gave carefully thought out opinions as to why it was important for both doctors and hospitals to measure their results and

---

185SHE, p. 6. All future footnote references to SHE refer to the 1917 edition of Codman's book *A Study in Hospital Efficiency*.

compare them to others, and included his thoughts on why doctors of his era resisted it.

> It is against the individual interest of the medical and surgical staffs of hospitals to follow up, compare, analyze, and standardize all their results, because:
>
> 1. It is seldom that any single individual's results have been so strikingly better than those of his colleagues, that he would desire such comparison and analysis. Perhaps the results as a whole would not be good enough to impress the public very favorably.
>
> 2. An effort to thus analyze is difficult, time-consuming and troublesome, and would lead, by pointing out lines for improvement, to much onerous committee work by members of the staff that would be still more time-consuming, difficult, and troublesome.
>
> 3. Neither Trustees of Hospitals nor the Public are as yet willing to pay for this kind of work.
>
> Therefore, if the trustees, the staff and the superintendent all avoid the analysis of results, and it is only for the interest of the patients, the public, and medical science, - why bother about it?
>
> The truth is, the patients and the public do not yet understand the problem. They suppose that of course somebody is looking into this important matter. They do not realize that the responsibility is not fixed upon any person or department.[186]

Though Codman was speaking of the resistance to the End Result Idea in the 1910s, he could as well have been speaking of the end of the 20th century.

What Codman wished to do was emulate Lord Kelvin and apply the scientific method to medicine. It would consist of making an intervention, measuring the outcome, and having concrete numerical

---

186*Ibid.* p. 5-6

outcomes to measure which outcomes were better. Although it could be considered experimentation, at least it was experimentation with an End Result in mind in which the scientist was attempting to find the best method of treatment. It was very similar to Taylorism but applied to the medical world.

Was Codman alone in his quest to reform medicine by use of the End Result Idea? To a degree, yes. Certainly, he was the only person for whom this quest was an obsession. But gradually, some of the other top surgeons in the country were becoming sympathetic to Codman's ideas, and foremost among them was Edward Martin. If Codman had to have a supporter, he could not have chosen a better one. Codman had known Martin since at least 1903. Though Harvey Cushing was Codman's closest lifelong friend, Codman and Martin struck up a strong friendship and mutual admiration. Their wives also became friendly, and it is possible that some of the affinity between the couples was that they were both childless.

In 1910, Codman and Martin spent time together during the meeting of the Society of Clinical Surgery in England. After one of the clinic visits, Martin and Codman shared a return ride to London. Codman recalled that throughout this visit to London, and especially during this cab ride, he spoke at length to Martin about the End Result Idea. He wrote of it, "From the day in the summer of 1910 on which Dr. Edward Martin of Philadelphia and I drove back to London in a hansom cab from the Tuberculosis Sanitarium at Friml[e]y this End Result Idea has taken the major share of my intellectual efforts."[187]

During this meeting Codman and Martin discussed the formation of the American College of Surgeons. Codman thought that the American College of Surgeons would be an important way to introduce the End Result Idea to the hospitals and doctors of the country, and Martin agreed with him. Codman quoted Martin as saying that, "The tail [End Result Idea] is more important than the dog [American College of Surgeons], but we shall have to have the dog to wag the tail."[188]

187Preface, p. xiii.

188*Ibid.*

Martin served as President of the Clinical Congress of Surgeons of North America in 1912. At the New York meeting in 1912, his first act was to appoint two committees—one to organize an American College of Surgeons to which he appointed Dr. Franklin Martin as chairman, and one to form a Committee of Standardization of Hospitals, to which he appointed Codman as chairman. Codman was delighted with this appointment, as he stated in the preface to his book on the shoulder, "This was proof enough for me of the result of my talk in England two years before, with Edward Martin, about the End Result Idea. He had recognized the zealot in me and had taken this opportunity to thrust on my Puritan conscience the duty to preach the doctrine I had expounded to him."[189] Franklin Martin informed Codman of his appointment as chairman of the committee in a letter dated 3 December 1912.

Be It Resolved By The Clinical Congress Of Surgeons In North America Hereby Assembled, That some standardization of hospital equipment and hospital work should be developed, to the end of these institutions having the highest ideals may have proper recognition before the profession and those of inferior equipment and standards should be stimulated to raise the quality of their work. In this way patients will receive the best type of treatment and the public will have some means of recognizing those institutions devoted to the highest ideals of medicine.

The following committee on standardization of hospitals was appointed by President Edward Martin, Ernest A. Codman of Boston, W. J. Mayo of Rochester, Minnesota, Allen B. Kanavel of Chicago, John G. Clark of Philadelphia and W. W. Chipman of Montreal. Martin also noted, "According to the names in this committee and precedent in such matters, you

---

189Preface, p. xvii.

will be known as the Chairman." This is, quite sure, as Edward Martin desired.[190]

Codman did note disappointment, however, that his obsession interrupted his work on the shoulder. For the next eight years his chief thought was to spread the End Result Idea to surgeons and hospitals of the country.[191]

The four other members of Codman's committee were Dr. Walter W. Chipman of Montreal, Dr. John G. Clark of Philadelphia, Dr. Allen B. Kanavel of Chicago and Dr. William J. Mayo of Rochester, Minnesota, all distinguished members of the medical community.

William James Mayo (1861-1939) was one of the two Mayo brothers responsible for forming the renowned Mayo Clinic in Rochester, Minnesota. He graduated from medical school in 1883 and then returned to Minnesota to take over his father's practice of medicine and, with his brother, Charles, helped establish the Mayo Clinic. His greatest recognition came for his work in abdominal surgery, especially for the treatment of ulcers and cancers. At various times he was President of the American Medical Association, the Society of Clinical Surgery, the American Surgical Association, and the Congress of American Physicians and Surgeons.

Dr. Walter William Chipman (1866-1950) practiced in Montreal, Québec, Canada, where he was a gynecologist and obstetrician at McGill University. The most politically influential physician of that era from Canada, Chipman helped found the American College of Surgeons, served as its president in 1925 and was a Governor of the College from 1938—1941.

Dr. Allen Buckner Kanavel (1874-1938) was a midwestern surgeon who received his medical degree from Northwestern in 1899. He joined the medical faculty at Northwestern in 1902 and served as an attending surgeon at the Cook County Hospital from 1913 to 1919. In 1905 he was

---

190This letter was published in the *Daily Bulletin of the Clinical Congress of Surgeons of North America, Third Annual Session*, November 11-16, 1912 in the minutes of the business meeting from Friday, 15 November at the Waldorf Astoria.

191*Ibid.*

appointed Associate Editor (under Franklin Martin) of the journal *Surgery, Gynecology & Obstetrics*, one of the leading surgical journals of the time. He is most famous today for his monograph, *Infections of the Hand* (1912), for which he is remembered by the eponym "Kanavel's Signs," which help with the clinical diagnosis of flexor tendon sheath infections in the hand.

Dr. John Goodrich Clark (1867-1927) was a Philadelphia surgeon who primarily practiced gynecology. He graduated from medical school at the University of Pennsylvania in 1891 and became a Professor of Gynecology at that school in 1899. He probably published more journal articles and books than any other surgeon of the era, and later served as the president of the Clinical Congress of Surgeons of North America in 1917.

As chairman of this committee, one of the first tasks Codman undertook was compiling a report for the Committee on Standardization of Hospitals. Concurrent with this, many letters circulated between Codman and the other members of the committee. Codman also corresponded extensively with Dr. Robert Dickinson, a gynecologist in New York who was a supporter of Codman's ideas. It should be noted that the Committee on the Standardization of Hospitals was not looking at End Results exclusively. The Committee was formed to evaluate the overall quality of hospital care, but Codman hoped to use the Committee to get hospitals to study their own End Results and thus perpetuate his goal. Surely, he also realized that quality could only be qunatified with the use of the End Result Idea.

The Committee on the Standardization of Hospitals was originally formed by the Clinical Congress of Surgeons of North America, but it was soon subsumed by the American College of Surgeons, and became a standing committee of the College. It was not the only such committee formed in this era. In fact, the idea of evaluating hospital care appears to have been somewhat "in the air." In the Codman Archives, there is a letter discussing this from Dr. John [Allen] Hornsby (1859-1939) of Chicago to Dr. Kanavel, dated 25 April 1913.[192] Hornsby told Kanavel, a member of the Committee on Standardization of

---

192CA 2/27.

Hospitals, that he was a member of the hospital section of the American Medical Association (AMA), which was a similar committee formed by the AMA at their Atlantic City meeting in 1912. He also mentioned that there was a third committee of five members, on which he (Hornsby) also served, that was appointed by the President of the American Hospital Association in Detroit in September 1912. He said that Dr. Henry M[ills] Hurd of Johns Hopkins (1843-1927) and Dr. Frederic A[ugustus] Washburn (1869-1949) of the MGH were members of both of the other committees and recommended to Dr. Kanavel that the three committees should work together.

Hornsby also mentioned that the Carnegie Foundation had become interested in Dr. Codman's work and was considering funding some of it. Codman attempted to interest the Carnegie Foundation to help force hospitals to study their End Results. There are several letters in the Codman Archives between Codman and Dr. Henry Pritchett of the Carnegie Foundation discussing this idea.[193]

Thus although Codman may have been somewhat a voice in the wilderness, the wilderness was becoming more crowded, and he was fortunate to be chairman of a committee made up of some of the most powerful physicians in the country and who supported his ideas.

Over the next year (1913), after the formation of the Committee on Standardization of Hospitals, Codman and these committee members worked to produce a report in which they hoped to establish standards by which to compare and certify hospitals. The members presented their report to the Clinical Congress of Surgeons at their meeting in Chicago on 11 November 1913. The report was well received by the Congress and they resolved that a copy of the report should be sent to all hospitals in North America.

Parts of the report read as follows:

REPORT OF THE COMMITTEE ON
STANDARDIZATION OF HOSPITALS

Your Committee on the Standardization of Hospitals begs to present the following report:

193CA 1/8

We have believed it to be the wish of this Congress, that we should examine the ways and means by which this body might best do its share in the general movement which the public is beginning to demand toward increasing the efficiency of hospitals.

We shall presently offer to you three definite suggestions for action by which you may materially aid this important movement, but first we should like to call your attention to the method by which we have approached this subject.

By what standards can we compare hospitals? It is obvious that there are many. There may be a standard of architecture, of cleanliness, of kindness to the patients, of nursing, of medical education, etc. To some persons the per capita cost, the number of patients annually treated, the success in private practice of their medical and surgical staff, the quality of the scientific papers produced, or the up-to-dateness of the laboratories may seem the important elements. Some hospitals seem satisfied with the famous contributions to medical science which some member of their staff made a hundred years ago.

We believe that you will agree with us that even cleanliness, marble operating rooms, famous physicians, and surgeons, up-to-date laboratories, and time-honored reputation do not necessarily mean that the individual patient will to-day be freed from the symptoms for which he seeks relief.

Even the standard of kindness cannot replace entirely the actual facts of the relief or prevention of symptoms or of the prolongation of life. Nor does a scientific paper written about the autopsy give the patient the satisfaction that a successful operation might have done.

The more time we have spent on this subject, the more obvious it has seemed to us that the only firm

ground on which we can compare hospitals is by the
actual results to the individual patient.[194]

The report then discussed hospitals' annual reports and how they
were quite variable. Usually the reports did not discuss actual End
Results of the patients' conditions, but merely gave financial and
economic summaries of each hospital's year. This format is similar to
that of many reports today, and unfortunately, echoes the modern
attitude of health insurance companies, which equate efficiency and
quality only with lowered costs and not better outcomes. Codman's
committee noted that:

> Further personal investigation of a number of the
> best institutions in the country developed the
> astounding fact that no effort is made to trace the
> patient beyond the gate of the hospital except such
> investigation as is individually made by members of
> the staff for their own interest. A patient might be
> operated upon, leave the hospital with the wound
> healed, and yet no effort be made to record the result
> of the operation. In other words, we have the paradox
> that neither the hospital trustees, the physician, nor
> surgeon, nor administrator consider it their business
> to make sure that the result to the patient is good.
>
> A factory which sells it products takes pains to
> assure itself that the product is a good one, but a
> hospital which gives away its product seems to regard
> the quality of that product as not worthy of
> investigation.
>
> In a way, trustees of hospitals who do not
> investigate the results to their patients do not audit
> their accounts.
>
> We believe it is the duty of every hospital to
> establish a follow-up system, so that as far as possible

194Codman EA et. al. Standardization of hospitals: report of the committee appointed by the Clinical Congress of Surgeons of North America, *Trans Clin Congress Surg North Amer*, 4: 3, November 1913.

> the result of every case will be available at all times for investigation by members of the staff, the trustees or administration, or by other authorized investigators or statisticians. We believe that the publication of such material in abstract by case numbers is practical and does not entail a disproportionate expense.[195,196]

Codman further discussed the consistency of hospital reports, and gave several methods by which hospitals could achieve this, always emphasizing that the reports had to include End Results. He then began a short discourse on how other medical groups could assist in this quest to better medicine. He also mentions the possibility of the Carnegie Foundation helping to institute the End Result System and assisting the Committee on the Standardization of Hospitals. This would eventually occur, but not as Codman visualized it, and not until 1917.

> It would be obviously inappropriate for this Clinical Congress of Surgeons to attempt any specific suggestion as to forms of hospital reports. Bodies such as the American Medical Association and the American Hospital Association are more fitted to do this since they represent general medical science and not a special branch.
>
> Your committee has been in touch with the various committees of these associations and has found them already actively working. The Committee on Medical Education of the American Medical Association whose chairman is Dr. [Arthur Dean] Bevan, has approached the Carnegie Foundation with a petition that it should investigate the efficiency of American hospitals after a similar manner to that in which they recently investigated medical education. Since such an investigation would entail great expense and require much time and effort it is unlikely that any unpaid

---

195The italics are mine.

196*Ibid.*, pp. 3-4.

board from the medical profession would be able to conduct it thoroughly. It is also probable that such a question of efficiency would best be studied by modern efficiency engineers—not by the medical men with preconceived ideas. For these reasons your Committee would favor any action you may see fit to take in adding the petition of this body to that of the American Medical Association and the American Hospital Association to broaden the scope of the investigation beyond that of medical education.

As it is highly probable that the Carnegie Foundation will undertake this matter at least so far as it concerns medical education, we may now consider what this Congress can do to aid them.

Representing as you do almost all the hospitals of the country, there is much which you may accomplish by a united, or rather a uniform, effort. It is safe to assume that those employed by the Carnegie Foundation will thoroughly investigate such matters as business efficiency, laboratory equipment, and the relations of medical education, etc.[197]

Codman further discussed the End Result System in the next section of the report, noting rather bluntly that, "When a follow-up system is once established it will do much toward weeding out the super-annuated, the lazy, and ill-trained surgeons of your community, even though they hold high places." It was further proof of Codman attacking the seniority system. Finally, the Committee's report gave three concrete suggestions as to how hospitals could improve their "efficiency."

Your Committee, therefore, has to offer the following three suggestions:

I. That this Congress give the stamp of its approval to an investigation of hospitals by the Carnegie

---

197*Ibid.*, p. 4.

Foundation and empower its representatives to urge the Foundation not to limit its inquiries purely to the bearings on medical education, but to classify hospital[s] according to their actual efficiency.

II. That each of us do what he can to induce the trustees of his own hospital to organize a follow-up system for all patients treated.

III. That each of us do what he can to induce the fellow-members of his staff to appoint efficiency committees who may look into present conditions in his own hospital, in order that we may as far as possible do our own housecleaning.

Such efficiency committees should be composed of a member of the trustees, a member of the staff and a superintendent.[198]

In closing the report, Codman left no doubt as to where his emphasis stood:

In closing this report, your Committee wishes to again state its conviction that the essential factor which will most contribute to raising the standard of American hospitals is the establishment in each hospital of a follow-up system of tracing the outcome of treatment give to each individual patient.[199]

The report was signed by all five members, led by Codman as the chairman. (Figure 9) It was purportedly from the entire committee, but it obviously was pervaded by Codman's philosophy. And just as surely, Codman made certain that the emphasis was on the End Result Idea by urging hospitals to begin implementing such a system.

198*Ibid.*, pp. 4-5.

199The italics are mine. The voice is, surely, Codman's alone.

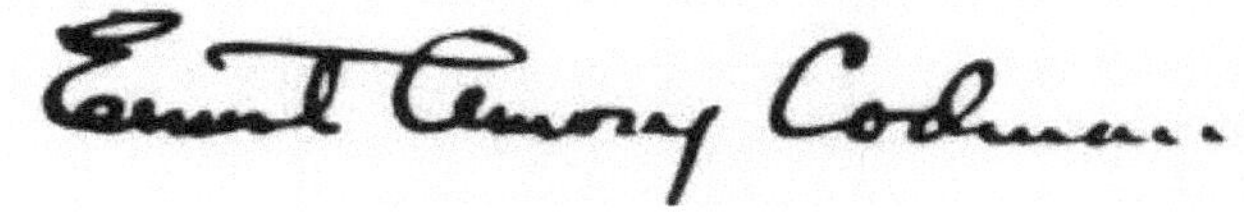

Figure 9—The signature of Ernest Amory Codman. (Courtesy Bill Mallon, M.D. Collection)

The Codman Archives contains telegrams and letters received from his fellow committee members as well as William Mayo's brother, Charles Mayo, congratulating him on the report.

> **Telegram from Allen B. Kanavel: "Congratulations Your report ought to be a landmark in hospital work No fault could be found with it We are delighted to have a report of that kind come from a member of the committee"[200]**
>
> **Telegram from W. W. Chipman: "Honestly think your paper is excellent Its chief strength is its personal note It is what cometh out of a man that is of value Congratulate you Very sorry cannot attend Boston meeting." [201]**
>
> **Letter from Charlie Mayo: "If I might give advice I would say that it would be well to publish this report as it requires something radical to call attention to the pressing conditions and creates an interest in discussion and brings about any change The report is most interesting." [202]**

Codman's report was well received by many people and, as Charles Mayo suggested, it was eventually published in *Transactions of the Clinical Congress of Surgeons of North America*, although it is now quite difficult to find.[203] However, it was probably best received by the man

---

200CA 1/10.

201*Ibid.*

202*Ibid.*

203Codman EA et. al., *op. cit.*, pp. 2-8.

who first entrusted him with the idea, Edward Martin. Martin's admiration for Codman is evident from the many letters he wrote him, which can be found in the Codman Archives. Though Martin received much credit for starting the Committee on Standardization of Hospitals he knew the philosophy behind it was Codman's and noted in a letter dated 8 May 1913, "You have put it up to me to 'create the phoenix' but I have no doubt this shall be considered your bird. She may prove to be a Vampire."[204]

This letter from Edward Martin followed a talk given by Codman in front of the Philadelphia Medical Society on 8 May 1913, as a result of an invitation received from Martin. Codman had warned the assistant administrator of the Massachusetts General in advance, "… If you know any trustee whom you would feel particularly glad to see insulted induce him to go to this meeting."[205] The talk, entitled "The Product of a Hospital," was his first public salvo in shocking doctors of the era, though its effect was mild compared to what he would achieve later with his cartoon. McLendon had this to say about Codman's speech, "Codman later wrote that this address was given to 'an enormous audience in the great hall of the Academy of Medicine' in Philadelphia, PA, on May 14, 1913, as the 'opening gun' of a national effort to standardize hospitals (an effort that resulted in the founding of the American College of Surgeons).[206] He related that 'there was much that seemed very radical in this address, and the audience showed itself [to be] not only interested, but stirred.' As a result, '…for a time, Pennsylvania was the shining light of this new form of hospital housecleaning.'"[207]

204CA 2/32.

205CA 2/36.

206McLendon has his chronology incorrect here. The American College of Surgeons was formed on paper in late 1912, well previous to Codman's talk in Philadelphia. Formal recognition came in May 1913 at a meeting in Washington, DC, but Codman's talk had no influence on that recognition. That work had already been completed.

207McLendon WW. Ernest A. Codman (1869-1940), the end result idea, and *The Product of a Hospital*. *Arch Pathol Lab Med*, 114: 1101, November 1990.

As it was given, however, without reading between the lines, the address seems rather tame. Following are some of Codman's conclusions:

> As a rule standards are raised by stimulating the best—not by whipping up the laggards. ... What then, are the products of a large hospital, ... The most obvious is the instruction of medical students receiving clinical experience as assistants or as graduates or undergraduates. ... Another product is the number of nurses graduating, and this product varies too, not only in number but in quality. ... The Massachusetts Hospital also furnished the community with a product of 18 trained house surgeons and physicians. ... I must confess that I have doubts as to whether the actual treatment carried out by these social workers during the past year has given real benefit, and yet I consider Dr. Cabot's exploitation of the social-service idea one of the most important products of our institution in the last decade. ... To my mind, ridden as it is by the end-result hobby, the social service department should be of greatest value as an instrument of recording the results of treatment. ... In 1912, 115 papers were printed by the staff of the Massachusetts General Hospital. All these papers are more or less products of the hospital—most of them entirely so. ... There remain many other by-products of a hospital, some of which are important. To my mind the influence of the hospital on the standards of medical practice in the community is of greatest importance. ... I therefore place the raising of the standard of professional honor—or shall I say accuracy—in a community as one of the most important by-products of a great hospital. ... We must formulate some method of hospital report showing as nearly as possible what are the results of the treatment obtained at different institutions. This report must be

made out and published by each hospital in a uniform manner, so that comparison will be possible. With such a report as a starting-point, those interested can begin to ask questions as to management and efficiency. (Italics mine)[208]

Edward Martin and Amory Codman began a vigorous correspondence, much of it contained in the Codman Archives. Much of it discusses the End Result Idea and Martin, older than Codman and a bit of a father-figure to him, often admonished him in the letters. Martin's letters display a wide-ranging, oft-amusing vocabulary, and he obviously delighted in addressing Codman by unusual, usually highly respectful, but occasionally deprecatory names such as "Jeremiah," "Wonderful Wizard," "Godlike," "Godlike Youth," "Joy of My Heart," "Martyr," and "Despair of My Mind."

> 1/21/14
> Dear Jeremiah; also Wonderful Wizard:
> How you forced through your admirable and galling regulations God alone, He know[s]; but you must have used some base means. Truly you have the knack of getting to the very heart of matters. I am taking your propositions very seriously. Also, my own little town has not been entirely idle. Socrates in the end was a civic pet. Jenner was blackballed by the College of Physicians of Philadelphia. Pasteur was scoffed and scorned in his own town. St. Peter's winning traits availed him nothing. Therefore supplication should be sent heavenward for the multiplication of enemies. Friends, true friends, frank friends are the hardest ones of all to endure, especially frank friends.
> As for your airy flight of fancy you surely have approached the subject of ptosis from a new angle. A novel method of treating. Doubtless the Bergeyon

apparatus, long since set away in attic and closets, will be brought out again and furbished and the biconcave neurasthenic blown to a condition of concavo-convexity will change her drag to a leap and her whine to a warble. In such a time a belch in place of being an embarrassing incident, will become a bereavement calling for letters of condolence. A favorite social amusement will take the form in arranging guests in the chromatic scale and percussing madrigals and roundelays on their ventral gipposities. Oh! happy, Godlike youth, I wish I had thought of it myself. Truly on the rare occasions when the Gods laugh the earth quakes in terror. Your dedication touched me deeply, a fitting tribute to a beautiful and blameless life.

My love and sympathy to the Haughty Lady.

Faithfully, nay fondly, yours,

Edward Martin

P.S. A person not unlike you in some ways, who occupies his own seat in history, when he came to be shot by the justly enraged humans, upon whom he had been inflicted by an all wise Providence, asked of his executioners, when he came to be destroyed, that they might not hit him in the face lest thereby the pleasure his beloved wife take in his demise, and the evidence thereof, might be marred. When your colleagues of the Massachusetts General see fit to exact their just due of you it might be well to make a similar request, or at least ask that the mutilation be confined within such limits as will make recognition possible. Think of the horror incident to an incomplete identification!

No more at present, excepting to tell young Cushing where he can go to, from

Faithfully yours,

EM[209]

In a letter of 23 February 1914, Martin mentioned, "We are now busy raising funds towards an efficiency study. The letters had gone out for the efficiency committee.[210] I am installing your system of follow on [End Results] at the University; starting at a number of other institutions. On the whole I am glad I met you."

Codman asked Martin to be a visiting professor in Boston on 10 June 1914, and made arrangements for this. A few months later, Martin replied, which contained his usual colorful comments:

> **13 May 1914**
> **Dear Codman:**
> **God bless you! I suppose I should hate you if I lived in the same town, but my feeling, being remote, is quite other. Indeed the very enemies who lurk in second story windows with muffled rifles are waiting your passing, are the ones who take off their hats in deepest respect as your cold, but beautiful, corpse is carried away.**
>
> **When a letter inviting me to come to Massachusetts came from an almost total stranger I had not thought but to tell him in three words to go to— —where he should. But when your communication came I had another think. If you truly want me to come of course I will. Martyrs are hell to live with but are delightful people to know and when they can be served and solaced without too much suffering upon the part of the server why go to! Man is a dog not to help. Therefore you shall behold me. Moreover, when a man says he wont do a thing and exhibits heat, it is quite sure he can be made to. The bitterness of denial is meant to conceal a fear of weakening. Also, you are entitled to your revenge and**

210The term efficiency was used frequently by Codman, and also by Edward Martin. Today we would interpret this meaning as "quality" and the "efficiency committees" of which they spoke are now termed "quality control committees."

I will do all the good I can, and incidentally, I will conceal much that I know of you.[211]

Letters continued to circulate between the two, with Codman always addressed by Martin with some unusual introduction such as "Dear God-like" or "Dear God-like Youth."

> 15 July 1914
> Dear God-like,
> … Before Mrs. Codman prostrate yourself in the form of a cross for three hours. Do this for me. In the presence of the Snail Lady, make seven genuflections, three salaams and respectfully suck in your breath eighteen times. Some day when you find an untrodden wilderness, without mosquitoes, ticks or thorny underbrush, ants or other troublesome denizens, trout streams environ by green meadows on which the grass grows short and the dew is in the early morning and a sandy bottom and a temperature at high noon of about 64, we will rough it together. I, however, to do the cooking, unless this sequestered spot is placed within easy sauntering distance of a French chef.[212]

Despite Martin's support the End Result Idea did not become the standard at hospitals and among doctors in the United States. In fact, it was hardly used at all, and still to this day, only some aspects of Codman's idea have been implemented. What were the reasons for this? This has been much debated. Mulley has these theories, "Now, back to the questions about Codman's frustration. Why was such a simple idea so strongly resisted? An answer might be that it was not so simple. Codman wanted to inform decisions and thereby improve the efficacy of medical care. However, outcome information is a necessary

---

211*Ibid.*

212CA 2/32.

but not sufficient element in any strategy to improve decision making."[213]

The longest discussion of why Codman failed to make the End Result Idea the norm has come to us from Berwick, who made these comments, "Ask a doctor about outcome measures; search a hospital for its end results recording system; study a nursing home for its continual improvement of process based on systematically acquired data from its patients. Nearly a century after Codman began, none will be found."[214] His fuller explanation for the reason was as follows:

> **Codman met in his time the resistance of arrogance, the molasses of complacency, the anger of the comfortable disturbed. Would he today find the same sources of resistance? I think he would find at least four, and we better honor his memory if we have the insight to see how we, too, resist the Codmans of today.**
>
> **Ambiguity in our objectives ... the outcomes of our care are not immeasurably complex, but they are complex. They are not 3-by-5, but 8-by-10. ... In our measurement tools we follow his spirit, but no longer his method. We have outgrown his method, even while we have not yet matured to his spirit.**
>
> **The myth of the physician as process ... It is not that physicians are never responsible for outcomes, but rather that we have so little to tell us when it is the doctors, and when it is the systems they work in, that make success and failure. Doctors are people acting in processes. Until responsibility for the process is fixed, and until we have sound theories of the sources of failure in those processes, we cannot expect enthusiasm for the study of outcome.**

213Mulley AG Jr. E. A. Codman and the end results idea: a commentary. *Milbank Quarterly*, 67(2): 259, 1989.

214Berwick DM. E. A. Codman and the rhetoric of battle: a commentary. *Milbank Quarterly*, 67(2): 263, 1989.

Money ... When Codman's light is turned on, only a portion of medical practices will be found effective, and we do not know in advance which ones they will be. Codman, like Wennberg, would be welcome today in the board room of the American payer, though not among those who make health care. In the doctor's cafeteria, Codman still might dine alone. He will cost somebody money.

Fear ... Codman would have about a 20 percent chance of being sued next year for malpractice ... Ernest Codman would be afraid today, not because he would doubt the wisdom of outcome measurement, but because he would doubt the wisdom of its use for censure, surveillance, accusation of the well-intentioned, and puffing of the proud. There is no hint of shyness in his character, but perhaps even he would hesitate. Perhaps even he would wonder, on the way to court, if the world he seeks to improve is showing the maturity to use the tools of improvement.[215]

Reverby has also speculated as to the reasons why Codman did not succeed in his quest. "More broadly, the E[nd] R[esult] S[ystem] broke the unwritten rules for tolerance and no open criticism considered necessary in the surgical world. ... Codman was exposing the limitations of its commitment to that excellence. ... It may well be that others in the profession knew far better than he that their understanding of the disease process was not advanced enough to withstand the scrutiny he demanded."[216]

By 1914, Codman had become the most powerful man in the country on the subject of standardization of hospitals and outcomes. With Martin's help he virtually controlled the topic in the United States but there was something further that he needed to do. He needed to publish his own outcome studies and let everyone know that he was willing to do this work himself. His only publications on outcomes

---

215*Ibid.*, p. 263-265.

216Reverby, p. 170.

were those describing Harrington's service in 1902 and 1904. He had alluded to the End Result Idea many times, but he had not yet published anything describing the results of his own outcomes, in which the article's primary emphasis was the End Result Idea. He would find a unique way to do this—enter the next stage of his life.

The Codman Hospital

In August 1911 Amory Codman left his full-time post as an assistant visiting professor at the Massachusetts General Hospital to open up his own hospital, which he called the Codman Hospital, located at 15 Pinckney Street in Boston. The Codman Hospital opened and begin treating patients in November 1911. It was a bold and risky move. He left the security of the best known hospital in Massachusetts, perhaps in the United States, for an unknown, unestablished hospital, whose main goal, to other surgeons of the era, seemed to be an attempt to analyze how often they screwed up.

Over the next few years (1911-1917) he used his hospital to follow the outcomes of every patient that he treated and those who were treated by the other doctors at the hospital. In fact, he openly sought to have other doctors help him at the Codman Hospital, although it was a small one with only 12 beds. However, he did require that anyone using his hospital was to report his own End Results and follow-up all of their own patients, however it is not clear how he enforced that requirement.

If Codman was a thorn in the side of other surgeons and physicians because he demanded that they follow their End Results, they could look no further than Amory Codman himself as an example of someone with the highest of ethics and the highest of ideals when it came to following his own patients. Nowhere is this more evident than in some of the advertisements which Codman developed to promote his own hospital, which are now contained in the Codman Archives.

Perhaps the most impressive promotional brochure is entitled, "Medical Ethics of the Codman Hospital". This is a short list of the ideals and goals of the Codman Hospital.. What we would now call a *mission statement*, it was unheard of at the time. It is reproduced here in full.

Medical Ethics of the Codman Hospital

This hospital stands for the following ideals which it desires to help to introduce into modern medical and surgical practice.

1. The best possible modern diagnosis should precede any form of treatment.

2. Diagnosis should be made impersonally for large numbers of patients for relatively small fees, whereas personal care and the friendly attention of the private physician should command relatively large fees, for it necessarily can be well given to but few people.

3. Skilled treatment, especially surgical treatment, should also be given to large numbers for small fees, for the attainment of skill necessitates constant practice.

4. Large fees are only justifiable when the profession has recognized the skill of the operator from the published reports of a recognized institution where his unexcelled ability in some particular kind of work has been demonstrated.

5. The prime function of the large charitable hospitals is the treatment of patients too poor to employ a physician, not to give diagnosis to physicians. Their secondary function is to contribute to medical science and to train doctors and nurses to serve the community.

6. It is an abuse of their function to allow men who neither contribute to science nor medical education, to serve on their staff, unless these men can <u>demonstrate superior skill by their results</u>.

7. It is an abuse of the confidence of a patient for a physician or surgeon to undertake his treatment unless the diagnosis is obvious or has been made authoritatively, or the need is urgent.

8. It is an abuse of the confidence of the patient for any physician or surgeon to undertake treatment which he knows he is not well qualified to give, even if the patient thinks he is.

9. Successful treatment is justifiable but the physician or surgeon who undertakes treatment which proves unsuccessful should be liable to the law to show that his diagnosis was authoritative and his experience justified thus undertaking the treatment.

Dr. Codman desires to announce that he has resigned from the Massachusetts General Hospital and will devote himself to his own hospital in the future with the hope of setting a practical and successful example to prove that the above principles are capable of actual demonstration.

If even a small fraction of the members of the profession of this community will help support this small hospital of twelve beds to make it a practical success the big hospitals will be forced to accept these ideas, or else see capitalized institutions take up their work.

The hospital is open for the use of other surgeons under the same conditions as those under which we use it ourselves, namely the strict observance of the End Result System.

When we know that any surgeon has demonstrated at any recognized public institution results in any branch of surgery which are superior to ours, we shall refer the case to him. If his fee is beyond the patients means the patient may return to us. Cases requiring expert diagnosis which only certain individuals can give will be referred in the same way.[217]

Note the emphasis in the above—it is all on the quality of care. "Large fees are only justifiable when the profession had recognized the

---

217CA 5/91.

skill of the operator ..." "...unless these men can demonstrate superior skill by their results." "... the physician or surgeon who undertakes treatment which proves unsuccessful should be liable to the law."

Codman needed help in getting his hospital started and he sought investors. Again, he produced a seven-page prospectus in an effort to interest investors in the project. He certainly must have scared many businessmen away with his emphasis on the fact that his hospital was based on getting the best patient results, and not making the most money. However, he discussed money at some length in this frank and unusual document.

An Opportunity to Invest in a Standard Hospital

People invest their money in real estate, railroads, mines, factories, industrial plants, and in all sort of securities, but very rarely in hospitals. The result is that there are very few good hospitals, where the patient is able to get his money's worth in service. If the public wants good hospitals, well run and conducted for their interest, they must invest in them, and ask a reasonable rate of interest in return. We hope that what follows will interest you enough to induce you to invest in the land, buildings and equipment of a standard hospital, run at standard rates for people of moderate means.[218]

What followed was a discussion by Codman in which he described "The Ideas for Which This Hospital Stands." Essentially, what he expected was that the hospital *not* be designed to make people rich - not the doctors, nor the investors. It was designed to improve the health of its patients. The product of the Codman Hospital would be the patient, nothing more, nothing less. If he was trying to attract financial investors, his candor surely frightened off many of them.

In the prospectus, he then listed his fees:

218*Ibid.*

MAXIMUM FEES

(Half of which will be used to maintain the Hospital and Clinic, and the other half divided among the Professional Staff)

Physical examination, diagnosis, and advice— $10.00

X-ray examination—$10.00

Later office visits for advice or treatment—$3.00

Calls at patient's homes—$5.00

(and $3 an hour after first hour)

Consultation with patient's physician at home— $10.00

(and $10 for each additional hour)

Care in Hospital (including operation and other professional services of Staff)

For first week—$100.00

For each week thereafter—$50.00

General Anesthetic—$10.00

Operations at patients' homes or at other hospitals—No fixed charges

MINIMUM FEES

(For patients who claim inability to pay the above).

One-half the above amounts (all used to maintain the Hospital and Clinic).[219]

Codman then described the advantage that would accrue to the patients who used his hospital. These were certainly the people who would benefit the most from his approach, and there was likely little reason to include this in the prospectus. But since he had by now likely scared off all potential investors by his earlier diatribes against the

---

219*Ibid.*

financial benefits of a hospital, there was probably no reason not to include this!

The Advantage to the Patient

The patient who comes to this hospital will first have a thorough physical examination, including perhaps several special examinations, e.g., those necessary for his eyes, teeth, nose, throat, etc. He, or his physician, if the patient delegates the responsibility, will be told in what respects he differs from the normal, and advice will be given as to how to obtain appropriate treatment for any disease or abnormal condition which may be discovered. If the patient has some trouble which our Staff is competent and equipped to treat successfully, we will accept the case; but if his trouble is obscure, or so difficult to treat that we do not care to undertake his case, we will refer him to a list of those specialists who have received the honor of appointments at our Charitable Hospitals, or the patient may engage the services of any member of our Staff privately, without having his case go on record. If he needs an operation, and we feel that we are likely to obtain a good result for him, we will undertake to operate at the rates shown in the fee table.

We believe that Insurance Companies, large industrial plants and even the State, may ultimately find that it will be less expensive in the long run to send patients to us under these conditions, than it is to send them to private physicians or to the Charitable Hospitals, as they do now.

The patient who seeks our aid will be assured, at least, that if we fail to give him relief, we shall not only refund our professional fees a year later, but will acknowledge the cause of error publicly in our

> **Hospital Report, and take what steps we can to prevent similar errors in future.. (Italics mine)** [220]

The last paragraph contains a statement that the medical profession still has never accepted to any degree—a warranty if the quality of care is found wanting. The vow to publish such failures to fulfill the warranty is also something which speaks of Codman's honesty in publishing his outcomes. You will not find this vow in any modern medical article, journal, book, or hospital report.

In the next section of this document, Codman described how he wished to finance his hospital. Basically, he solicited investors at $100 per share, hoping to raise $30,000 equity for start-up costs. It was a slightly dry section, addressed to doctors, giving financial details of how the hospital would be financed, and how the investors would be reimbursed. After that description, he returned to the subject of how he would manage the hospital, and the advantages it would offer, now emphasizing the advantages to the members of the professional staff, that is, the doctors. He noted, "Those physician, surgeons, or specialists who accept appointments on the Staff of this hospital, put themselves on record as approving the idea that the End Result System should be used in our Charitable Hospitals." But Codman never made it easy. He discussed the advantages that would come to the doctors at his hospital, but even these ideas may have scared off potential staff members.

> **There will be this advantage, then, to those who accept appointments at this hospital: that the records, which they will make of their reputations here, will be established by an exquisite test of their ability. This will be a far more delicate test than is customary in any other hospital, for in most of our Charitable Hospitals, at any rate, there is no standard whatever demanded, in regard to the actual competency of the individual members of the Staff, to successfully diagnose or treat the cases assigned to them.**

220*Ibid.*

> Of course, there will be a considerable percentage
> of error in the record of each member of this Staff, but
> this percentage of error will be far less than will be
> found in the private practice of other doctors, because
> as a rule, doctors do not select cases which they
> undertake to treat. Under present conditions of
> practice, there is no obligation for a doctor to refuse to
> treat a case which he knows he is not qualified to
> relieve. The patient is usually satisfied to have him
> say, "I do not know just what your trouble is, or
> whether I can relieve you, but I will try to do the best
> I can." [221]

Codman then returned to monetary matters, discussing what financial advantages would accrue to the doctors who operated at his hospital. He described in detail how the hospital staff would be formed. He proposed that he would invite the first member of the staff and from there, the staff would invite other members to join them. Always, he stated, they would try to find the "best" surgeons, those who had demonstrated some special expertise. He also noted, in direct contrast to the Massachusetts General, that the members would be re-appointed annually on a merit system. He finished this long advertisement by mentioning how his hospital would benefit many people, not simply the doctors, the investors, and the patients. And he ended it with the following summary, which contained some of his philosophy concerning End Results:

> We plan to have the coordination of our Staff so
> thorough, that no single physician or specialist can
> compete with us, but that every individual can
> cooperate with us, and use all that we can give him for
> the prices mentioned in the above Fee Table. This
> hospital is not a scientific institution except in so far
> as Simple Truth is Science. It is an eminently practical
> hospital, but it admits that to be truly practical it must

---

[221]*Ibid.*

> **necessarily be scientific in its methods of using facts.**
> **This is Efficiency.**
>
> **If you are interested in further details, send us**
> **word.** [222]

It was "classic Codman." Forthright, blunt, yet honest. He offended his "womb"—the MGH—by his attack on Charitable Hospitals. He offended all doctors who did not desire to participate in his hospital. He had to have offended almost the entire medical community of Boston and Massachusetts with the publication of the Codman Hospital goals. But at the core of his belief was an honest effort to start a new system of hospitals, one where the only goal was the betterment of the patient's condition by studying the outcome of medical interventions. The goal was not financial success, reputation, nor scientific fame. Paraphrasing a recent political catchphrase, Codman was saying, "It's the patient, stupid!"

Using his hospital, Codman was able to begin publishing and analyzing his own End Results. His first paper on the topic, based on his work at the Codman Hospital, was published in *The Modern Hospital* on 14 February 1914 and was entitled, "Money Spent on Hospitals for Cure of Patients". In April 1914, he published "The Product of a Hospital" in *Surgery, Gynecology & Obstetrics*. These two papers, which were basically summaries of his May 1913 talk in Philadelphia, argued that the product of a hospital was the patient and the successful outcomes of the patient's problems. His thesis was that financial matters were not terribly important and that the hospitals needed to be studying patient's outcomes and patient satisfaction more than publishing hospital reports that only examined financial statements, and the number of patients treated, rather than the number of patients treated successfully. He urged hospitals to standardize their annual reports so that they could compare their results.

Unfortunately Codman was never able to publish a large number of significant articles in medical journals on his own End Results from the Codman Hospital. The reason for this was that Codman wished to study the results of *all* patients with *all* problems, a goal that did not

---

222*Ibid.*

lend itself to grouping one or two isolated topics into simple articles. However, he did publish the complete results of his own outcomes, and the outcomes of the doctors in his hospital, but these would be in monographs and books which would come out between 1914 and 1917. The books and monographs were exhaustive, often giving case reports on every single patient treated. The information contained in these works could never have been contained in a journal article. Notably, and probably quite disappointing to Codman, other than Codman's descriptions in the monographs, no other doctor who used the Codman Hospital published their own End Results in journal articles. Again, it is not known how Codman tried to enforce this requirement for staff participation at the Codman Hospital.

Although Codman began working at his hospital in 1911, he also remained on the part-time staff of the Massachusetts General for a few years. For several years before his official resignation he attempted to get them to use the End Result System. Many letters went back and forth between Codman and the administration in which he urged them to lead the movement in the country by instituting a follow-up system. In 1912, certainly somewhat due to Codman's urgings, and probably also because of the Flexner Report's criticism of its seniority system, the MGH did adopt the basics of the End Result System, and abandoned its promotion system based only on seniority. After several frustrating years, and with his own hospital established, he withdrew from the Massachusetts General Hospital in the first week of March 1914. On 7 March, Dr. Joseph B[riggs] Howland (1873-1970), the assistant administrator of the hospital wrote to Codman after receiving his letter of resignation.

> **... they learn with regret of your resignation. I feel that the Staff and the Hospital have lost a good deal in your resignation. I realize that a large part of improvement in our methods following cases and recording results is due to your initiative and persistence in having these matters improved.**

I can only repeat that personally I regret
exceedingly that we shall not have you to prod us on
the things we should do.[223]

Codman replied to Howland two days later, continuing to urge him
and the Massachusetts General Hospital to institute the End Result
Idea.

9 March 1914
Dear Dr. Howland,
It was very kind of you to write me such a nice
personal letter regarding my resignation.

You have made one mistake in your letter which I
am afraid you will find troublesome. In your last
sentence you said you "shall regret that we shall not
have you to prod us up in the things we should do".
The reason for my resignation is largely you put me in
a position to do this with some effect. There are certain
things which I shall be able to do now which I could
not do before:

(1) to have personal talks with the Trustees when I
meet them;

(2) to speak in public straight from the shoulder
about the seniority system in motion;

(3) to tell people that although not so brilliant an
operator or so financially successful, I have done more
successful cases on really difficult stomach surgery at
the hospital than even the great Dr. [Maurice]
Richardson;

(4) and that the records of the M.G.H. will show
that with the exception of Accident Room cases (which
should be done by older men), I have never lost any of
the ordinary surgical cases such as hysterectomies, pus
tubes, joints, hernias, kidney cases, and all the other
routine things. In fact, I have magnified my own

223CA 2/36.

accordance to the horrible extent that feeling it is an excellent thing for the hospital to get rid of me in time to do the hospital some good!

Sincerely yours,

Codman[224]

These letters are contained in the Codman Archives, but unfortunately, Codman's resignation letter to the administration which had to have been dated just before Howland's letter of 7 March 1914 is no longer available to us. But Codman apparently mentions the above letter in the Preface:

> In order to attract the attention of the trustees of the M.G.H. I resigned from the staff in 1914 "as a protest against the seniority system of promotion," which was obviously incompatible with the End Result Idea. On the day on which I received the acceptance of my resignation, I wrote again, asking to be appointed Surgeon-in-Chief on the ground that the results of my treatment of patients at their hospital during the last ten years, had been better than those of other surgeons. I had tabulated my results in case they should ask to see them, but as no one had ever inquired into the results of other surgeons, there was of course nothing with which to compare mine. Thus, as I had planned, this fact was brought to the notice of the trustees, although at some personal sacrifice on my part. Naturally, my letter was ignored, and I was not appointed Surgeon-in-Chief.[225]

Codman's return letter requesting that he be appointed as Surgeon-in-Chief also has not survived, if he was indeed discussing his reply of 9 March 1914 to Howland (above). If so, he exaggerated somewhat in

---

224CA 2/36.

225Preface, p. xx-xxi.

the Preface, published 20 years later, as nowhere in that letter did he specifically make this request.

Between 1911 and 1914 Codman made a slow, grudging success of his hospital. Other prominent Boston surgeons, notably Harvey Cushing, were operating there, and financially he also did reasonably well for the era. He appeared to be busy, based on his increasing income. He noted in the Preface that his salary for 1911, $7,000, was his highest ever up to that point. It increased over the next few years to approximately $9,500 in 1913, with a small dip to $8,000 in 1914.[226]

By all accounts, at the end of 1914, Amory Codman had to be considered one of the most successful surgeons in the country. He had attended one of the nation's top college and medical school, and trained at one of the leading medical centers in the country. He had already published 63 journal articles, was the leader of one of the most powerful committees of the largest organization of surgeons in the country, had started and managed his own hospital, was a pioneer in shoulder surgery and abdominal surgery, and was the main proponent of a revolutionary idea that could possibly change the course of medicine. Surely, he was among the best and the brightest. But January 1915, in what Edward Martin later described as "his own lust for self immolation," lay just ahead.

226Based on inflation figured via the consumer price index, Codman's 1913 salary was equivalent to $145,000 in 1996 dollars, and his 1914 salary was worth about $122,000 in 1996. Both figures would be considered low for surgeons today, especially when one considers that Codman was among the elite doctors in a era when there was a large discrepancy between the best-trained and the poorest-trained doctors.

CHAPTER 7

THE MEETING AT THE BOSTON MEDICAL LIBRARY

There is a tide in the affairs of men,
Which, taken at the flood, leads on to fortune;
Omitted, all the voyage of their life
Is bound in shallows and in miseries.

William Shakespeare, *Julius Caesar*, [1599], Act IV, Scene iii, Lines 217-220

He had been to the medical manor born; schooled at a prestigious prep school, Harvard College and Harvard Medical School, a leading professor of surgery at one of the three or four most renowned hospitals in the country. The first 15 years of his practice had done nothing to diminish that career, so full of potential and hope. Though in the last five years, Amory Codman had sown the seeds of his discontent, he was still a member of all the best surgical societies, highly published in the medical literature, and a pioneer in several areas of medicine. But if one single night can effectively ruin a surgeon's career, it is likely that this happened to Codman on a Boston winter's eve in 1915.

What could he have been thinking? Surely he must have known that what he was about to do would possibly end the brilliant career which he had so carefully nurtured over the last two decades, but he seemed not to care. To Codman, it was the End Result Idea that mattered, and only the End Result Idea. He would do everything in his power to get the surgeons of Boston and the Massachusetts General

Hospital to realize how important the idea was, to the point of risking personal, professional, and financial ruin in the attempt.

In 1915, Codman was the chairman of the Surgical Section of the Suffolk District Medical Society.[227] As part of his duties, he was to chair two meetings to be held in the winter of 1915, both at the Boston Medical Library. The first meeting was to be held on 6 January 1915 and Codman planned it as a meeting for the discussion of hospital efficiency, which was the generic term in that era used to describe the improvement of medical care. However, he viewed it primarily as an opportunity for him to promote the End Result Idea to the physicians of Boston. The second meeting was to be held on 3 February 1915 and the topic of discussion was to be the treatment of femur fractures. Unfortunately, because of the events of the first meeting, Codman would never chair that second meeting.

Prior to the 6 January meeting Codman went to great efforts to organize it and enlist speakers whom he thought would support his views. He asked the president of Harvard, A[bbott] Lawrence Lowell (1856-1943), to speak but received a regret letter from him.[228] He was unable to get a commitment from Charles H[enry] W[heelwright] Foster (1859-1955), the administrator of the Massachusetts General Hospital, who cited a previous engagement. Codman was contemptuous of these refusals and so stated in the Preface, "Unfortunately the president of the university had an engagement for a small social dinner far in advance of the date of the meeting, and so on down the line. Nobody in any position with authority in our medical school cared to take the responsibility of answering these simple direct questions. They all knew the answer was, that nobody was responsible for examining the results of treatment at hospitals, and that the reason was MONEY; in other words, that the staffs are not paid, and therefore cannot be held accountable. Furthermore, I knew that even the speakers whom I did succeed in obtaining, could not, as guests of our SOCIETY, be as frank as perhaps they would like to be, and would not

---

227Suffolk County is the county in which Boston is located.

228CA 3/47.

suggest the reason for it, although they might admit the fact that there is no analysis of results in most hospitals."[229]

However, several influential people in the Boston medical circles in the Boston medical circles did accept Codman's invitation, as did two highly influential people who supported his ideas on reforming medical care, Dr. Robert Dickinson of Brooklyn, New York, and Frank Gilbreth of Providence, Rhode Island.

In addition to Dickinson and Gilbreth, the Mayor of Boston did agree to speak, and he would be the first speaker that night, as he had to leave before hearing the other speakers. Mayor James Michael Curley (1874-1958) was in his first term as Mayor of Boston, but he would eventually become one of the most powerful politicians in Boston and Massachusetts history. He was also quite controversial. A biography of Curley describes him as a, "Twice-jailed scoundrel and the people's champion, builder of hospitals and schools and shameless grafter, pioneer of the New Deal, 'Kingfish of Massachusetts,' compelling orator and master of political farce, James Michael Curley was the stuff of legend long before his life became fiction in Edwin O'Connor's classic novel *The Last Hurrah*. As mayor of Boston, as congressman, as governor of Massachusetts, Curley rose from the Irish slums in a career extending from the Progressive Era of Teddy Roosevelt to the ascendancy of JFK."[230]

Curley was of the appropriate Irish descent for that most Celtic of American cities. He served in the House of Representatives from 1912 to 1914, resigning when he was elected Mayor of Boston in 1914. He eventually served four terms as Mayor of Boston, 1914-1918, 1922-1926, 1930-1934, and 1946-1950. He also served as Governor of Massachusetts from 1935-1937. Curley was an appropriate politician to be on hand for a medical meeting, because he established much of his reputation by building and enlarging hospitals, often hospitals used mainly by the poor. He added many new wards and beds to the Boston City Hospital during his terms as mayor. After one of his construction improvements to this hospital, Boston had its lowest tuberculosis rate in years.

229Preface, p. xxiv.

230Beatty J., *The Rascal King*, (Reading, MA: Addison-Wesley, 1992), back cover text.

Demonstrating his knowledge of, and interest in, medical problems, Curley was noted to have said that he was always of the opinion "that tuberculosis was an economic disease, rather than a medical one."[231]

Although Curley would not stay that night to hear Codman's diatribes and the censure that Codman received, he was surely made aware of them. However, he remained a big supporter of Codman with several later letters from him lauding his work contained in the Codman Archives.

Dr. Robert Latou Dickinson (1861-1950) was a gynecologist who practiced in Brooklyn at the Women's Hospital. Although Codman has always received most of the credit for starting the End Result Idea in this country, Dickinson was his greatest disciple, and the Women's Hospital of New York was really the first hospital in this country to institute the use of the End Result Idea, and implement it more fully than any other hospital. He was a prolific writer, publishing over two hundred research papers on obstetrics and gynecology. He was also the first gynecologist in this country to devote time to studying sexual activity, and worked on the early research into birth control along with Dr. Margaret Sanger. Dickinson and Codman corresponded frequently, although their letters were never as verbose as those of Edward Martin.

Frank Bunker Gilbreth (1868-1924) was not a physician, but was one of the most important and influential engineers in the early part of the 20th century. Neuhauser has noted, "Gilbreth had once thought of becoming a surgeon but could not afford the education; instead, he went to work for a brick company, where he developed his theories on efficiency. As a patient, he concluded that hospitals were inefficient, and by 1913 he was taking movies of surgical operations in order to analyze the motions and speed of team members to see whether he could improve their efficiency."[232] He had taken his own engineering studies and principles, many of them based, at least initially, on Taylorism, and tried to apply them to the practice of medicine. This interested Codman, who wished to make similar contributions to the

---

[231] *Ibid.*, p. 230.

[232] Neuhauser, p. 312.

improvement of medical care. Wrege described Gilbreth's rationale as follows, "Because Gilbreth had once planned to be a surgeon, he decided surgeons were the 'high-brows' he should study. He began his studies by observing a large number of operations conducted by a surgeon friend and then criticizing his work from the point of view of scientific management. At the conclusion of his observations, Gilbreth told the surgeon: 'If you were laying brick for me, you wouldn't hold your job ten minutes. One sample of work like that and you would be fired. If you are a first-class surgeon, and this first-class hospital service, it doesn't take a clairvoyant to see where the undertaker gets his.'"[233]

Gilbreth lived only forty miles from Boston, in Providence, Rhode Island, and followed the early work of Frederick W. Taylor, and the precepts of Taylorism, in an attempt to establish principles by which workers could do their job better and more efficiently. At the time of the meeting in the Boston Medical Library, he was attempting to apply these principles to the practice of medicine and, as a result, Codman had become interested in Gilbreth's work. Unfortunately, Gilbreth ran into many of the same difficulties that Codman did, and was never terribly successful in modifying surgeons' and physicians' practices so that they became more efficient, both in terms of time spent and improved ergonomics.

Codman, Dickinson, and Gilbreth became the "great triumvirate" who attempted to radically change medicine and its efficiency in the second decade of this century. Dickinson first began studying ways to improve the efficiency of the operating room as early as 1902, but his ideas were greatly influenced by Gilbreth's publications, and Dickinson put into practice Gilbreth's idea of charting the organization of a hospital. In an early paper by Dickinson on his attempts to improve surgical efficiency, he quoted Gilbreth, "Use few tools. Imagine yourself operating out under a tree. Hunt out the best experience, measure it, make it a standard, write it down on an instruction card. Above all get your people thinking in terms of elementary motions."[234]

233Wrege CD, "Medical men and scientific management," *Proc Acad Mgt*, 114-118, 1980, referencing Nock AJ, "Efficiency and the High-Brow: Frank Gilbreth's Great Plan to Introduce Time-Study into Surgery," *The American Magazine*, March 1913, p. 50.
234Wrege CD, "The efficient management of hospitals," p. 117, quoting Gilbreth from RL Dickinson's paper, "Standardization of surgery: an attack on the problem," *JAMA*, 63(5): 763-765, 29 August 1914.

The triumvirate would not last, possibly self-destructing due in part to Codman's actions in January 1915, although Wrege had other ideas. He described the dissolution of the team, "The outset of World War I caused the team of Codman, Dickinson, and Gilbreth to dissolve. Codman closed his hospital and entered the Army Medical Corps, Dickinson went to China for the U.S. Public Health Service, and Gilbreth joined the Army Corps of Engineers. After the war, the team did not reassemble. Codman was financially unable to reopen his hospital, Dickinson turned to development of birth control devices, Gilbreth had a heart attack during the war and was not well."[235]

The other people who spoke that January night were Herbert Burr Howard (1855-1923), Walter Wesselhoeft (1838-1920, and Joel Ernest Goldthwait (1866-1961). Howard was termed by Codman as the "superintendent" of the Peter Bent Brigham Hospital in Boston. Today, he would be called a hospital administrator. Howard was a doctor, having practiced at the Massachusetts General Hospital until 1908 when he took over as administrator. He held the post until 1919 and never again practiced medicine.

Wesselhoeft and Goldthwait were also physicians. Born in Germany, Wesselhoeft first established his practice in North America in Halifax, Nova Scotia. In 1873 he came to the United States and in the same year helped found the Boston University School of Medicine. By 1909 he was professor emeritus at the University and later devoted much of his time to the Massachusetts Homeopathic Hospital, first as a visiting physician and later as a consulting physician and trustee.

Goldthwait was an orthopedic surgeon who was Harvard trained. He graduated in 1888 and, as had Codman, began his practice at the Massachusetts General Hospital. He resigned from the Mass General in 1907 to begin practicing at the Robert Breck Brigham Hospital. Although he continued to practice orthopaedic surgery at Robert Breck Brigham, and an influential orthopedic surgeon, he also became involved in hospital administration. Goldthwait spoke in January 1915 not as a surgeon, but as a trustee of the Robert Breck Brigham Hospital.[236]

235*Ibid.*, p. 117.

236Goldthwait and Codman did have a common interest in the shoulder. Goldthwait published an early

After he had organized the preceding group of speakers, Codman was eventually able to produce the following circular announcing the meeting.

A Meeting for the Discussion of Hospital Efficiency
At the Boston Medical Library,
Wednesday, January 6th, 1915, at 8.15 P.M.
under the auspices of
The Surgical Section of the Suffolk District Medical Society

Up to the present time the public and the medical profession have regarded Hospitals as places for the treatment of the sick, but not necessarily for their efficient treatment. Attention had been paid to the cleanliness of institutions, to the architectural arrangement of the buildings, to the kindliness of the staff and nurses, etc., but no attempt has even been systematically made to determine whether the treatment so freely given has been efficient—that is, as successful as possible.

In most hospitals there has been no official or department whose duty it has been to ascertain the results of treatment at all, much less to compare the results attained by different members of the staff in any one institution, or even to make a collective comparison of the results attained by the whole staff, with those of another similar institution.

Evidently, Trustees, as a rule, have felt that the best they could do was to appoint respectable men on their staffs and then to leave the degree of efficiency of the treatment given the patients to the individual conscience and ability of the physician or surgeon on

---

paper on sub-coracoid bursitis, similar to sub-acromial bursitis, and a topic which has found renewed interest only recently. Goldthwait's article was entitled "An anatomic and mechanical study of the shoulder-joint, explaining many of the cases of painful shoulder, many of the recurrent dislocations, and many of the cases of brachial neuralgias or neuritis," and was published in the *American Journal of Orthopaedic Surgery*, 6: 579-606, 1909.

duty. The terms of duty have been arranged by the calendar or by seniority.

Obviously, if there is any difference in the value of the services of one surgeon or physician and another—which the public seems to admit by its willingness to pay large fees—this difference must be capable of demonstration by some comparative test, so that the distribution of the cases may be made more rationally than by the calendar or by seniority. No physician or surgeon nowadays can be expected to be proficient in all the branches of even a single specialty.

Has the time come when hospital organization can be based on the idea of giving the patients successful and effective treatment as well as care and kindness? Is it possible to compare therapeutic results in medicine and surgery, or must we admit that no matter how much we read, study, practice and take pains, when it comes to a show-down of the results of our treatment, no one could tell the difference between what we have accomplished and results of some genial charlatan or some less painstaking and energetic colleague?

Comparisons are odious, but comparison is necessary in science. Until we freely make therapeutic comparison, we cannot claim that a given hospital is efficient, for efficiency implies that the results have been looked into. Hospital efficiency is mainly therapeutic efficiency.

The meeting on January 6th is to stimulate thought on these questions. Has it occurred to you that no person or department in a charitable hospital is responsible for the medical and surgical efficiency?

The speakers will discuss the questions of who should be responsible.

The following is the provisional Programme:

Hospital Efficiency from the standpoint of an efficiency expert.

Mr. Frank B. Gilbreth, of Providence, R. I.

Hospital Efficiency from the standpoint of a hospital surgeon.

Dr. Robert L. Dickinson, Brooklyn, N. Y., Surgeon to the Brooklyn Hospital (Gynaecology)

Hospital Efficiency from the standpoint of a hospital superintendent.

Dr. Herbert B. Howard, superintendent of Peter Brent Brigham Hospital.

Hospital Efficiency from the standpoint of hospital trustees.

Dr. Walter Wesselhoeft, trustee of the Mass. Homeopathic Hospital.

Dr. Joel E. Goldthwait, trustee of the Robert B. Brigham Hospital

Hospital Efficiency from the standpoint of a public servant.

His Honor Mayor James M. Curley.

General discussion.[237]

The six speakers who preceded Codman spoke for several hours, but Codman's talk lasted for only a few minutes. As with Lincoln's Gettysburg Address, which was preceded by a now-forgotten two-hour speech by Edward Everett, nobody remembers a word said that day other than those brief few spoken by Codman.

The speeches of Goldthwait, Howard, and Mayor Curley from that January night have not survived, but abstracts of the lectures of Gilbreth, Dickinson, and Wesselhoeft were later published in the *Boston Medical and Surgical Journal*.[238]

As mentioned above, Curley spoke first, and then left without hearing the other speakers. Gilbreth followed and began his talk by

---

237CA 3/50. The announcement is typeset, so it was printed, but its source is not given, and I cannot recognize it.

238BMSJ, 172(21): 774-779, 27 May 1915.

defining an efficiency expert, calling him someone who substituted accurate measurement for personal opinion, judgment, and unscientifically derived conclusions. He termed a hospital a "happiness factory," implying that its job was to produce patients who were happy with their medical care. Gilbreth finished by urging all in attendance to apply accurate measurement, recording what they were doing, how they were doing it, and why they were doing it. With a call to supporting Codman and the End Result Idea, he stated, "The first step in all improvement is an accurate record of present practice. But where is there such a record of hospital practice?"[239]

Dickinson followed Gilbreth and spoke on "Hospital Efficiency from the Standpoint of a Hospital Surgeon." He outlined the features of a hospital that he considered amenable to standardization, measurement, and improvement. Among these he considered the training and qualifications of the workers and heads of the departments, which included the doctors and nurses; the tools and equipment; the organization of the workplace; and finally, the procedures. Dickinson was using the principles espoused by Taylor and Gilbreth, and attempting to apply them to medicine and especially, to the operating room.

Dickinson emphasized that the procedures of medicine and surgery could be improved, stating, "As to the procedure, there is no frequently repeated act in hospital work, from the taking of the histories up to the team work in the gravest operation, that cannot be plotted out to standard made up from a study of the best methods, and printed on instruction cards."[240]

His talk was very concrete, giving specific examples of how hospitals and doctors could improve their methods and their efficiency. He presented a detailed form that he entitled "Suggested Form of Report on Efficiency of Each Member of Professional Staff," and in which he called for the professional staff to begin using "Codman's Method of End Results."[241]

239BMSJ, 172(21): 774-775, 27 May 1915.

240BMSJ, 172(21): 776, 27 May 1915.

241Ibid.

Wesselhoeft's talk was a bit unusual and probably frustrated Codman a great deal. Wesselhoeft spoke, not as a doctor, which he was, but as a hospital trustee, which he also was, representing the Massachusetts Homeopathic Hospital. He agreed with much of what had already been said by Gilbreth and Dickinson and the other speakers, but he felt that some of it could not be instituted, "I believe that sooner or later the profession will wake up to the need of this reform; but for obvious reasons the trustees cannot be asked to introduce innovations of so far reaching and difficult a nature." That was clearly not what Codman wanted to hear and echoed his earlier battles with the Massachusetts General administration.

Near the end of his lecture, however, Wesselhoeft made a comment that likely endeared him to Codman, "So long as doctors differ (and in our hospitals as elsewhere, they will always claim the right to do their best in their own way) there must be found a way of differentiating the better from the good and the good from the bad."[242] And that was clearly what Codman wanted all in attendance to hear.

After the other speakers finished, Codman stood up to speak. Almost immediately after he had begun his speech, he had Gilbreth unveil a large cartoon that he had commissioned from a friend.[243] The cartoon showed a picture of an ostrich with its head buried in the sand kicking out Golden Eggs to the Back Bay physicians who gladly accepted them while the administrators of the Boston hospitals sat by oblivious to any results of the medical care as long as Golden Eggs were produced by the ostrich. (Figure 10) Codman explained the cartoon in detail:

Now I want to say that there are two classes of people in this audience; one class is those who believe in humbug[244] and who are afraid to say so and the

---

242BMSJ, 172(21): 778, 27 May 1915

243The cartoon was drawn for Codman by an artist friend of his, Philip D. Hale.

244Humbug is a favorite adjective of Codman's, and actually was quite famous in medical history. The first public demonstration of anesthesia, then exclusively ether, occurred at the Massachusetts General Hospital. The ether was given by William T[homas] G[reene] Morton () to a patient of Dr. John Collins Warren, while Warren removed a tuberculous gland from the patient's neck. After finishing the operation, Warren turned to the audience and noted, "Gentleman, this is no humbug." Humbug, hardly ever heard used today, is defined in *Webster's Third International Dictionary* as "Something designed to deceive and mislead;

other class does not believe in humbug and is afraid to say so. Now, the speakers have approached the subject of humbug as nearly as I should expect them to. Now, I have with the assistance of a friend who is more of an artist than I, illustrated the subject of "Humbug." I will try to explain it and then after the meeting you can come up a little close. Now, may I ask those in the audience to raise their hands if they believe in humbug and now will those in the audience who do not believe in humbug raise their hands. Then there are those who believe in humbug and are afraid to say so and there are those who don't believe in humbug and are afraid to say so. Now, I will explain this picture, and I will say that I take the responsibility upon my own shoulders for its production and introduction here tonight and say that the Trustees didn't know about it and in fact nobody but my friend, the artist, and myself. Now, we have all heard of the Goose that laid the golden eggs. Now, in this case it is an ostrich with her head buried in the sand eating humbugs and she is kicking the golden eggs over to the Back Bay physicians across the bridge; and here is the Harvard Bridge and over there is the Harvard Medical School and on the left are the professors who are reaching out to grab the golden eggs as they fall; and over here to the right are three or four or five Trustees. I couldn't get them all in. When I was connected with that institution years ago I never found or could find even that number and I could rarely get at them at the Massachusetts General and I had to see some of them at the club and some of them at other social functions. The likenesses are not like anybody in particular and I trust that they are not enough like anybody here to be embarrassing. Now, if you will

---

quackery, hoax, fraud, imposture."

look closely enough, you will see what the Trustees are saying. The clinic group was originally taken from the Massachusetts General Hospital. We are all there too. There are only a few represented here.

As I pointed out in the announcement of the meeting this discussion was to be upon whose shoulders the responsibility for the efficiency in a hospital rest. Now, in this city of Boston there in this sketch there is the Harvard College, Harvard Medical School and the Harvard Medical professors. We are taken in hand by the physicians and the surgeons take out our appendix. We all admire the man who works for the title of surgeon.

Now, here you see President Lowell standing on the bridge and just this side of the bridge in the doorway of the Harvard Medical School you see the Dean of the Harvard Medical School standing and you see the Memorial Hospital there, and the Dean is wondering why those throngs of students don't come to the Harvard Medical School for we know that the Harvard Medical School hasn't as many students as they should have. What will bring them here? These Medical records and the clinic system. Now, I ought to have said and I suppose that I did say that on the West is put a little figure, that is Dean Badger who is heading so that he has his back to us. Now, I may be very wrong and dreadfully wrong and honestly I may be dreadfully wrong but I am sure that I wouldn't have taken hold of this unless I thought it was a great purpose.

Now, Dr. McL[a]ughlin has possibly something that he wishes to say and possibly there are others who have convictions as to whether or not they believe in humbug.[245]

245CA 3/48.

[Joseph Ignatius] McLaughlin's (né 1861) comments are not recorded, but he was a prominent surgeon at the MGH and it is certain that they were not adulatory. After fielding a few other comments, also not left to us, Codman took back the floor to close the meeting.

> **Gentleman, I am glad there are two gentlemen in the audience who are of the belief that there are humbugs in hospital efficiency and who are not afraid to speak.**
>
> **Are there others who wish to speak on this subject before us tonight? If not, the meeting is adjourned.**[246]

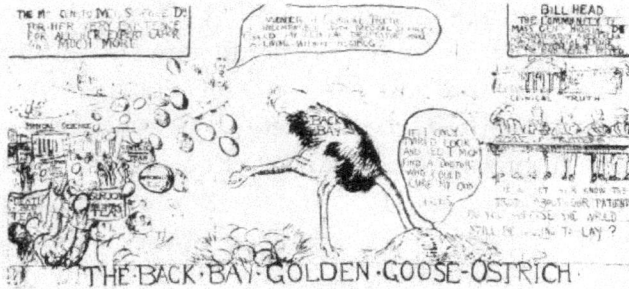

Figure 10—The famous, yet controversial, cartoon which Codman displayed at the Meeting of the Surgical Section of the Suffolk District Medical Society on 6 January 1915 at the Boston Medical Library. It was drawn by Philip D. Hale, and unveiled that night by Frank B. Gilbreth. (Courtesy Francis A. Countway Library of Medicine, Rare Books and Special Collections Department)

At the end, many of the doctors sat there stunned by Codman's presentation, and nobody really knew what to say. Codman had essentially insulted almost everyone in the room, as well as almost every doctor in Boston. He described the reaction in his Preface.

> **The audience held its mouth open while I explained the meaning of the picture, and even after I had finished, continued to be aghast for a minute or two. Then there was as near an uproar as ever I have**

246Ibid.

seen at a Medical Meeting. Some fine old men who had loyally worked for the university, and whose careers I respected, got up and walked out with bowed heads. Other younger ones of the same type rose together to seek the floor, with anger but with nothing practical to say. The great majority, however, were amused more than they were shocked, and a few even risked their reputations by coming publicly forward and shaking hands. For weeks some of my friends did not speak to me, and if I entered a room where other doctors gathered, the party broke up from embarrassment or changed their subject. I was asked to resign as Chairman of the local Medical Society.[247]

The response to his talk was immediate. Codman did resign, as requested, as chairman of the Surgical Section of the Suffolk District Medical Society, in a letter dated 11 January 1915. The resignation was accepted — probably unanimously. Within a few days[248] the Boston papers devoted extensive coverage to the meeting which was almost unheard of at the time for a medical meeting. The *Boston Daily Globe* story, which was on the first page of the paper, was headed by, "Cartoon Raises Surgeons' Ire: Dr. Codman Stirs Up Medical Society," while the *Boston Herald* carried the article on an interior page, with the headline, "Doctor-Critic Stirs Wrath."

247Preface, p. xxv.

248For some (unknown) reason, the articles in the Boston papers did not appear until Monday, 18 January 1915, 12 days after the meeting.

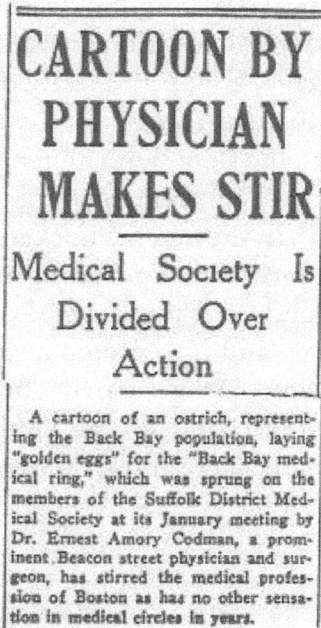

CARTOON BY PHYSICIAN MAKES STIR

Medical Society Is Divided Over Action

A cartoon of an ostrich, representing the Back Bay population, laying "golden eggs" for the "Back Bay medical ring," which was sprung on the members of the Suffolk District Medical Society at its January meeting by Dr. Ernest Amory Codman, a prominent Beacon street physician and surgeon, has stirred the medical profession of Boston as has no other sensation in medical circles in years.

Figure 11—Headline in the *Boston Post* from 18 January 1915, detailing the reaction to Codman's cartoon and the meeting at the Boston Medical Library. (Courtesy Bill Mallon, M.D. Collection)

The articles in the Boston papers were very similar, with the longest one contained in the *Boston Post*, and entitled "Cartoon by Physician Makes Stir." (Figure 11) The *Post* article stated that Codman had stirred up a hornet's nest and described his resignation:

Resigns as Chairman

The cartoon and certain "personalities" indulged in by Dr. Codman in an effort to awaken his colleagues to the importance of prompt action in establishing a system for hospital efficiency aroused such resentment among some of the members that Dr. Codman has resigned as chairman of the surgical section of the society of which he had arranged for a series of discussions on this topic.

The resignation has been accepted by the committee of supervision of the Medical Society, and

the president, Dr. Horace D. Arnold, has been placed in charge of the future lectures in the series.[249]

Throughout this article, however, Codman is quoted as defending himself multiple times. He said that he had intended the cartoon to be humorous and that his criticism of men in institutions was friendly.[250] When asked what he meant by humbug, Codman replied, "By 'humbug' I mean the immemorial habits of the community of insisting on being deceived to a greater or less extent by the medical profession. For instance, there is hardly any surgical operation simpler and surer than the removal of the appendix, if the patient is not sick. Yet the community insists on paying high prices for this comparatively simple operation and permits any surgeon to explore any of their vitals if he merely mentions the possibility of appendicitis. One of the first things which a lay trustee and efficiency committee would discover would be the fact that all the hospital reports of Massachusetts show that simple appendectomy in earlier chronic cases has practically no mortality."[251] He would not back down. Surely the newspaper articles served only to alienate more of the Boston medical community.

Codman insisted that he had not resigned from the Suffolk Society altogether but only as Chairman of the Surgical Section. He also stated that he, in no way, would be deterred from his eventual goals. He noted, "When the twelve hundred surgeons representing the American College of Surgeons meets in Boston next October, I hope to take personal pride in the efficiency of the Boston hospitals."[252]

In the same article, the President of the Suffolk Medical Society, Dr. Horace [David] Arnold (1862-1935), in an early 20th century example of spin doctoring, pointed out that the general public should not mistake the cartoon incident as meaning that Boston physicians and the society in general did not favor the hospital efficiency movement:

249*Boston Post*, 18 January 1915.

250*Boston Post*, 18 January 1915.

251*Ibid.*

252*Ibid.*

Fears Misunderstanding

I regret that the incidents of the recent meeting of the Suffolk District Medical Society should be brought up for public discussion, for I fear that they are likely to be misunderstood, and that the attempt to secure better efficiency in our hospitals may suffer a setback. The members of the medical profession are a unit in their desire to improve the service given to the public at our hospitals. Any difference of opinion lies only in the details by which this end may be attained.

The subject of the meeting was hospital efficiency. It was a meeting for the impartial consideration of the merits of this subject. The chairman's enthusiasm for the cause led him to speak of certain institutions and individuals in such a way that the audience interpreted it as a personal criticism. The introduction of the personal element, as it was understood, into a scientific meeting was resented by many of the members of the society. On learning the extent of this feeling, Dr. Codman tendered his resignation as chairman of the surgical section, expressing the view that the two remaining meetings of the section would be more likely to be successful under other leadership. This resignation was accepted.[253]

At the end of the article, Arnold stated that he supported Codman's goals but not his methods of achieving them, further noting:

That the committee of supervision, acting for the Suffolk District Medical Society, approves of the movement to secure greater efficiency in our hospitals.

That it believes the adoption of the principles of the "End Result System" in hospitals would be conducive to greater efficiency of those institutions.

253*Ibid.*

That the president of the society is authorized to appoint a committee which shall inquire into the practical application of this system and shall later make a report and recommendations to the society.[254]

Even Edward Martin, Codman's close friend and inspiration, had difficulty with Codman's methods of trying to introduce the End Result Idea, and expressed these feelings to Codman shortly after the meeting.[255]

> **Dear God-like Youth,**
> **Your cartoons I thought did little good and much harm. Of course the wheels of progress must hurt and bruise someone but the chariot should be driven with some thought as to reducing to its minimum the crop of crippled. Your thought of a showdown is good. If this College of Surgeons can accomplish in part or in whole an efficient follow-on system, it will have justified its creation, proved its reality and given assuring promise for its future ... Having already the crown of thorns and nails, why should not you have the spear thrust? But remember drive carefully and hurt as few as you can.**
> **Yours faithfully,**
> **Edward Martin[256]**

However, Martin still supported Codman, as evidenced in two later letters:

> **Your winged thoughts are incubating and countless thousands of lives shall be sweeter and longer and more useful because you are now hanging on the martyr's cross. Consider for a moment the case**

254*Ibid.*

255CA 2/34.

256CA 2/34. There is no date on the letter, but it was certainly either January or February 1915.

of Sapphira. Doubtless, earnest, able and devoted to the cause, to whit her husband for which she did not step forth no way and outlie him in the face of the Lord and does not her name now sound through the generations not because of exemplary life and devotion, but because of the whopping lie which thunders through history.[257]

Dear Martyr:

As usual your dreams are quite wonderful and were you only human[258] entirely applicable, with a beneficent affect both upon the laity and the profession beyond belief. I had hoped you would quietly sneak in and raise hell after you were placed, but you are proposing to do a thing which only the best really want and the best, alas! are not in the majority. Perhaps they may so leaven things that the opportunity may come. In the meantime I have been ordered to Oglethorpe in the Main, probably because I am a friend of yours.

My love to the lofty lady. This from,

Yours more in sorrow than in anger,

Edward Martin.[259]

Martin's letters were far from the only ones that he received after the meeting. The day after the meeting, one of the speakers, his great supporter Robert Dickinson, wrote him.

He is the best political actor who can call the best nicknames. Whether "humbug" was the best is the question. There is no question somebody has got to be "the gadfly of the Republic."

Yours to help,

257CA 2/34. Again, no date is on the letter.

258The italics are mine.

259CA 2/35.

Dickinson.[260]

It seems that Dickinson was supporting Codman, but even he had to admit that Codman may not have chosen the best method to force-feed the End Result Idea on the Boston medical community.

But on the day after the meeting, Dr. Frederick [Cheever] Shattuck (1847-1929), an influential Boston physician wrote a very disapproving letter.

> 7 January 1915
> Codman:
> I told your wife downstairs last night, before the meeting, that I came to applaud. I am sorry that I left the meeting in a very different frame of mind. Your cause is good, and as you know, has my sympathy. Whatever possessed you to damage your cause by personalities, insults and a picture on the level with the yellow journal Sunday editions, I don't know. I am awfully sorry. Is it not conceivable that a person should differ from you without being a knave or a fool? Your cause is too good to fail, but, as it seems to me, you retarded it instead of advancing it last night.
> Most sincerely and sorrowfully,
> Your friend, F. C. Shattuck[261]

Shattuck was a very powerful man in Boston medical politics. He had trained at Harvard, graduating from college there in 1868, and medical school in 1873. He also earned an honorary LL.D. from the University of Cincinnati in 1908, and practised medicine as a professor at Harvard from 1888-1912, and served on the emeritus staff until his death in 1929. Bringing on his wrath was definitely a sign that Codman had angered doctors at the highest levels in Boston.

260CA 3/48.

261CA 3/45.

Within the month, Codman also received a letter from Dr. M[arsena] P[arker] Smithwick (né 1867) criticizing his tactics.

> **The sad thing is your determination to separate you from you the friends you have by a course which strikes me as too radical in points and too naïve—in fact your diplomacy or lack of it seems quite Teutonic.**
> **Sincerely yours,**
> **Smithwick**[262]

Though Smithwick did not have the influence of Frederick Shattuck, his displeasure with Codman probably ended a long friendship—they had been medical school classmates at Harvard.

Finally, although it took two years to reach him and is not signed, a letter dated 23 December 1917 reflected the sentiment of many of the doctors of Massachusetts towards Codman:

> **My dear Dr. Codman ...**
> **It is very unfortunate my dear Codman, that a man of your great and acknowledged ability could not have possessed a temperament to enable him to get on with his fellow men more comfortably than you do, particularly with his fellow doctors. Your failure to be recognized as one of the leading surgeons in Boston is largely due to your habit of never being willing to recognize the rights of others. Under such circumstances one never has his own rights respected ...**
>
> **After having quarreled with the Trustees of the Massachusetts General Hospital the wretched appearance you made with your cartoon at the medical meeting was enough to break your standing with the medical profession, unless one was charitable enough to think you mentally deranged. It is certainly hard to believe that anyone of sound mind could have made**

262CA 3/46.

so stupid a blunder as you made on that occasion. However, if you have learned better manners from that experience you may in time gain the confidence of the profession.

I have great sympathy with a man who possesses so unfortunate disposition as you have shown for you deserve better things and they can never come to you.[263]

But Codman never admitted in any of his writings that he regretted his actions at the Boston Medical Library, nor that they merited any reprobation. In a letter to Kanavel he defended his tactics, although he admitted that they initially ostracized him from his colleagues:

15 February 1915
Dear Kanavel:
You have perhaps heard rumors of the meeting which I got up here to arouse interest in the End Result System and Hospital Efficiency. I enclose one (the programme), two (a leaflet which was distributed), and three (a newspaper clipping showing the excitement it produced.) My cartoon attained the desired effect. It made every physician in Massachusetts ask: "What in the hell is this End Result System and what do they mean by Hospital Efficiency?"

At first, I was hardly spoken to; now almost everyone grins and some congratulate ...
Codman[264]

Though many of his peers may have grinned, there is no evidence in the Codman Archives that any local physicians congratulated him on his actions. There are supportive letters, though they are rare, but all are from national colleagues far removed from the Bay State. One

263CA 5/91.

264CA 2/30.

was from Dickinson, as described above, while another was from Allen Kanavel:

> **23 February 1915**
> **My dear Doctor,**
> **I want to congratulate you on stirring up the End Result System and Hospital Efficiency in Massachusetts. I congratulate you on your dare and your success.**
> **Kanavel**[265]

Even the doctors who supported Codman, however, usually expressed disapproval with his tactics, but they did not disagree with what he hoped to achieve. Later in the year, Kanavel wrote him on 22 December 1915, concerning a letter he had received from a Dr. Stephen Tracy (né 1875):

> **My dear Doctor:-**
> **Many things we pay for greatness. Among them is the privilege of answering the enclosed. I told Dr. Tracy that I had referred the letter to you as the author, the Father, Son and Holy Ghost of the chart.**
> **Sincerely yours,**
> **Allen B. Kanavel**[266]

Financially, the events of 6 January 1915 may not have completely destroyed him professionally, but they certainly caused hardship. From an income of $9,500 in 1913 and $8,000 in 1914, his income plummeted in 1915 to just over $5,000 (a 47 percent drop in income in two years). At his own hospital he relied on the referrals of other doctors and, with most of them now angry at him, these referrals were hard sought. He rebounded somewhat in 1916 and 1917, with his salary getting up again over $9,000, but inflationary pressures artificially inflated that figure.[267]

265*Ibid.*

266CA 3/52.

267The 1917 salary of $9,000 was probably worth no more than $105,000 in today's dollars. Though

It was not only the doctors and hospital administrators in Boston who were mad at Codman for the meeting at the Boston Medical Library. He had hired a woman named Mary A. Fisher to type the notes of the meeting. She did so, but he considered her work substandard and refused to pay her the entire sum. She then brought suit against him for the remainder of the payment which was listed as $27.24. In the Codman Archives, Codman has letters to his lawyer in which he noted that he was thinking of trying the case himself, but his lawyer, Robert Shaw Barlow, recommended against this. Barlow also recommended that Codman not attempt to fight the case, probably thinking it indefensible, and recommended that Codman pay her. Nothing further is mentioned of it in the Codman Archives. Apparently, Codman found the End Result of her work less than satisfactory.

It is hard to fathom exactly why Amory Codman chose this inflammatory attack upon the doctors of Massachusetts as a means of presenting to them his insistence on the importance of the End Result Idea. He was obviously intelligent, and he had stated many times that he knew had been somewhat "of a thorn" in the sides of his fellow doctors. He must have known that what he would do that January night could cause him grief. Perhaps he felt he had no choice? The Massachusetts General Hospital had not supported him. He had been corresponding with the Carnegie Foundation, looking for their support, to no avail. Though many doctors had given lip service to the End Result Idea, few seemed willing to support Codman with their actions. Perhaps he was seeking publicity via the lay public in the press, hoping that this publicity would stimulate the medical profession to start using the End Result Idea.

Though the meeting at the Boston Medical Library effectively ended his ascent up the surgical ladder, there is no indication in any of his writings that he ever regretted his actions that night. He paid a heavy price for his recalcitrance, but it seemed to be one he was willing to pay.

Codman's salary increased in 1916-1917, this was likely due to the inflation in the American economy caused by World War I. The consumer price index increased by 33% in those two years alone. Thus, his "recovery" financially was probably more an illusionary one. In fact, he was certainly not doing as well as he had in 1913-1914.

It was then up to Codman himself to resurrect his once meteoric surgical career. He had to re-establish his reputation and bolster his financial status. Despite the Boston Medical Library meeting, his mind never wandered from his goal of establishing the End Result Idea as a fundamental principle of American medicine. Over the next few years he would publish profusely on this topic, using the Codman Hospital and its End Results as the source of those publications.

CHAPTER 8
A STUDY IN HOSPITAL EFFICIENCY

In order to swim one takes off all one's clothes—in order to aspire to the truth one must undress in a far more inward sense, divest oneself of all one's inward clothes, of thoughts, conceptions, selfishness, etc., before one is sufficiently naked.

Søren Kierkegaard, *The Journals of Søren Kierkegaard*, entry 4 [1854]

In his search for the truth, Codman was exposing more and more of his true self. But if he was discouraged by other doctors' opinions of him and his actions at the Boston Medical Library meeting, there is no evidence of this in his writings. He continued to operate only at his own hospital at 15 Pinckney Street, gathering data so that he was able to begin publishing papers and books on the End Result Idea and outcome studies.

As mentioned earlier (Chapter Six) his first two articles in the literature on his own End Results came out in 1914. Almost concurrent with those he published a small monograph which came out on 10 May 1914 entitled, *A Study in Hospital Efficiency: The First Two Years of a Private Hospital*. He followed this shortly over one year later, with the publication of a follow-up report with the same title on 19 October 1915. It was essentially a second printing of the first monograph but did include a few more case reports. In both the monograph and the follow-up report, Codman listed the results of every case treated at his hospital since its opening in November 1911. In addition, he looked at the poor outcomes and tried to find the causes of all of them, setting the causes up into separate categories.

Medical communities are not isolated, and reputations, good or bad, are spread easily. Even in 1915, this was certainly true. After his harangue at the Boston Medical Library, Codman's national reputation waned dramatically. His declining reputation made him decide to resign as Chairman of the Committee on Standardization of Hospitals of the American College of Surgeons, and he did so in a letter to the president of the American College, Dr. John [Miller Turpin] Finney, (1863-1942) on 27 December 1915:

> **27 December 1915**
>
> **Dear Dr. Finney:**
>
> I am thinking over the question as acting as Chairman of the Hospital Standardization Committee of the American College of Surgeons, I have concluded it would be much wiser for me to resign. My chief reasons for this are twofold:
>
> First, Harvard University and the Mass General Hospital—my own Alma Mater and Pater—have shown no enthusiasm in backing me up. In fact they have sat on me and obviously intend to suppress me.
>
> The second reason is that my hospital is a financial failure. The public do not care for ideas from a man who is a self-confessed failure as far as money is concerned.
>
> I could get along without the backing of Harvard and the M.G.H., provided that I have the truth on my side and could prove the public is ready to pay for it, but that is not yet the case, so, for the present, it seems to me that I can do more by trying to make my own hospital a success than by criticizing other hospitals all over the country.
>
> Sincerely yours,

Dr. Ernest A. Codman[268]

Finney replied to him a few days later, accepting the resignation.

Despite Finney's comments, Codman then heard from the Mayo brothers, who were members of the Committee which he had chaired and with whom he had great mutual admiration.

> 21 January 1916
> Dear Codman:—
> I have gone over your letter with sincere regret and while I have every faith in Dr. Finney's judgment as well as your own, I think it is a mistake. No man can bring out a new and important idea without opposition. Men who pride themselves on being conservatives really are contented, a do nothing and satisfied type from whom no progress ever comes.
>
> Your career as a hospital re-organizer has been vivid, to say the least, in spots. It has already accomplished a great deal of good ...
>
> Personally, I can only realize that I am making progress when I am being stepped on, I am proud to be stepped on because it means there is movement that the conservatives want to check before it disturbs their positions. Cultivate a smile, don't take the thing too seriously, and keep at it, because you are right. Dr. Charlie joins me in kindest personal regards.
>
> Yours sincerely,
> W. J. Mayo[269]

His brother, Charles H. Mayo, then responded:

> 24 January 1916
> My dear Dr. Codman:

268CA 1/1.

269CA 2/40.

I have just read your letter to Will concerning your proposed resignation from the Hospital Standardization Committee. This is a tremendous undertaking. It looms up larger than ever each time I try to consider it. It must come, but it is a great problem as to how best to undertake it. It is going to stir up the same ill feeling all over the country that has been stirred up in Boston. The fact is men must be, for the most part, driven to this thing; of course, many will accept it as the natural progress of medicine, it benefits appealing to them as a necessity. Until it is a settled fact you will not receive recognition in Boston, or you will receive recognition but not gratitude, however, you would not in New York or Chicago.

Why not let it drop and slide along until necessary changes demand it in the Committee if it should be, by arriving at some new method. Don't quit because you are under fire. Remember you have had the most active part in this work and such things are appreciated by the professional in general but not by those in your own city.

Very truly yours,

C. H. Mayo[270]

Charles Mayo's letter supports the thesis that Codman's diminishing reputation among Boston physicians had been spread throughout the medical community on a broader, nationwide scale.

At about the same time as his resignation, his report from the Committee on Standardization of Hospitals appeared in *Surgery, Gynecology & Obstetrics*[271] It was also published almost concurrently in the *Transactions of the Clinical Congress of Surgeons of North America*.

Although Codman was no longer the leader of the nationwide medical efficiency movement, he was certainly the man still

---

270*Ibid.*

271*SGO*, 22(1): 199-120, January 1916. All future footnote references to SGO refer to the medical journal *Surgery, Gynecology & Obstetrics*.

responsible for it, and he never abandoned it. He published several other papers over the next few years on hospital standardization and efficiency, including: "The Dividing Line Between Medical Charity and Medical Business,"[272] "Uniformity in Hospital Morbidity Reports,"[273] "Case Records and Their Value,"[274] "The Value of Case Records in Hospitals,"[275] and "A Wise Preliminary to the Adoption of Any Compulsory Health Insurance Act."[276] Of note, in the article on a compulsory health insurance act, he proposed that evaluation and follow-up—the End Results System—were necessary pre-conditions to adoption of national health insurance. It was a further example of Codman's prescience, as the article on compulsory health insurance presaged much of our current thinking about the possibility of instituting a national health insurance system in the United States.

But despite his resignation from the Committee on Standardization of Hospitals, Codman was still considered the leader of the movement, even if he no longer held the political power. In 1917 John Hornsby wrote him, supporting this thought, and seemed to be offering support to Codman in what was certainly a trying time for him. At this time, Hornsby was then the editor of the journal *The Modern Hospital*, one of the leading journals of the era.

> **18 December 1917**
> **My dear Dr. Codman**
> **I want you to know now that I fully appreciate what you have done for the hospitals for this country, for the medical profession and through them, for the public at large, during your propaganda for better reports and records.**
>
> **Any man who follows a single thought to its ultimate conclusion and insists upon getting that**

272*Medical Record*, 89: 868-872, 13 May 1916.

273BMSJ, 177 (9): 279-283, 30 August 1917.

274*Bul Amer Coll Surg*, 3: 24-27, 1917.

275*The Modern Hospital*, 9: 426-428, 1917.

276BMSJ, 176 (12): 435-438, 22 March 1917. This article presaged by 75 years Hillary Rodham Clinton's committee which attempted to institute a national health insurance program.

thought registered in the public mind is going to be considered a nuisance by many people; I myself am just such a nuisance and you are another, but just the same you have done more to get recognition of the value of follow-up records than all the rest of us combined and I want you to know that I feel that way about it. I shall look with much interest to the coming of the report and it will give me pleasure to review it for the Modern Hospital.

    Very sincerely yours,
    John A. Hornsby[277]

The esteem with which Codman was still held can be seen in a series of letters contained in the Codman Archives from Dr. G[eorge] Paul La Roque (1876-1934), of Richmond, Virginia. La Roque was a great admirer of Codman's who also attempted to study the End Results of his own cases, and he published four small monographs that are contained in the Codman Archives. They all have the same main title, *Abstracts of Records (Standardization of the Surgery)*. However, the four monographs carry different subtitles as follows: 1) Operation on the Upper and Lower Extremities (The First One Hundred Cases), 2) Operations on the Urethra, Bladder, Prostate, Ureter and Kidney (The First Seventy-six Cases), 3) Operations on the Head, Neck and Trunk (The First Seventy-eight Cases) and 4) Operations for Diseases of the Anus and Rectum (The First Ninety-seven Cases).

La Roque once wrote Codman and said, "Permit me to say that I have said to others, that my inspiration is Codman and while my plan is not Codman's because it is not as good as Codman's, yet my ideal is Codman of Boston."[278]

Still his loyal supporter, Codman received a letter from Edward Martin after the publication of his first two monographs on hospital efficiency (1914 and 1915):

Dear Joy of My Heart and Despair of My Mind:

277CA 2/27.

278CA 2/31.

I have read your study in Hospital Efficiency with dazed amazement. Also your estimate of the value of case records in hospitals. I am in accord in much that you write and say and nearly all that you do. But being essentially human where we stop at the brink of a precipice over which you blindly plunder the perfectly fool idea it would get you somewhere, that it would do someone else good, which it does not; which is as a rule destructive to yourself and somewhat trying to others ...

... I would be profoundly grateful if I could have as vivid an appreciation of my own clarity of vision and infallibility of judgment as have you. It ought to make one very happy. Curiously enough it does not seem to have this effect upon you. Your proposition at the end of the book is an absolutely frightful one doomed to entire failure in its inception, a failure which incidentally would do you some harm, a matter of minor moment, except for some people have your good traits, few though they be, a very tender affection. Among those remains,

Edward Martin[279]

Codman followed his series of articles in the literature and his two monographs from on his own hospital's end results with his first book, *A Study in Hospital Efficiency: As Demonstrated by the Case Report of the First Five Years of a Private Hospitals.*[280] Codman charged one dollar ($1.00) for the book but sent it free of charge to any member of the American College of Surgeons or of the Massachusetts Medical Society who requested it. He dedicated the book to Richard C. Cabot with whom he had had correspondence for years concerning the End Result Idea.

279CA 2/35.

280Codman EA. *A Study in Hospital Efficiency: As Demonstrated by the Case Report of the First Five Years of a Private Hospital*, Boston: Thomas Todd Printers, *circa* 1918.

Richard Clarke Cabot (1868-1939) had been a Harvard medical student, like Codman, who obtained his M.D. degree in 1892. He then joined the staff of the Massachusetts General Hospital and also attempted to reform medicine in this country. However, Cabot took a different approach than did Codman, and presented his ideas with more tact. Cabot is really known as the Father of Social Medicine and Social Work in this country. He was the President of the 1st National Conference on Social Work in 1931, and was awarded a gold medal by the National Institute of Social Service in 1931, for his work in that field. Although Codman dedicated his book to Cabot it was not in his character, even in the dedication of a book, to be less than totally honest:

> **This volume is dedicated to Richard C. Cabot because I respect his motives, admire his courage and energy but hardly disapprove of some of his opinions and methods for he seems to want to reform the bottom of the profession while I think the blame belongs at the top.**[281]

The resulting book is a tremendous effort that could not be written today by a *sane* person, for fear of immediate malpractice litigation. First of all, Codman listed the results of every patient treated at his hospital between August 1911 and July 1916. It included 337 cases treated by multiple doctors, but mostly Codman himself. It did not matter if the results were poor, the full outcome of each case was still presented along with various suppositions about the reasons for the poor results. Neuhauser described the audacity which it took for the publication of the book, "It is hard to imagine anyone admitting that he had made a terrible error resulting in a patient's death, putting that fact in print, paying out of his own pocket to publish it, and making sure that the information was available to anyone who might wish to know what happened, including some prospective patients trying to decide what surgeon and hospital they should choose. Codman

---

281SHE, Dedication page.

challenged others to do the same. He sent free copies of his report to the notable hospitals across the country asking them to do the same."[282]

Codman also described herein the full use of what he called End Result Cards to implement his End Result Idea. An End Result Card was a card that he kept for every patient. On each card he listed the following information: 1) the symptoms or conditions for which the patient sought relief, 2) the diagnosis for the pathologic conditions which the doctor who gave the treatment believed to be the cause of the symptoms and upon which he based his treatment, 3) the general plan or important points of the treatment given, 4) complications that followed before the patient left the hospital, 5) the diagnosis which proved correct on final discharge and 6) the result each year afterward. After keeping track of every patient via the End Result Card, Codman then produced a large chart, which today would be called a spreadsheet. He recommended filing each End Result Card numerically and then giving each patient one single number for record keeping. The rows of the chart were based on anatomic regions and the columns were based on pathologic conditions. Each patient's record number would then be entered into a single row and column based on the pathologic condition affecting a certain anatomic region. Thus, if a doctor wished to look up cancerous lesions of the abdomen, or tubercular lesions of the extremities, he simply needed to look in the appropriate cell in the chart, retrieve the numbers of the End Result Cards, and then look up each End Result Card for the results of the treatment. No patient was excluded.

A Study in Hospital Efficiency: The First Five Years is far more than a simple description of how Codman ran his hospital and how he used the End Result Cards. Throughout the book his candor and bluntness are remarkable and would result in him immediately being sued countless times if he were to produce this same book today. On page 11, he noted that all the results of surgical treatment that were less than perfect could be explained by one or more of the following causes:

All Results of Surgical Treatment Which Lack Perfection May Be Explained by One or

---

282Neuhauser, p. 310.

More of the Following Causes

Errors due to lack of technical surgical knowledge or skill—E-s

Errors due to lack of surgical judgment—E-j

Errors due to lack of care or equipment—E-c

Errors due to lack of diagnostic skill—E-d

These are partially controllable by organization.

The patient's unconquerable disease—P-d

The patient's refusal of treatment—P-r

These are partially controllable by public education.

The calamities of surgery or those accidents and complications over which we have no known control.

These should be acknowledged to ourselves and to the public, and study directed to their prevention.[283]

His honesty was remarkable. Realize that the book came out within a year of some of the operations and subsequent complications described in it. And yet Codman admitted, for all the world, and all the lawyers, to see, "I made an error in surgical technique or judgment." He asked a lot of other doctors, and often offended them by the way he asked for their support, But he always asked more of himself. I suspect that no surgeon has so forthrightly admitted, and published, his own shortcomings, as did Amory Codman.

Codman noted that the End Result System was not complicated but that it was difficult to have it implemented by a hospital staff:

There is nothing complicated about the End Result System. It is merely a plan for giving accurate, available, immediate records of each case which the hospital undertakes to treat. Its unit is an ideal result for each individual patient treated. It subordinates the individual interests of the staff, if those interests are incompatible with the ideal, it boldly encourages

them, when they are not. It demands an analysis of the final result in each case treated and the fixation for responsibility of failure or success on the individual who undertakes the treatment. Such a system is truly scientific. Science is simply a record of truth.

The really difficult thing about the End Result System is to induce the staff in any hospital to be willing to make a truthful acknowledgment of the personal part which contributes to the success or failure of the cases. It is here that we meet the conflict between man's insatiable desire to ascertain the truth and his supposed necessity to deceive his fellowmen for the sake of his own self-preservation or ambition.[284]

Although Codman emphasized its simplicity, it still involved work for the doctors, work they had never had to do before. And it was not catching on at many hospitals, and Codman was not blind to this. There were good reasons why other people did not use the End Result System, and Codman realized this as well. He listed seven reasons that he knew of which people would list as objections to the use of the chart and then tried to answer the objections himself:

Objections to Use of Chart

1. It is too complicated.
Answer. Try it for one month and really see if it is.
2. It is too expensive.
Answer. Try it for one year and see if it does not save the cost in the elimination of waste products.
3. It is too difficult for a house officer to decide which squares to put the diagnosis in.
Answer. Then let the senior surgeon do it, for it is the most important work in a hospital to make sure of a good Product.

284SHE, pp. 112-113

4. Members of the Staff themselves would not know which square to put a given diagnosis in, and would not use it after it is done.

Answer. Then get a staff who can do it, and who will use it.

5. A large hospital would use up the sheets too rapidly.

Answer. Large hospitals should use the charts as a basis for a card index system.

6. Special hospitals would fill up some squares to overflowing and have few in the rest.

Answer. Each special hospital could use one sheet for all its diagnoses except those in the squares of its specialty, and devise a still further subdivided sheet for its special cases.

7. It does not give the sex or age.

Answer. No, nor the birthplace, nor the color of the hair and eyes. Nevertheless, it is practical, if you are in earnest.[285]

Despite these difficulties, and the excess paperwork that doing any outcome study entails, Codman still thought that the End Result System was essential and important. He listed five uses for the End Result Cards, all contributing to what would today be used for outcome studies:

Various Uses

As An Index
For Morbidity Statistics
For Mortality Statistics
For End Result Records

285SHE, pp. 121-122.

As An Efficiency Study [286]

Continuing, Codman inserted some of his own philosophical thoughts concerning the End Result Idea and his own attitude toward it.

Working for This Generation or for The Next

Selfishness and unselfishness differ merely in the time-return of the reward.

The man whom some call selfish, demands immediate reward for his labor; he works for this generation and is paid by it. The man who may be called unselfish, works for the next generation, and necessarily cannot be paid by it, - except in honor, which is often misplaced. The man who works for this generation is the practical, successful, beloved person who backs up his friends and fights their enemies. The man who works for the next generation is the dreaming, unsuccessful, often embittered person, who fights the faults in his friends and backs up the virtues of their enemies.

Some persons honor as unselfish the man with tact enough to make no enemies, and who values the love of this generation more than the honor of the next. Others regard that man as unselfish who seeks truth so sternly, that he will not permit a lie which will damage the next generation, to exist, even among his friends in this generation. [287]

He was obviously describing and defending himself. Codman believed that the End Result System could reform medicine by improving the standards of treatment. By looking at all the outcomes, and analyzing where outcomes were less than optimal, people could

---

286SHE, p. 121.

287SHE, p. 85.

search for different or better treatments that might improve those outcomes. He described his vision and how the End Result System could see it come true:

> I look forward to the day when endowed institutions, by the publication of their clinical results, will perform a part of their duty to their communities in letting people know what physicians and surgeons have proved themselves competent to cure or relieve every pathologic condition, and just which surgeons and physicians are devoting themselves to the study of each incurable condition.
>
> The End Result System will give Trustees the means to do this, and it will establish definite Standards, so that each pioneer can demonstrate that his added knowledge actually enables him to relieve cases which others have not relieved. Trustees can say to the man who has original ability: "Here is a class of cases which has hitherto been unsatisfactory in its results. Study the pathology and natural history of this disease. Devise new methods of treatment, and if you have conviction that the knowledge you have acquired will enable you to demonstrate that you can relieve our patients with this condition, you may take charge of them. But be sure that the next series of cases clearly excels the standard we already have. If it does, we want you to continue to treat such cases for us; and we will let our Community and the Scientific World know it, through our Hospital Report."[288]

What were these standards which Codman was describing? Did any exist at the time? They did not, although some would very shortly, as we will see, and they were Codman's work, as we might expect. His *Study of Hospital Efficiency* further discussed the need for standards.

288SHE, p. 86.

Standards

The exponents of scientific management constantly tell us that standards are necessary, if we wish to attain efficiency.

Is it possible to standardize the treatment of disease, or the work of the hospitals, or the work of individual members of hospital staffs? Is it possible to standardize knowledge, skill, judgment, and diagnosis, or curable and incurable diseases, calamities and mortality? It is possible that we can have standards for cases like appendicitis, cleft palate, pneumonia, hernia and fibroids of the uterus?

It is the opinion of the writer that such standards can be established, and one of the aims of this hospital is to establish standards; even with the few cases we have already had, we can in a measure set up standards, because no such standards of consecutive operations have heretofore been offered.

Is there a standard of judgment?

Is there a standard of skill?

Are there standards of care?

Are there standards of curable and incurable conditions?

Are standards of results possible?

Is there a standard of mortality from anaesthesia?

Finally, let us remember that the object of having standards is to be sure to raise them. The standards which we are establishing may be low ones, but we are making them to raise them.[289]

Although Codman may have thought that the standards were low, they were the only ones available in 1917—nobody else was proposing such standards. And he stated above, certainly he expected to eventually raise the bar.

289SHE, 91-93.

Pages 98 through 107 in the book contain a remarkable section entitled, "Analysis of Our Total Errors in Five Years With a View to Future Improvement." This section has various subsections: 1) Total errors due to lack of technical knowledge or skill in five years, 2) Errors possibly due to lack of judgment, 3) Errors due to lack of care or equipment, 4) Errors due to incorrect diagnosis, 5) Cases in which the nature and extent of the disease was the main cause of failure, 6) Cases who refused to accept treatment, 7) Deaths and 8) Calamity.[290] His candor was stunning, as can be seen in the following.

Analysis of Our Total Errors in Five Years With a View to Future Improvement

Total Errors Due to Lack of Technical Knowledge or Skill in Five Years

Cases 39, 80, 114, 186, 250 were trivial. Case 31—I probably missed a small gallstone, but one of the Mayos missed the same one, and the patient has since passed it. Cases 50, 220, 275—Perhaps lack of skill resulted in these symptomless hernias, or bulging scars following acute appendicitis with drainage. Case 103—Possibly the errors of skill resulted in orchidectomy. Case 138, 255—Small, symptomless hernias in the epigastric wounds in patients who were relieved of lifelong discomfort. Case 124—I may have missed an ulcer of the stomach. Case 241—S[amuel] J[ason] Mixter, J[ames] G[regory] Mumford, H[enry] O[rlando] Marcy, M[aurice] H[owe] Richardson, and C[harles] A[llen] Porter also failed in this case.

290Berwick has noted (p. 265) that Codman would have a 20% chance of being sued today because of this section of the publication. As a practicing physician, I would state that Codman would have a 100% chance of being sued today by publishing this 10-page section. In fact, my publication of this section in itself probably will stimulate several plaintiffs' lawyers to attempt to track down the heirs of Codman's patients who sustained the complications that he described in an effort to sue Codman's heirs. They will soon discover, to their certain dismay, that Codman died without issue, and this had no direct heirs.

Logical conclusion: If my analysis has been self-searching and accurate, and it is true that in five years these are the only errors due to lack of technical knowledge or skill, it may be fairly concluded that what we need for the success of this hospital is not more skill, but more patients.[291]

I know of no other medical article or book, before or since, in which a doctor blatantly admitted that his errors were due to a lack of technical knowledge or skill.

The last half of his book is a separate section entitled, "Part Two: The Financial Report; An Illustration of the Money Value of a Surgeon's Services and Influence of the Charitable Hospitals Upon It." Codman went into great detail here about the cost of surgery at his hospital and other hospitals in Boston, equating and determining the value of his own time and the value of an operation. Much of this section anticipated a great deal of what is done today with capitated payments. He also hypothesized somewhat in this section about how he could do better financially and increase his own income.

Oddly, Codman devoted several of these pages to argue with the man to whom he dedicated the book, Dr. Richard Cabot, in the section. "A Few of the Things on Which I Do Not Agree with Richard Cabot."[292] Although, given the backhanded compliment in the dedication, perhaps it was no so odd, but simply Codman being Codman.

Even though Codman seemed to be doing better financially by 1917, he noted that he had run the hospital at a loss for the first four years:

The Concept of This Hospital

As may be seen in the first statement, my loss for running the hospital, including my Professional Fees, in the first four years was $3,367.94. In this last year alone (owing largely to the hospital's having been

---

291SHE, pp. 98-99.

292SHE, pp. 113-115.

closed for two months) it was $2,216.60. This means that in five years I have lost $5,584.54 and a fraction of my labor.

I am quite willing to pay $1,116.91 a year to force the End Result System on these Hospital Surgeons, because I rely on my own results to give me the position to which I am entitled. He notes, however, "I have a ten bed hospital, and have been able to only keep four and half beds full on the average."[293]

Codman then discussed whether or not his hospital had been a success in spite of financial losses. He began by defining Success as "the attainment of an object," and then noted that the main object of his hospital has been to "force the great Boston Hospital affiliated with the Harvard Medical School[294] to adopt the principles of the End Result System."[295] He described how his hospital was necessary as a demonstration of the End Result Idea and the End Result System. However, he admitted that, financially at least, he had not done well.

Why This Hospital Has Not Been a Financial Success

The following five reasons occur to me:
1. I have exhibited a Cartoon at a local medical meeting, ... Is it any wonder that after this, my former colleagues do not patronize my hospital?

Do you blame them for spreading and exaggerating the unfortunate facts that I am not a skillful operator, that I am hard to get along with, aggressive, independent, idealistic, and a monomaniac on the End Result Idea? Even my friends damn me with faint praise.

293SHE, p. 126. Codman has earlier described his hospital as a twelve bed-hospital. It is not certain if he closed two beds but another author (Donabedian) has also noted the same discrepancy.

294Quite obviously, the Massachusetts General Hospital.

295SHE, p. 126.

2. But as they have not yet reappointed me, and until then, therefore, I have no right to the rich patients, I must lower my prices and try for those of moderate means ...

3. There are also, perhaps, some personal reasons,—perhaps I have not worked hard enough, been gracious enough, or taken enough personal interest in my patients.

4. I have been inefficient in my advertising.

5. Last year the deficit was caused by shutting down the hospital for two months, so that I could take some vacations, write the last Report, and prepare the Report of the Committee on Hospital Standardization of the Clinical Congress of Surgeons.

Having thus considered the reasons for our lack of Financial Success, we can make the following good resolutions for the future, and thus increase our business:

1. To publish no more cartoons.

2. To advertise directly to the laity.

3. To continue to employ the same superintendent.

4. To issue no more Reports, unless they are paid for.

5. To shirk committee work for national medical associations. In other words: To Mind Our Own Business. [296]

Amory Codman did not show great concern over the fact that neither he nor his hospital was a great financial success. He knew all too well what a surgeon's true reward was and he described it in the book, "The surgeon's reward is the daily pleasure of seeing the proof of his knowledge and skill as revealed in his convalescent patients."[297] He went on to defend his own record, claiming that his results were as good as any other surgeon's and because of this, he deserved not only

296*Ibid.*

297SHE, p. 135.

an appointment at a charitable hospital in town, "Such as the Massachusetts General," but that he also deserved to be the Chief of the Surgical Service. In making this claim, however, he emphasized that he was not abandoning his claim that hospitals should reform the method by which they selected the members of their staff, urging institutions not to select staff members based on seniority but based on their results, or outcomes, namely to base their hiring decisions on the End Result Idea.

The Proof That the Writer Deserves an Appointment at a Charitable Hospital

I claim that I had a minimum number of preventable fatalities, and I challenge any one to show that any other surgeon who operated at the hospital during these fifteen years has as few in proportion to the number of difficult cases which were successful.

I claim that in almost all of the cases in the following list, the cause of death was the patient's condition or disease, and not my errors of diagnosis, skill, judgment, or care. 107 of the 141 were grave emergencies.

If not, I claim the appointment as Chief of Staff under the same ruling that caused my resignation.

Resolved, that in making appointments the Trustees will consider the fitness of the applicant for the special services which he will be called on to perform, and will seek to secure the best service available, without being bound by any custom of promotion by seniority.[298]

But the first paragraph highlights a problem that still exists today with outcome studies. Codman could show what his End Results were. But could anyone else? If only one pioneer is willing to perform

---

298SHE, p. 186.

outcome studies, there is nothing to compare him to. No one can really tell how good or bad the outcomes are.

Within a few years, though the End Result Idea did not become a force in medicine, the Committee which Codman started and first chaired, the Committee on the Standardization of Hospitals, did. In 1917, the American College of Surgeons authorized the Committee to begin a Hospital Standardization Program, and in March 1918, the ACS published a "Minimum Standard for Hospitals" in their *Bulletin*:

> 1. That physicians and surgeons privileged to practice in the hospital be organized as a definite group or staff. Such organization has nothing to do with the question as to whether the hospital is "open" or "closed," nor need it affect the various existing types of staff organization. The word STAFF is here defined as the group of doctors who practice in the hospital inclusive of all groups such as the "regular staff," "the visiting staff," and the "associate staff."
>
> 2. That membership upon the staff be restricted to physicians and surgeons who are (a) full graduates of medicine in good standing and legally licensed to practice in their respective states or provinces, (b) competent in their respective fields, and (c) worthy in character and in matters of professional ethics; that in this latter connection the practice of the division of fees, under any guise whatever, be prohibited.
>
> 3. That the staff initiate and, with the approval of the governing board of the hospital, adopt rules, regulations, and policies governing the professional work of the hospital; that these rules, regulations, and policies specifically provide:
>
> (a) That staff meetings be held at least once each month. (In large hospitals the departments may choose to meet separately.)
>
> (b) That the staff review and analyze at regular intervals their clinical experience in the various departments of the hospital, such as medicine,

surgery, obstetrics, and the other specialties; the clinical records of patients, free and pay, to be the basis for such review and analyses.

4. That accurate and complete records be written for all patients and filed in an accessible manner in the hospital—a complete case record being one which includes identification data; complaint; personal and family history; history of present illness; physical examination; special examinations, such as consultations, clinical laboratory, X-ray and other examinations; provisional or working diagnosis; medical or surgical treatment; gross and microscopical pathological findings; progress notes; final diagnosis; condition on discharge; follow-up and, in case of death, autopsy findings.

5. That diagnostic and therapeutic facilities under competent supervision be available for the study, diagnosis, and treatment of patients, these to include, at least (a) a clinical laboratory providing chemical, bacteriological, serological, and pathological services; (b) an X-ray department providing radiographic and fluoroscopic services.[299]

To a surgeon of the 1990s, these standards are next to nothing. In 1917, however, medical records contained almost no information. Doctors presumably admitted and treated their patients, keeping the results and outcomes of the treatment only in their heads. In an estimated 75 percent of American hospitals in 1917, patients were not examined upon admission, no history was taken nor diagnosis made, and no follow-up work was performed to determine the results of treatment. As a result, medical records were useless.[300] The hospitals were glorified rest homes. However, Dr. Franklin Martin eventually called this the Minimum Standard, and noted that "... the *Minimum*

299*Bull Amer Coll Surg*, 4(1): 6, March 1918.

300*Committed to Quality: An Introduction to the Joint Commission on Accreditation of Healthcare Organizations*. Oakbrook Terrace, IL: JCAHO, 1990, p. 11.

Standard had 'become to hospital betterment what the Sermon on the Mount is to great religion.'"[301]

The Hospital Standardization Program was financed by the Carnegie Foundation, which had finally come to see the wisdom of the idea, and gave the American College of Surgeons (ACS) $30,000 to start the program. The results of the first program were unexpected and caused a dramatic outcome for the data it produced:

> **The results of the field trials were announced by [John Gabbert] Bowman (1877-1962) [director of the American College of Surgeons] at a conference on hospital standardization in New York on Oct 24, 1919. Bowman told the audience that 692 hospitals of 100 beds or more had been surveyed and that only 89 hospitals had met the [minimum] standards. While these results are not surprising when one considers conditions in hospitals at the time, the results were nevertheless shocking.**
>
> **Although the College made the numbers public, it burned the list of hospitals at midnight in the furnace of the Waldorf Astoria Hotel, New York, to keep it from the press. ... However, 109 hospitals corrected deficiencies after their initial surveys and were subsequently approved.[302]**

In fact, only 12.9% of the hospitals surveyed were approved by the Committee in 1918. This percentage rose slowly to 58.8% in 1920, and did not reach 80% approval until 1944.

Eventually the standards would expand dramatically from these five simple points of the "Minimum Standard," some would say transmogrify, such that in 1970, they took up 152 pages, and now take up several volumes.[303] The Committee that founded them, and which

---

301*Ibid.*, p. 937.

302*Ibid.*

303Roberts JS et. al. A history of the joint commission on accreditation of hospitals. *J Amer Med Assoc*, 258(7): 938, 21 August 1987.

Codman chaired and essentially fathered, also has changed dramatically. On 15 December 1951, the American College of Physicians, the American Hospital Association, the American Medical Association, and the Canadian Medical Association joined with the American College of Surgeons to form the Joint Commission on Accreditation of Hospitals (JCAH), although the Canadian Medical Association withdrew in 1959, to participate in the development of its own program, the Canadian Council on Hospital Accreditation.[304] In 1987, the JCAH changed its name to the Joint Commission on Accreditation of Healthcare Organizations (JCAHO).[305]

Thus, at least one of the "babies" which Codman "gave birth to" would prosper and grow into a major force in American healthcare, though with the changes that have been implemented, he would hardly recognize it today. And on a personal level, Codman appeared to have survived the events of 6 January 1915, and actually overcame somewhat the opprobrium of his peers. Though after December 1915, he was no longer the leader of the American College of Surgeons' Committee on Standardization of Hospitals, it was obvious he was still considered the Godfather of the End Result Movement—perhaps we should call him Don Codman. As he himself compared his quest to Don Quixote, he probably would have enjoyed it.

Unfortunately, just as his career seemed on the rebound, the events of 1917 would prevent him from continuing to pursue the End Result Idea at his own hospital. There was a war going on in Europe, and American and Canadian soldiers were becoming involved in it. Codman could not know it early in 1917, but it would involve him as well, because of his own altruism. His efforts on behalf of his principles would require great personal sacrifice, causing him to abandon, even if only temporarily, his quest of reforming medicine through the End Result Idea. But he accepted that sacrifice, and that acceptance tells us a great deal about Codman's character.

304Ibid., p. 937.

305*Committed to Quality*, p. 14.

CHAPTER 9
HALIFAX, INFLUENZA, AND WORLD WAR I

Then leaf subsides to leaf.
So Eden sank to grief,
So dawn goes down to day.
Nothing gold can stay.

Robert Frost, *Nothing Gold Can Stay* [1923]

At the end of 1917, despite his difficulties and the alienation from his peers, Codman continued to operate at his own hospital and use it as a source to test his End Result System. Despite the War in Europe, like most Americans, Codman's life was little different than it had been in the past few years. That would soon change with the events of December 1917.

Thursday, 6 December 1917, was a beautiful early winter's morning in Boston. The sky was cloudless and a brilliant blue. The morning was cold, as always for that time of year in New England, but the air was crisp and clear as people prepared to start work that morning. Codman probably walked the ¾ of a mile from his Beacon Street brownstone to his Pinckney Street hospital.

In Halifax, Nova Scotia, it was a similar morning. Halifax sits on the west coast of Halifax Harbour, on the southeastern shore of Nova Scotia, almost directly east of Maine, and about 360 miles north of Boston. An important center for commercial fishing, Halifax was founded in 1605 by Samuel de Champlain and was settled in 1749 by

Edward Cornwallis. Its access to the North Atlantic has made it a vital strategic port in times of war.

On that December morn, the Halegonians started their day by preparing for work, or for school. A holiday atmosphere was in the air, and although World War I was raging in Europe, Halifax was a happy city that Thursday. The war actually brought business to Halifax, as the strategic port city was used for the movement of warships to carry troops, to refuel supplies and to carry munitions.

That morning, two ships started their fateful course in the Halifax Harbour. One was the Belgian relief ship *Imo*. The *Imo* had spent the night before harbored in Bedford Basin in the northwest corner of Halifax Harbour, only because the dockworkers were overworked by the excess business caused by the war. The *Imo*'s captain, Håkon From, had wished to leave the harbour on the previous afternoon, but needed to be supplied with tons of steam coal. The coal tender was supposed to be there by 3:00 P.M., which would allow the *Imo* to leave the harbour but did not get to them until after 5:30 P.M. by which time the harbour boom was closed and the *Imo* was forced to stay overnight. Captain From, and his pilot, William Hayes, would have to wait until the next morning to start their voyage.

The *Imo* had recently arrived in Halifax from Rotterdam, in The Netherlands, and was returning to Belgium at this time. Though it served now as a Belgian relief ship, the *Imo*'s original name was the *Runic*, and it was a Norwegian ship of the White Star Line, the same line which produced the ill-fated *Titanic*. Even a worse fate would soon await the *Imo*.

At the entrance to Halifax Harbour, at approximately 8 o'clock in the morning of December 6th, the *Mont Blanc* began her entrance into the harbour. She was led by her captain, Aimé Le Medec, and her pilot, Frank Mackey. Both Le Medec and Mackey were nervous because of the cargo carried on the *Mont Blanc*. The *Mont Blanc* had come up from New York where they had been loaded with the cargo for their return trip to Europe. The French government agent in New York told him rather reluctantly, "It's explosives, I'm afraid, on this trip."[306] Indeed,

---

[306]Bird MJ, *The Town That Died*, (Toronto: McGraw-Hill Ryerson, 1967), p. 15.

the ship's manifest of the *Mont Blanc*, later examined closely, listed her cargo as 2,300 tons of picric acid, 200 tons of TNT, 35 tons of benzol and 10 tons of gun cotton. (Picric acid is a highly deadly explosive, even more unstable than TNT.) Essentially the *Mont Blanc* was carrying 2,545 tons of high explosive in her cargo holds.

The Halifax Harbour has a tight narrows after ships bound for the sea exit Bedford Basin. The piers, where many of the ships docked, were on the southwestern side of the basin, bordered by the Richmond neighborhood of Halifax and by an army barracks, Fort Needham. On the northeastern side of the Harbour lay the sister city of Dartmouth.

On that morning the two ships entered the narrows at around 8:30 a.m. The *Imo* was a much larger and faster ship than the *Mont Blanc*, was traveling very fast, and later was felt to be too close to the Dartmouth side of the harbour when first seen by the *Mont Blanc*. The *Mont Blanc*, though she was traveling in her correct channel, was not flying a red flag, then required by all ships to indicate that she was carrying explosives. As they approached each other, the *Imo* signaled that she intended to bear further to port, even closer to Dartmouth and even more into the *Mont Blanc's* channel. The *Mont Blanc* replied that she wished to pass to starboard, although she was, by this time, very close to the Dartmouth shore and almost at a dead stop.

Captain Le Medec and Pilot Mackey of the *Mont Blanc* expected the *Imo* to swing towards Halifax but she did not do so. Instead she maintained her course and Le Medec and Mackey saw only one possible course available to them to avoid collision, and that was to swing sharply towards port, towards Halifax and across the bow of the *Imo* to pass starboard to starboard. The *Imo*, seeing what was happening, signaled full speed astern as did the *Mont Blanc*, but, by now, a collision could not be avoided. The bow of the *Imo* ripped into the side of the *Mont Blanc* igniting sparks and starting what would be a deadly harbour fire.

The crew of the *Imo*, having no conception whatsoever of the cargo on the *Mont Blanc*, remained on board their boat. The crew of the *Mont Blanc* immediately took to their lifeboats, and headed for the Dartmouth shore, which allowed their burning ship to drift towards Halifax and Pier 6. At just about 9 A.M., as the fire raged on board the

Mont Blanc, the entire crew of the *Mont Blanc* reached shore on Dartmouth just south of Tuft's Cove.

The *Mont Blanc* continued to burn, starting a brilliant fire in the harbour that attracted the interest of many Halegonians that morning. Unfortunately, many of them came down towards the Harbour to watch the ongoing blaze. As the *Mont Blanc* drifted by the Halifax pier, it broke Pier 6 and set it ablaze. Shortly after 9:04 A.M., the fire aboard the *Mont Blanc* reached the explosives in the cargo hold, igniting the largest man-made explosion in the history of the world, prior to the August day in 1945 when Hiroshima was incinerated. The explosion was huge, and could really only be appreciated by someone outside the town looking towards the city with some sense of perspective. Such a person was Captain Campbell, aboard the *Acadian*, who was fifteen miles outside of Halifax that morning observing the scene. Bird describes the scene in his book on the explosion, **The Town That Died.**

> **Suddenly the scene was thrown into relief by a flash brighter than the sun. An immense cloud of smoke shot up into the air above Halifax crowned by an angry, crimson ball of rolling flames. Almost at once the flames were swallowed up in the black-grey smoke but from time to time they reappeared, boiling in its midst.**
>
> **The billowing mass rolled higher and higher and then, after a few seconds, Campbell heard two thundering reports in quick succession.**
>
> **The captain's sextant lay near at hand and, grabbing it, he took an observation of the summit of the smoke, now flattened and spreading outwards. His rapid calculations showed that it had risen to more than 12,000 feet.**
>
> **Fifteen minutes later the vast cloud was still visible. Now it hung, almost motionless, like an open umbrella over the funeral pyre of the town that died.[307]**

307*Ibid.*, Prologue, p. 10, reprinted with permission.

Nothing could have prepared the citizens of Halifax that morning for what had just happened. The French ship, *Mont Blanc*, absolutely vanished, having been disintegrated in the explosion. The explosion was of such force that one of her cannons was found 3½ miles away from the site of the explosion and part of her anchor shank, which weighed over half a ton, flew two miles in the opposite direction. In Truro, which was over fifty miles away, windows were shattered by the shock wave, which was even felt in Sydney on Cape Breton Island, 270 miles to the northeast.

Bird's description of the hideous explosion is the most vivid.

> **With a thundering, staccato roar the blast waves from the exploding chemicals struck out at Halifax and Dartmouth with the violence of a hundred typhoons. The earth shook and the bed of the Harbour was split open ...**
>
> **With a scream of rending metal a bridge spanning the railway was swept away and the tracks were plucked from the earth, bent and corkscrewed ...**
>
> **Up from the water's edge and into the town raced the air wall of destruction. Roads trembled into a thousand running fissures; tramlines buckled; trees were uprooted; telegraph poles snapped like matches and the overhead power cables, torn from their supports, whip-cracked in the air, sparking fiercely. Close to the explosion center street after street was obliterated with savage force as churches, schools, shops, factories and houses alike caved in or burst into clouds of flying wreckage ...**
>
> **As the air was pressed out with such tremendous force so, almost immediately, it was sucked in again to fill the vacuum that the explosion had created, eddying the glass and other still-airborne debris backward, sucking nails from woodwork to fly like shrapnel, dragging down walls and buildings which had withstood the initial shock and the falling hundreds of tons of wreckage before it ...**

Rocks, many of them huge, which had been scooped up from the sea bed and hurled into the air by the explosion now crashed back to earth and with them descended a shower of more than three thousand tons of red-hot metal fragments—all that was left of the Mont Blanc ...

Following the explosions came the fury of the sea. As it rushed in to fill the chasm that had opened in the Harbour bed, a monstrous wave, thirteen feet high, reared up in a gigantic bore to foam outwards at incredible speeds ...

When the wave had gone, and the air wall and the earth tremor had fled out into the Province to set church bells swinging and booming in towns more than sixty miles distant, a widening column of smoke and burnt-out gases rose for three miles into the sky above the North End. It hung there for many minutes, turning from black to grey and then to cotton-wool white, and it looked for all the world like some enormous, mutated mushrooms.[308]

It was the worst explosion in North American history, dwarfing the 1995 destruction of the Federal Building in Oklahoma City.[309] Within minutes of the explosion, over 1,900 people were killed. The eventual devastation was listed as over 3,000 dead, and over 20,000 injured, many of them permanently. The flying shrapnel and flying glass caused thousands of people to sustain serious eye damage. Three hundred and twenty-five acres, or almost the entire north end of Halifax, was destroyed.

Immediately after the explosion, the city set into motion to rebuild and recover. They were not without help. In addition to local efforts, many countries, and especially the United States, quickly started relief

---

308*Ibid.*, pp. 63-65, reprinted with permission.

309 This was written before 11 September 2001.

efforts to help the Halegonians. Money came in from as far away as China and New Zealand. The Canadian government donated $18 million, the British government almost $5 million dollars. But to this day, Halifax has never forgotten the generosity of the state of Massachusetts that donated $750,000 in money and goods the next day, but gave even more in volunteer assistance via what was known as the Massachusetts-Halifax Relief Committee.[310]

The Massachusetts relief effort was led by Dr. A[braham] C. Ratshesky (1864-1943), who boarded a train on the day of the explosion with twelve surgeons, ten nurses, an anesthetist and a representative of the American Red Cross. Ratshesky was a wealthy banker from Boston, but he was well qualified for his task. He had been part of a relief group that had gone to San Francisco in 1906 after the famous earthquake and fire in that city. The group also brought with them a large supply of dressing, bandages, anesthetics, beds and blankets or essentially a portable MASH[311] unit to help the people of Halifax.

Codman had many friends in Halifax and had visited there many times over the years, both for hunting and fishing trips, and also as a visiting speaker to the doctors of that Nova Scotia city. Within one hour of hearing the news of the explosion, he made plans to travel to Halifax. Codman left Boston on the same day as the disaster, but not as a part of the official Massachusetts relief effort. He traveled on his own, and offered his assistance with no request for publicity or assistance.

Later in the afternoon of 6 December 1917, one of the worst blizzards in recent history raged through New England and the Maritime Provinces of Canada, completely blanketing Nova Scotia and Halifax and hampering the relief efforts. It also delayed many of the trains transporting the Massachusetts doctors and relief committees to Halifax and thus delayed Codman's trip north. On Friday, 7 December 1917 the Codman Hospital on 15 Pinckney Street did not open. With Codman on his trip north to Halifax were several nurses from his staff,

---

310Every year since 1917, and continuing to this day, on December 6th, the Mayor of Halifax, Nova Scotia travels to Boston, donating and lighting an annual Christmas tree to that city in gratitude for the Bostonian and Massachusetts relief efforts.

311Mobile Army Surgical Hospital, or MASH Unit, popularized by the movie and television show of the same name.

and as many supplies as he could gather from his hospital. That day should be remembered as a landmark day in Amory Codman's life. It was the day that his beloved hospital, to which he had devoted so much, and which meant so much to the End Result Idea, closed forever. Surely he did not know it at the time, but it would never re-open.

Codman arrived in Halifax on Saturday, December 8th and quickly began working to help the injured. The amount of trauma sustained by the citizens of Halifax was a hideous sight and one that could turn the stomach of anyone not used to caring for the injured. One young volunteer doctor, Dr. Nathan Shacknove (1885-1917), who had come from Hamilton, Ontario to offer his help, was not used to the sight of so much death and misery. He worked on Friday morning but became ill from the sight of the injured and the dead, and was unable to handle the mental anguish that he suffered. He hanged himself that night. [312]

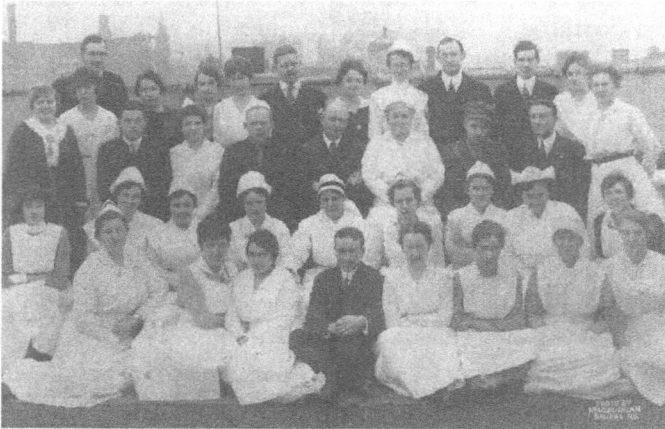

Figure 12—Amory Codman and his staff at the Halifax YMCA Emergency Hospital, which he supervised after the Halifax Disaster of 1917. (Codman is directly in the middle of the photo—the first row standing, with his arms crossed, and a nurse in all white on his left.) (Courtesy Maritime Museum of the Atlantic, Halifax, Nova Scotia, Canada)

Codman worked long and hard in Halifax, tending to the sick. (Figure 12) On December 11th he sent a telegram to Katy stating, "No

---

312Bird, p. 151.

time to write home about week Shall stay while clearly useful Well but weary" The time on the telegram was 5:36 A.M.

Codman set up his small mobile hospital in the YMCA building in Halifax and was later joined by several physicians and nurses from the other maritime provinces. He brought with him a small X-ray apparatus from Boston, which was one of the few functioning X-ray machines in Halifax after the explosion. As one might expect, Codman used the Halifax explosion to test his own theories and promote them. For every patient he treated in Halifax, he made an End Result Card, exactly like the End Result Cards that he used at his own hospital. Each card listed a detailed diagnosis, treatment given, and eventual outcome of the case.[313]

One Halifax doctor, Dr. David Fraser Harris (né 1868), of Scottish birth, was assigned to be the medical historian of the Halifax explosion by Lieutenant Colonel F[rederick] McKelvey Bell (né 1878) of the Medical Relief Committee. Harris produced a report that, unfortunately, was not well received by Bell and was never published. In fact, this report was only unearthed in 1989 by the efforts of Dr. John Fisher, then a third-year medical student at the University of Ottawa.[314] However, since the discovery of the Fraser Harris report, Codman's report is also now available to us.

In *Ground Zero*, a book containing essays about the Halifax Explosion, Murray, who has written of Fraser Harris' missing report, discussed Codman's recently discovered report and noted that it "... showed his meticulous administrative management."[315] Harris's report also discussed Codman's contribution, as follows:

The labours of Sunday, December 9th, were not yet ended for late that evening it was ascertained that Dr. E. A. Codman of Boston had arrived in the city with

---

313The fate and current location of Codman's End Result Cards from Halifax is unknown. In fact, much of the medical report and records from the Halifax explosion are somewhat of a mystery.

314Murray TJ, "Medical Aspects of the Disaster: The Missing Report of Dr. David Fraser Harris," In: *Ground Zero Reassessment of the 1917 Explosion in Halifax Harbour*, Ruffman and Howell, editors, co-published by Nimbus Publishing Limited and the Gorsebrook Research Institute for Atlantic Canada Studies at Saint Mary's University, Halifax, NS, 1994.

315Murray TJ. p. 239.

certain members of the staff of his private hospital. By Monday, the tenth, Dr. Codman's Unit was installed in the Y.M.C.A. building, which had been rapidly prepared as a large emergency hospital. Under Dr. Codman was serving besides surgeons, nurses, and a radiologist, three obstetricians, Dr. [Robert Laurent] De Normandie, Dr. [Foster Standish] Kellog and Dr. [John Baker] Swift[, Jr.], all of the Red Cross Unit, Boston. It was therefore resolved that the Y.M.C.A. hospital should have wards set apart for obstetrical cases, a class of case which from the day of the explosion had urgently needed proper housing. These wards were soon filled. Dr. Codman acted as Senior Medical Officer, Lieut. F. A. Reid acted as Adjutant, Captain H. Barratt, A.M.C. supplied equipment and stores, Dr. W[illiam] [Richardson] Woodbury and Mr. Dawson (the physical instructor at the Y.M.C.A.) proved themselves valuable assistants. So popular, indeed were Mr. Dawson and Lieut. F. A. Reid, that two babies born there a few days later were named after them. Mrs. J. C. MacDougall and a committee of ladies had from the day of the disaster taken charge of all the domestic arrangements at the Y.M.C.A., which they had carried out so satisfactorily that the committee was asked to continue, and Mrs. MacDougall was appointed temporary matron. To the great regret of everyone, Dr. Codman had to return to Boston on December 19th. Dr. Codman's own account of his arrival and inaugurating of the Y.M.C.A. hospital will be found in section nine of this narrative.

Codman's report of his work in Halifax, never before published, is now available to us and is reproduced here in full:

The situation at the Y.M.C.A. Hospital on the evening of December 14, 1917, with a brief statement concerning the use of the Y.M.C.A. Building since the accident on Dec. 6th.

Dr. Codman's connection with the Hospital

"On Thursday, December 6th, after hearing of the accident from the Boston newspapers, I telegraphed to Dr. Thomas Walker of St. John to say that I would gladly give my help if needed at Halifax. On Friday I received a telegram from Dr. Walker saying that Halifax needed my help, and at a little over an hour's notice I took the 7.30 train from Boston with Dr. H[arold] V[irgil] Andrews, Miss W. L. Stevens, Miss M. Adams, of my own hospital staff. On the way I was joined by Miss L. Allen, formerly of Halifax, now a trained nurse working in Massachusetts, and a Miss Bridges, who was recommended to me by Dr. [Thomas] Walker of St. John and who, though not a regular trained nurse, had had experience for a year at a military hospital in Leeds, England. On the train, I was joined by Dr. L[eander] M[arshall] Crosby and Dr. C[harles] W[entworth] DeWolf.

When I arrived in Halifax early Sunday morning, I reported as directed by Dr. Walker of St. John to the Victoria General Hospital. At the suggestion of Dr. McDougall of the staff of the Victoria, I came to the Y.M.C.A. Building, and finding medical service was needed, applied to Colonel Weatherbe at the City Hall for authority to take charge there. I accordingly went to the Y.M.C.A. Building, and since then have continued to direct the hospital without any further written authority but with the consent of the directors of the institution and the various emergency committees. During this period a number of doctors have served temporarily under me, namely—Dr. [Theodore Rupert] Ford of Liverpool, N.S., Doctors [Robert Laurent] Normandie, [John Baker] Swift[, Jr.], [Foster Standish] Kellog (Obstetricians of the Red Cross Unit from Boston) Doctors [William Alfred] Rolfe and [Kenneth Llewellyn] Dole of the Surgical

Red Cross Unit, Dr. [George Clowes] VanWart of Fredericton, and Dr. E[benezer] R[oss] Faulkner of New York. Most of these gentlemen have now returned home, so that my present staff consists of the following: -

H[arold] V[irgil] Andrews, Surgeon

C[harles] W[entworth] DeWolf, Assistant Surgeon

L[eander] M[arshall] Crosby, Specialist, Eye, Ear, Nose & Throat

E[benezer] R[oss] Faulkner, recently assigned to me to do general surgical work and nose and throat.

This staff has to care for fifty-eight patients, eight of whom are obstetrics, nine are eye, and the rest surgical or trivial.

In addition to these patients, we now have fifty empty beds.

Female Ward—15 beds, 2 of which are vacant.

Eye Ward—12 beds, 4 of which are vacant.

Male Surgical Ward—45 beds, 28 of which are vacant.

Obstetric Ward—48 beds, 14 of which are at present vacant.

The obstetrical ward is composed of single rooms, some of which have two beds in them, and the reason why there does not appear a larger number of vacant beds is that some are occupied by doctors and nurses.

In addition to the beds which we have now ready to receive patients, we have the beds and equipment for about thirty more, which could be set up in the present dining room if this seems best to your committee. I have decided not to put up these beds until it has developed that there is a real need for their use.

X-Ray Apparatus

We have installed on the floor near the operating room and large male surgical ward, a first-class X-ray apparatus which was brought from Boston by the Medical Red Cross. This X-ray apparatus is now in operation, and owing to the fact that Miss Twombley, radiologist of my own hospital in Boston, is here to do the work, we could probably take care of any demand there may be for X-ray work from other hospitals. Male patients with fractures or foreign bodies needing X Rays can readily be admitted to the 28 empty beds in the surgical ward for X Rays and the necessary surgery afterwards.

The Relation with the Military Authorities

I suppose that I must have received some informal military appointment to temporarily fill the place of senior medical officer, but I have received no formal appointment. During transformation of the Y.M.C.A. Building into a hospital, I have been acting in this capacity and have been greatly aided in getting the hospital into condition by Lieutenant Reid, who, from the date of the accident to the present time, has rendered invaluable service, at first as a volunteer and later as Adjutant. Captain Barratt has given most satisfactory and efficient service in helping us obtain equipment and stores.

Housekeeping Situation

At the time I took charge of the hospital, I found a committee of ladies under the informal charge of Mrs. McDougall and Mrs. Henry, who had seen to it that the some twenty odd patients who had been admitted during the emergency should be able to get their meals and the necessary bedside care. Up to the present, these ladies have served with the greatest skill and diligence, and no patient or member of the personnel has gone away hungry. For the last few days it has been evident that the strain has begun to tell on these volunteers, and it is necessary now to constitute a more regular kitchen service. Lieutenant Reid has engaged two cooks and plans to engage one more in order to put the Quartermaster Department on a definite military basis. I have gladly signed his suggestion for this work, as he has shown great ability in meeting the needs of his office.

Nursing Situation

When I arrived at the hospital I found that Miss Stewart of Fredericton, N.B., who is an extremely capable woman, had already attended to the nursing of the emergency patients. She has worked in the capacity of Superintendent since I arrived, although my own Superintendent, Miss Stevens, has nominally been head. Miss Stevens has confined most of her work to the operating room and the large surgical ward. My other nurse, Miss Adams, has worked under Miss Stewart and the various nurses who have been assigned from your office and with those who came from Fredericton with Miss Stewart.

Orderlies

The orderlies have worked well under the direction of Lieut. Reid, and have taken their meals in the building at the same mess which has been served by the Halifax ladies, but from now on Lieut. Reid plans to have them given a separate mess downstairs and the cooking done by one of the chefs he has engaged. Owing to the occasional crowding in the dining-room, I have made a lasting arrangement with the proprietor of the Green Lantern, so that members of the personnel can go in there for meals and sign slips as coming from the Y.M.C.A.

Quarters

Through the efficient work of Mr. Dawson of the Y.M.C.A. staff, arrangements have been made with some of the citizens of Halifax to quarter some of the nurses and doctors outside the hospital. This arrangement could be increased if there were a greater demand for patients' rooms and all nurses were thus displaced.

Housekeeping

During all this period Mrs. McDougall of Halifax has taken the best of care of the housekeeping arrangements and has seen to it that many patients who were destitute have been supplied with clothing. In many other respects also Mrs. McDougall has given much needed service.

General Direction of Institution

This part of the work has largely been done by Dr. Woodbury, one of the directors of the Y.M.C.A., who has been on hand all the time, except a few hours, since the catastrophe.

Future Outlook

The whole hospital is now in fairly good order and can go on expanding or contracting according to the wishes of the Medical Committee. It is well equipped to take care of eye cases, surgical cases needing X Ray and operation, and even maternity cases.

We have a card catalog of the important facts about each patient received since I took charge, but this is the only system of record.[316]

I feel that the work that I have done so far in the institution has been the best that I could give it, but my own office at home renders it necessary for me to return unless it is very clear that there is no one to take my place as administrator.

316These are Codman's End Result Cards.

It seems to me that the time has come when it should be decided whether this hospital should be a proper-going military institution or whether it should be taken over by some of the local surgeons and doctors as a civil hospital.

I should be greatly obliged if you will give this whole matter your consideration and let me know your decision.

Dr. Andrews, Miss Stevens, Miss Adams and Miss Twombley should return when I do, and I know that their circumstances are such that they need compensation for work which is not distinctly emergency or philanthropic. Up to the present time they are in my own employ, but as I need them in my work at home, I should have to make some financial arrangements if I am to leave them to continue the work of the institution until their places can be taken by others.

Dr. DeWolf, Dr. Crosby, and the other nurses, are thoroughly independent of my part, and it is time that some definite arrangement should be made with them.

E. A. Codman, M.D.
S[enior] M[edical] O[fficer][317]

The report was typical Codman—complete, well written, describing in detail what he had done, why he had done it, and what further remained to be done. Codman left Halifax on Wednesday, 19 December 1917, returning to Boston. In the Codman Archives there is only one reference in which the Halifax explosion is mentioned at all. It is a letter written in French from the French General Council of Canada, based in Halifax, which thanks Dr. Codman for his efforts in

---

317Codman EA. "The situation at the Y.M.C.A. Hospital on the evening of December 14, 1917, with a brief statement concerning the use of the Y.M.C.A. Building since the accident in Dec. 6th. Dr. Codman's connection with the Hospital," *In:* Harris DF. "Report of the Halifax Medical Commission," Unpublished document held at the Public Archives of Nova Scotia, Call Number MG36c, #118-119.

going to Halifax and helping with the survivors of the *Mont Blanc* explosion.[318]

It is not exactly clear why, but the Codman Hospital never re-opened. Codman could have resumed operating at 15 Pinckney Street in early 1918, but he did not do so. The reasons have not been left to us. But other factors would prevent Codman from resuming work at his hospital from mid-1918 onwards.

As mentioned, Codman had many Canadian friends, from his frequent trips to the Maritimes for hunting, fishing, and medical meetings. He had actually enlisted in the Canadian Army shortly before the Halifax explosion and was preparing to help the Canadians in England when the disaster occurred. But returning to America after the disaster, he was drafted into the Medical Corps of the United States Army and, in September 1918, was appointed Senior Surgeon of the Coast Defenses in Delaware and Virginia. In November 1918, he was made a regimental surgeon in the artillery and began treating the many sick army recruits. He kept End Result Cards on all his patients, setting up his own End Result System. In January 1919 he was transferred to be Surgeon-in-Chief at the base hospital in Camp Taylor, Kentucky. He continued his work with End Result Cards, using them to provide better care for the soldiers. In May 1919, he wrote his niece, Maria, the following letter,

> **Dear Maria,**
>
> **It occurred to me tonight that of the 250,000 American wounded, over 2,000 have passed through my hands. I have notes on practically every one. That is, it would have taken only 125 surgeons like me to see them all. Put this in the paper to compare with the Cabots who each took care of one-sixth of the wounded. What did those other surgeons do?[319]**

Although it may have seemed unusual that Codman would be so busy during World War I, while stationed in Kentucky and Delaware,

---

318CA, 3/59, letter of 22 December 1917.

319CA 8/155.

it was because of one of the worst disasters in American and world history, which followed only a few months after the Halifax disaster.

In March 1918 at Fort Riley, Kansas, a solider complained of fever, muscle aches and a sore throat. Within a week, more than 500 soldiers at Fort Riley were sick with influenza. The flu spread to other nearby army camps, and thus began what many considered to be the worse pandemic in the history of the world. The worldwide influenza pandemic would last approximately one year, but before it was over, it would infect over 1/5th of the world's population, by conservative estimate, including 25 million Americans. Medical historians are still puzzled by the fact that the majority of the people who were infected, and died from the influenza, were young healthy people between the ages of 20 and 40, usually an age group best able to ward off illness. This, unfortunately, included many of the soldiers in the American army that Codman ended up treating.

The influenza pandemic has been described thusly: "The only specific event in history that compares with the world wars of this century as a reaper of human lives is the influenza pandemic of 1918-19. Like the world wars, the pandemic killed tens of millions of people, but it was vastly more efficient: it did so in less than a year whereas the wars took four or five years to accumulate the same toll."[320]

It is considered that the influenza pandemic began in the United States and then was spread to Europe by American soldiers landing in France in the spring and summer of 1918. By the fall of 1918, 20 percent of all American soldiers stationed in the United States were sick, an enormous number given the huge numbers of young men had been enlisted or drafted into the military service. The spread of the disease was likely aided by the war: "The most apparent threat that influenza portended was that the war had produced optimum conditions for the development of new variants of influenza viruses. Millions of people of the ages most susceptible to severe influenza infection were jammed together in industrial cities, military camps and ships, and were shifting about the world in immense numbers."[321]

320Crosby AW Jr. "The influenza pandemic of 1918,", In: *History, Science, and Politics: Influenza in America 1918-1976*, edited by JE Osborn. (New York: Prodist, 1977), p. 5.

321*Ibid.*, p. 7-8.

In addition, medical science at that time was barely able to treat the sick. People all over the United States were inoculated with various vaccines, but none of them worked to any extent. Across the country people began to wear anti-flu masks; in some cities it was against the law to board a bus or trolley without wearing a mask. Laws were enacted prohibiting coughing, sneezing, shaking hands, and spitting in public places.

By the late spring of 1919, the worldwide influenza pandemic abated as mysteriously as it had begun. In the United States it was estimated that more than 500,000 people died from influenza. Throughout the world India suffered the worst of the disaster, as influenza claimed 12 million dead in that nation. Crosby noted, "The full history of the pandemic cannot be encompassed by the human mind."[322]

Codman himself described the difficult times caring for the sick soldiers during the influenza epidemic.

I had more soldiers under me than had the general in command of the three old forts. At the end of my endurance, I stood one night in the upper ward of the old hospital in which had been concentrated those whom I judged to be hopeless. My other medical officers were sick abed—even my tireless and capable junior, Captain Ellis, was on that night exhausted. The floor was slippery with bloody sputum; there were no nurses; no petticoats of any kind; no bedpans; no gauze and few medicines; in fact, there was no medical or nursing care. Those that were able lurched to a toilet with the aid of some other soldier who had yesterday been a recruit and now found himself an orderly in this death house, mopping up bloody slime from the floor or cleaning the bed of another boy after he had helped to dump the body and the soiled blankets in a box. I turned and said good-night to those boys who were facing their dangerous duty as bravely as those

---

322*Ibid.*, p. 9.

> who fought in the trenches. After a few hours I was
> able to get up and go on with the "paper work,"
> reporting the numbers of sick and dead, filling out the
> death certificates, making applications for transfer of
> insane recruits and otherwise obeying the orders of
> my competent subordinate, a Sergeant of the Medical
> Corps.[323]

Codman described his use of the End Result System during his time at Camp Taylor, as we would expect of him. Although the time Codman spent at Camp Taylor was difficult and many people were overworked and overburdened, he saw this not as an obstacle, but as an opportunity to test the End Result System.

> Five hundred hospital beds and some 300
> convalescent soldiers in barracks gave an excellent
> opportunity. An orderly carrying my box of cards
> attended all visits or operations. The cards were not
> substituted for the regular records, but served to keep
> in touch with them when desirable. The senior
> surgeon of a hospital of 500 beds, if he worked eight
> hours a day, could give less than one minute to each
> patient, even if he did no operating or executive work
> (60 minutes x 8 hours = 480 patients), yet, with the aid
> of my catalogue and of a good orderly, who has since
> become Dr. Fraasch, I kept a certain amount of
> supervision over every patient, operated on many,
> dressed difficult wounds, and made personal notes on
> the condition of nearly every soldier at entrance, and
> again at discharge. At least once a week I inspected
> each serious wound and often had consultations in the
> Medical Wards as well. My cards were of the greatest
> help, for I could talk over his cases with each ward

---

[323]Preface, p. xxxi.

officer as often as seemed desirable. However, I must admit that my day was often longer than eight hours.[324]

Codman did not spend all of his time in the Army tending to the sick and injured, finding time even then to indulge in his hobby of hunting and fishing. Simmons later noted, "While in the army, stationed in [Kentucky] during the war, he carried on his hobby to such good effect that he was given the honorary title of 'Fish and Game Officer to the General in Command.'"[325]

In June of 1919, Codman left the Army and returned to Boston. His hospital was closed, and he was deeply in debt. He was considered a poor credit risk at this time, and he himself commented that he had "no borrowing capacity."[326] He made only $2,700 in 1919 and he and Katy were probably surviving on her own trust monies.[327] Although his leanings were altruistic, and he had devoted his life to an attempt to reform medicine for the good of others, even he saw the need at this time to focus on himself and his family, and improve his financial situation. He noted, "I steadfastly abstained from embarking on any new adventures for the benefit of coming generations."[328] In fact, Codman did something that was quite unlike him, especially when one reads the mission statement of the Codman Hospital—he raised his fees! He explained his reasons near the end of the Preface:

I had patched up too many fine young men to feel much enthusiasm about keeping the aged and infirm alive, or to listen with any pretense of sympathy to even the nicest lady's description of the daily behavior of her digestion. I determined to be a money-maker, at least until I had paid off my debts, and for two years

---

324Preface, p. xxxii.

325Simmons CC. Ernest Amory Codman. 1869-1940. *Trans Amer Surg Assoc*, 59, p. 613, 1941.

326Preface, p. xxxii.

327For a surgeon, this equates, in today's dollar equivalent, to far less than a resident's salary. Codman's income of $2,700 in 1919 would now be worth no more than $20,600.

328Preface, p. xxxii.

charge most of my patients three times as much as formerly.[329]

The Codman Hospital at 15 Pinckney Street was now an apartment house, although Codman still owned it. As stated above, it never reopened, though he did solicit investors in an attempt to resurrect the hospital.

> **The Codman Hospital has been closed during the time that Dr. Codman has been in the Army. It will be opened again if others feel enough sympathy with the principles for which it stood, to help bear the financial risk.**
>
> **Ten thousand circulars, similar to this, will be sent out to former patients, personal friends, neighbors, members of the Massachusetts Medical Society, and others who have shown an interest in the End Result Idea. If five hundred persons reply that they will loan one hundred dollars or more, each, at 5 per cent, the hospital will be reorganized on the basis published in the last "Study in Hospital Efficiency."[330]**

The appeal did not work, however, and his hospital ended up like the End Result Cards from Halifax, which were "scattered like a Cumæan Sybil, at the time, they served to keep my finger on every pulse in the hospital and illustrate the simplicity of installing the plan, even in a city paralyzed by calamity."[331] His End Result Idea would also now be scattered, and drift off with less direction. It, too, had felt the effects of the disaster in Halifax and the brutality of the war.

His once promising career now lay scattered as well, set adrift first by his own obsession with the End Result Idea, and his refusal to

---

329Preface, p. xxxii. The Cumæan Sibyl was a prophetess of Greek legend. Legend relates that a famous collection of prophecies, the Sibylline Books, was offered for sale to Tarquinius Superbus, the last of the seven kings of Rome, by the Cumæan Sibyl. The King refused to pay the offered price, so the Sibyl burned six of the books, and then sold the remaining three at the original price.

330CA 5/93.

331Preface, p. xxx.

compromise in his efforts to implement it on a wide-scale basis, and now by the loss of his hospital. Almost 50 years old by the end of the War, a pariah to his medical colleagues in Boston, riven from the security of the Massachusetts General Hospital, his prospects for recovery were far from bright.

CHAPTER 10
THE REGISTRY OF BONE SARCOMA

Finish every day and be done with it. You have done what you could. Some blunders and absurdities no doubt crept in; forget them as soon as you can. Tomorrow is a new day; begin it well and serenely and with too high a spirit to be cumbered with your old nonsense. This day is all that is good and fair. It is far too dear with its hopes and invitations to waste a moment on the yesterday.

Ralph Waldo Emerson, *Essays, First Series. Self-Reliance.* [1841]

Codman returned to Boston in late 1919 and set about attempting to resurrect his surgical career. As always, the End Result Idea would never be far from his mind. Now, at age fifty, and surely learning the lessons of maturity, perhaps he realized that his previous antagonistic methods of attempting to convince others of its merits were not the best way to proceed.

The years from 1919-1925 are a bit of a mystery in Codman's life. The Codman Hospital was closed and he no longer was a member of the staff at the Massachusetts General Hospital. Where did he operate and see patients? The *American Medical Directories* for these years list over 35 hospitals in the city of Boston, many of which no longer exist. There are some hints in the Codman Archives that he operated at the Boston City Hospital, but beyond that, it is uncertain where he did surgery during this period. As to seeing patients, his office was in the first floor of his home at 227 Beacon Street, and he saw patients there from 1919-1925. He did have a practice for these years; in the preface to

The Shoulder, he lists his income for these years in the chart in the Preface. He did well in 1920 and 1921, possibly from rentals of 15 Pinckney Street, which he converted to an apartment house. But in 1922-1925, he made less than $6,000. Practicing completely on his own, without a strong hospital affiliation, alienated from his fellow physicians, his own income declining, these had to be difficult years for him. He found solace in the next great project of his life.

Shortly after his return to Boston, Codman began treating a patient from a wealthy family with a presumed sarcoma of the ilium (part of the pelvis). The family of this patient gave Codman $1,000 asking him to make an attempt to acquire all possible knowledge of bone sarcoma, so that it might be applied to cure their relative. The attempt eventually failed, as the patient died from his cancer on 27 November 1920, and ironically, at autopsy the disease proved to be a metastatic carcinoma rather than a true bone sarcoma.

The important point, however, was that this stimulated Codman's interest in bone sarcoma and the family's gift enabled him to begin a more detailed study of the problem. In August 1920 he addressed a circular letter to the individual members of the American College of Surgeons and sought out the advice of the two recognized experts on bone tumors in the country, the pathologists Dr. James Ewing (1866-1943) and Dr. Joseph C[olt] Bloodgood (1867-1935). In the letter he asked the recipients to provide examples of bone sarcoma patients who were still alive after five years. Codman, Ewing and Bloodgood then decided to form a Registry of Bone Sarcoma to tabulate all cases of the problem in the United States, especially those that had been cured, in an attempt to find the best methods of cure.

Following is the complete text of Codman's letter, which was sent to the members of the American College of Surgeons:

> **Dear Doctor: Have you any living cases of bone sarcoma? I include in this question, recent cases which are now under treatment and also any cases which you may consider as having recovered.**
>
> **I have a patient with a sarcoma of the ilium, who is having treatment with radium, and I am most anxious to get in touch with other surgeons who have similar**

cases, whether of the ilium or of other bones, or whether their treatment is by surgery, by Coley toxins, by radium, or by other agencies.

Dr. Bloodgood and Dr. Ewing are joining me in this investigation, and it is our intention to keep a file of all living cases in which the diagnosis is reasonably certain, and to send to each surgeon who contributes a case, a duplicate file of all the others. In this way each case will have the benefit of the experience of the rest. We feel that surgery has perhaps been a failure in such cases, and that today, radium should be considered as offering more hope than surgery, at least in some cases where the position of the growth makes amputation too great a sacrifice.

Cases known to have died cannot be included in the investigation at present, but we should be glad to correspond with any surgeon who has (or is willing to do so) collected data about the past cases in his clinic or neighborhood, for it is important to confirm or disprove the conclusions from Bloodgood's series, i.e., that the periosteal infiltrating form has an almost universally bad prognosis, and the giant-cell medullary type an almost universally good one. We must also standardize the pathological nomenclature.

For the purpose of this investigation, cases which are diagnosed as sarcoma from the clinical data and the X-ray, without the removal of a pathological specimen, must be accepted, for, as in our case, it may seem best not to incise on account of the danger of provoking metastases. It may prove best to make this a rule, for apparently radium cures the benign forms and the limb is not needlessly sacrificed; and if the malignant forms, almost as a rule, recur rapidly in the lungs, whether amputation is done or not, it may be well to save the limb, if the growth can be held in check by radium.

We feel that these cases are too rare for each individual clinic to work alone, and that the plan outlined will bring before surgeons in general, in the most rapid possible manner, the facts as they develop.

If you can contribute one or more cases please send me a very brief description of each, and I will write you in greater detail about the plan above suggested.

(Signed) E. A. Codman, M.D.[332]

Codman, Ewing and Bloodgood presented the idea of their Registry of Bone Sarcoma to the American College of Surgeons at their annual meeting in Philadelphia in October 1921. The American College was so impressed that they made the committee a standing one of the College. With further contributions from the College, over $8,000 became available to Codman's committee for research into bone sarcoma.

Initially, Codman did not receive much of a response to his entreaties for information on bone sarcoma. In addition to the above letter, which was mailed in August 1920, he later (February 1922) published a similar letter in the *Boston Medical and Surgical Journal*. At that time, the *Journal* was sent to all members of the Massachusetts Medical Society, in addition to other subscribers.

Registry of Bone Sarcoma

February 2, 1922

Mr. Editor:

I wonder if you would give me your help in obtaining some statistics for the Registry of Bone Sarcoma. It is desirable to know the frequency of occurrence of cases of this lesion and there are no statistics by which we can obtain it. It occurred to me that a pretty accurate estimate could be made in the following way:

332CA 3/59.

According to the Directory of the American Medical Association the population of Massachusetts is 3,662,329 and the number of physicians 5,494. If each one of these physicians should drop me a postal saying, either, "I do know or I do not know of a case of bone sarcoma at present alive in Massachusetts," we should have almost by return mail the best information in the world on the percentage of this disease per capita of population.

Of course, I realize that your Journal, interesting and instructive as it is, by no means reaches every physician in the state and that many of those whom it does reach do not read everything in it. Nevertheless, there seems to be a way to counterbalance that discrepancy. If every physician who does read this letter will constitute himself a local committee for a week and ask every other physician he meets during that week whether he knows of a living case of bone sarcoma, and obtains their signatures, I believe we should reach nearly every physician in the state. These could be checked off in the Directory and I could make a personal appeal to the remainder.

I believe that every doctor in Massachusetts would be glad to contribute his bit to medical science, if the doing so did not involve too much time and expense. This plan would involve but a minute of time and a cent apiece, so the main thing would be to get the plan to them. Will you try it? They will each do their bit if you do.

A few words about the Registry may not be out of place. The Registry of Bone Sarcoma aims to be a combined national study of the diagnosis and treatment of this lesion.

Although organized independently by Dr. Bloodgood of Baltimore, Dr. Ewing of New York and the writer, it is now a Committee of the American

College of Surgeons. Our object is to register every case of bone sarcoma and by following the cases (through their medical attendants) to learn what the result of each was and what, if any, forms of treatment are effective. At present, these cases are too rare for any one surgeon or clinic to obtain a sufficient number for study. We do not expect to find an excessive number in the whole country. In fact, during the year and a half in which we have been collecting cases, we have only found four five-year cures by amputation, and altogether only under one hundred cases which are now living, including those known to be moribund.

If the physicians of Massachusetts will promptly send in the postal cards, negative and positive, as above suggested, we shall at least know what the problem is in this state. All supposed-to-be bone sarcomas should be reported, including giant-cell tumors, except epulis [a tumor or tumorous growth of the gum]. We want to know of all cases now alive whether cured, under treatment or moribund. We want negative answers as well as positive.

When we once know who has charge of each case in Massachusetts we can communicate directly with him and perhaps by showing our collection help him to treat his particular case more satisfactorily. We can, at least, give him expert pathologic opinion on sections of tissue. We should be glad to demonstrate our collection to anyone interested.

I hope, Mr. Editor, you may see fit to publish this letter, although I fully realize that it may be a precedent you do not care to establish. I ask the favor because our Committee represents a great national association which has undertaken this intensive study of a rare and singularly fatal disease. The work of the Committee consumes a great deal of time and I hope that you and your readers will help us out.

The American College of Surgeons holds its Clinical Congress in Boston next October. I hope we shall then be able to state the exact number of cases of bone sarcoma in Massachusetts, with pathologic proof of each case if it is obtainable.

Should this letter be read by physicians outside of Massachusetts, I may repeat this investigation is a national one, and we should appreciate any positive reports of cases. It is only in Massachusetts that I am trying to get negative as well as positive replies.

Sincerely,

E. A. Codman, M.D.

[Note.—Here is an opportunity for the profession to contribute to this study of an important subject. Let everyone do his part and send in his postal card.—Editor.][333]

A few weeks later Codman sent another letter which was also published in *the Boston Medical and Surgical Journal* in which he gave his readers information concerning the responses he had received.[334] He noted at that time he had received only 19 responses from 5,494 physicians, seventeen negative and two positive (meaning that they could report a case of bone sarcoma). Further, he then requested that the readers who had not responded send him a letter stating why they had not done so, listing the following reasons from which to choose: 1) inertia, 2) procrastination, 3) disapproval, 4) opposition, 5) not interested, 6) specialist, 7) retired, 8) economy, 9) personal and 10) other reasons. Codman was still adept at irritating his fellow physicians!

He did not stop there. The letter above, which appeared in the 3 March 1922 issue of *the Boston Medical and Surgical Journal*, was reprinted in the 30 March and 6 April editions of the same year.[335] In the latter two re-printings of his letter, he again requested the physicians of Massachusetts to respond to his original letter and, if they

---

333BMSJ, 186(5): 161, 2 February 1922.

334BMSJ, 186(10): 335, 9 March 1922.

335BMSJ, 186(13): 441, and BMSJ, 186(14): 489.

had not, to please give the reasons why. An addendum to his letter in the last two issues included a note from the editor of the *Journal* stating that he had received 40 reports since the publication of his first letter, one positive and 39 negative.[336]

In March 1922, Codman published two articles in *Surgery, Gynecology & Obstetrics*. The first article was a highly unusual one entitled, "A New Instrument to be Called the Registry of Bone Sarcoma Scissors."[337] Codman had developed these scissors which were an interesting attachment that could be put over the fingers. The scissors clipped on to adjacent fingers and had blades intervening which would be held in the web space between the digits. After tying a surgical knot the surgeon could then cut the knot simply by pulling the remaining strands up between his fingers and closing his fingers, using the scissor blades to cut the suture.

Codman noted that he wished to make some money on this, " ... partly to control the name of the instrument and partly to make a fortune out of it, should its use extend to industry and the household sewing basket, a patent has been applied for."[338] Codman did, in fact, receive patent #1601560 for his registry of bone sarcoma scissors, but it does not appear that he made any money from these. Codman hoped to use the scissors to stimulate his fellow surgeons to report their cases of bone sarcoma: "It is my hope in presenting this instrument to the profession that it will become the fashion to make it socially uncomfortable for any surgeon who is found using this appliance, if he has not recorded his cases of bone sarcoma to the best of his ability. He must be 'jollyed' into registering or 'jollyed' out of using the scissors."[339] His altruism and devition to the Registry of Bone Sarcoma extended to the point that he offered to obtain them for any surgeon at cost if they would simply use them as a reminder to register their cases of bone sarcoma.[340]

336I cannot resolve the fact that his letters state that he has two positive answers and the editor's note states there was only one positive answer.

337SGO, 39: 127-128, March 1922.

338*Ibid.*, p. 128.

339*Ibid.*

340The exact same article also appeared in BMSJ, 190 (17): 710, 24 April 1924.

The other article in the March 1922 issue of *Surgery, Gynecology & Obstetrics* was a far more important one, entitled, "The Registry of Cases of Bone Sarcoma." In this article he summarized the first year and a half of the Registry of Bone Sarcoma as well as giving details of its early formulation. The article noted that up to that time 171 surgeons had given descriptions of cases of bone sarcoma and another 345 had replied in the negative. In this important article, Codman gave the philosophy behind the Registry, the plan of the Registry, the future plans and the early results and analysis of the Registry of Bone Sarcoma.

In describing the workings of the Registry, Codman pointed out that bone sarcoma was so rare that few doctors saw cases of it and that the purpose of the Registry of Bone Sarcoma was to have all the registered cases of bone sarcoma sent to the various experts on the problem throughout the country. This procedure would then allow the Registry to acquire a large database of information, hopefully to eventually standardize the classification and treatment of the problem. Codman stated that all cases of bone sarcoma, rare as they were, essentially constituted an experiment and that it was important for them to record the results of their experiments in this difficult disease.[341]

The plan was for every physician to record all their cases of bone sarcoma with the Registry. With each case sent to the Registry, the physician was asked to include slides of tissue, copies of X-rays, and a short history of the cases. The Registry requested that the consulting surgeon send reports of the success or failure of whatever treatment was performed. Codman also noted that the Registry would make suggestions and give advice as to treatment, if requested, but stated correctly that, at the time, treatment of bone sarcoma was so unsatisfactory that no authoritative advice could be given in most cases. All of the slides of tissue, after receipt by the Registry of Bone Sarcoma, were to be forwarded to both Ewing and Bloodgood for their pathologic analysis.

341SGO, 34(3): 335-343, March 1922.

Codman then went into several pages of description of the nomenclature of bone sarcoma. Eventually the early results of the Registry of Bone Sarcoma would deal extensively with this nomenclature, including a book that Codman would later publish. This instance was really the first mention of it.

In the analysis of the cases reported to the Registry by 1 January 1922, Codman cited the following:

Cases Reported and Registered

Total cases about which we have had correspondence—454

Cases excluded for lack of X-rays, slides, or tissue or obviously incorrect diagnoses—317

Cases which we have little doubt are instances of osteogenic sarcoma—41

Cases of giant-cell tumor—43

Cases still undetermined or other tumors—53

Cases of osteogenic sarcoma living over 5 years—4

The article ended with a further call for help from all surgeons, asking them to register their cases of bone sarcoma. Codman listed the cases which were eligible for registration as any case which had been diagnosed as sarcoma of bone with sufficient certainty to justify beginning any kind of treatment on that basis. He requested four typewritten copies of the information, one to be retained by the referring physician, one to be retained by Codman, and two to be sent off, one each to both Ewing and Bloodgood. The data requested for registering a case of bone sarcoma was as follows:

Data for Registration of a Case of Bone Sarcoma

Name and Address—
of doctor registering case
of patient
of friend, with permanent address, who would be likely to answer follow-up letters

of family physician

of surgeon operating

of roentgenologist

of pathologist

of hospital. Record reference or hospital number

Dictate history so as to cover following headings, and typewrite four copies on standard typing paper.

Clinical note. Date it was made. Age at this time. Race. Sex. Bone involved—part of bone. Date of trauma, if any, character of trauma—date and duration of pain, swelling, tumor, fracture, loss of function. Any other important clinical data.

Examination. Date and by whom. Notes on local disease, especially as to swelling, tenderness, loss of function, involvement of joint. Presence or absence of bone shell. Pulsation. Size and extent of swelling.

Brief note on examination. Especially blood, Wasserman. Urine, Bence-Jones bodies. Physical examination of chest. Date and diagnosis of first X-ray. From X-ray whether considered central or periosteal. If there are no X-rays or prints to be sent, give as complete a description of the X-rays as possible. Note as to whether X-rays of other bones and chest were made, and results.

Treatment. Date or dates of treatments. Operation—exploratory incision. Piece taken for diagnosis. Curetting. Partial excision. Complete excision, extend. Bone transplantation, from where. Amputation, exact position. Coley serum. X-ray. Radium. Any other treatment.

Gross pathology. Description at operation of specimen.

Microscopic. Description and diagnosis.

Condition at date of last examination or report. Date of this.

> Have sections been preserved by you? Sent to
> registry with this? To be returned or preserved?
>
> Have X-rays been preserved by you? Sent to
> registry with this? To be returned or preserved?
>
> Has gross material been preserved by you? Sent to
> registry with this? To be returned or preserved?
>
> Make four typewritten copies, keep one and mail
> three to Dr. E. A. Codman, 227 Beacon Street, Boston,
> Mass.

In his discussion of the Registry, Codman always included a call for its use as a method of employing the End Result Idea. Near the end of this article, he commented, "Another great reason why we have not been successful in finding more living cases is because hospitals, as a rule, have no follow-up systems."[342] He had not given up on the End Result Idea. Perhaps by now, somewhat chastened by the events from 1915-19, he realized he would never be able to incorporate it to all of medicine in its entirety. The Registry of Bone Sarcoma was a perfect example of a rare disease, to which the End Result Idea could be applied, demonstrating to the medical world that it could work on a small scale. Certainly, Codman hoped for more than that with the End Result Idea. But he had probably begun to realize that he was not going to be able to reform all of medicine by himself, and get every physician to register all of their End Results. Even here, as can been seen from the above comments, he met the same resistance from physicians and initially had the same difficulty that he did with the End Result Idea. But it was, to Codman, at least a beginning.

A few months after these two articles appeared in *Surgery, Gynecology & Obstetrics*, Codman had another letter published in the *Boston Medical and Surgical Journal* which included his original letters of 2 February and 27 February 1922. The article also included additional comments from Codman. He noted the indifference with which his letters had been met, including samples of some of the comments he had received from other doctors:

342*Ibid.*, p. 341.

Undoubtedly, in sending this questionnaire I have added to many annoyances which afflict the modern practitioner. One writes as follows, expressing his "amusement at the solemn earnestness with which a statistical study of bone sarcoma developed into an intensely serious tabulation of physicians. No serious soul with a burning missionary zeal appreciates that when he asks a general practitioner of pause and give him his facts he is one more of a horde of modern complications that are wearing on our patience. We are beset by telephone, by mail, by interviews, by social service sleuths, family welfarers, accident and health insurance certificates, worker's compensation documents, lawyers' letters, etc. These time-consuming, insistent nuisances have multiplied most horribly in the last ten years. The end is not yet, because now the soldier and, especially, the almost soldiers, are just beginning to drive for bales of affidavits to bolster up claims, many of them bogus." However, he did his bit and said he did not know of a case of bone sarcoma!

Another wrote that he was no more interested in bone sarcoma than I was in knowing "how many flies could light on a golf ball." But he, too, did his bit and said that he did not know of a case. There were other interesting replies, but none were so depressing as those who did not reply at all, for they spoiled the statistics.

Evidently the postals were received in very different spirits by different individuals according to their views of life in general. Dark suspicions of the intentions of the writer were probably held by some who promptly dropped the postal into their waste basket.[343]

343BMSJ, 187 (6): 209, 10 August 1922

In late October 1922 Codman published another article in the *Boston Medical and Surgical Journal* entitled, "Bone Sarcoma; Prevalence in Massachusetts." This article documented the results of the replies to his letters to the many physicians in Massachusetts. He noted that by then the Registry had located 71 possible cases and had found only nine cases of survivors of osteogenic sarcoma,[344] and he gave details of those nine cases. He also stated that there were four practical points that could be deduced from the information gathered to that date.

1. **That the diagnosis should be made with great caution.**

2. **That Bloodgood's claim of the benign character of giant-cell tumors (erroneously called sarcoma) is confirmed by experience in Massachusetts.**

3. **That true osteogenic sarcoma is almost always fatal (the rare exceptions being cases where early amputation is performed).**

4. **That since only nine living cases could be located in a population of 4,000,000 there are probably only 225 in the whole United States (100,000,000). It certainly is not likely that there are more than double this number at any rate.**

The last point was extremely important and one of the early significant findings of the Registry. Bone sarcoma is a rare disease and no single medical center, working alone, could possibly have compiled a large number of cases, even over years of study, even today. This was an early example of what is now called a "multi-center study," where clinical data from various centers is combined to obtain numbers that may be used to reach conclusions concerning the diseases which have clinical and statistical significance. And it was really the first time that

---

344Codman at times used osteogenic sarcoma and bone sarcoma interchangeably. However, there are many types of bone sarcoma, of which osteogenic sarcoma (now usually called osteosarcoma) is only type, albeit a very deadly one.

Codman had shown that the End Result Idea could be used to make important contributions to medical knowledge.

Although Codman was certainly one of the country's top experts on bone tumors by this point, he was modest enough to demean his own abilities both in lecture and in print. He gave a talk on pathologic fractures at the Clinical Congress of the American College of Surgeons in Philadelphia in October 1921,[345] which he opened by stating, "Since I have had little personal experience in treatment of pathologic fractures, my function has been to review the literature of this subject in order to give you in ten minutes a résumé of present recorded knowledge concerning it."[346] Between 1924 and 1926 Codman published three journal articles and one book on bone sarcoma. These writings contained complete summaries of the work of the Registry, and of what was known about bone sarcoma to that date.

The first article was entitled, "The Method of Procedure of the Registry of Bone Sarcoma" and appeared in *Surgery, Gynecology & Obstetrics* in late 1924.[347] The article made several important points. Codman included pictures and details of the forms that were sent to the members of the American College of Surgeons. In the first sentence of the form for the Registry of Bone Sarcoma, he again brought up the End Result Idea: "The Registry of Bone Sarcoma is an activity of the American College of Surgeons to stimulate the study of cases of Bone Sarcoma to keep before the Medical Profession the End Result Idea which is the basis of the minimum standard of the College."[348]

Codman noted that bone sarcoma needed studying because there was no agreement as to nomenclature or treatment of the problem. He further stated, "The American College of Surgeons expects something more of its Fellows than annual dues. It expects any Fellow who has undertaken the care of a case of bone sarcoma (or has discovered a case accidentally as more often happens) to give the other members of the

---

345This was the conference at which the Registry of Bone Sarcoma was accepted as a committee by the American College.

346SGO, 34: 611-613, 1922

347SGO, 38: 712-721, 1924.

348*Ibid.*, p. 713.

College and through them to the rest of the profession the benefit of the experience gained."[349]

Codman also discussed the medico-legal problems inherent in treating rare diseases such as bone sarcoma and how surgeons might protect themselves from litigation by registering a case.

> **One sentence in the paragraph on the envelope refers to the medicolegal responsibility in these cases. It is well recognized in court that no individual physician is liable for such errors as the failure to recognize a rare disease or the failure to cure a notoriously intractable one. On the other hand, in any disease frequent or rare, neglect or the failure to seek advice from colleagues, when in doubt, may at times be prejudicial. Any surgeon who promptly registers a case of bone sarcoma as soon as he suspects the diagnosis certainly shows his good faith and his willingness to seek advice.**[350]

On the envelope for the form that the Registry sent to all the consultants, Codman requested further information from any doctor registering a case. On the back of the envelope was a space to provide a brief typewritten abstract of the case history, with a space for noting the date of registering the case, the condition of the patient, and when the date of the last follow-up occurred. On the underside of the flap was a list of the contents of the envelope. Every item in the envelope was numbered with the case number assigned by the Registry of Bone Sarcoma. Inside the main folder was a small manila envelope to be used for the slides of the tissue, as well as providing a typewritten, more detailed history of the case; prints or photographs of the X-rays, and all correspondence relating to the case. Finally, a large classification sheet was included, which contained a detailed description of the pathological entities that the Registry admitted as possible diagnoses. By 1924 the Registry considered there were only eight possible

---

349*Ibid.*

350*Ibid.*, p. 714.

pathological diagnoses of tumors of bone: 1) metastatic tumors, 2) periosteal fibrosarcoma, 3) osteogenic tumors, 4) inflammatory conditions, 5) benign giant-cell tumor 6) benign angioma, 7) Ewing's sarcoma, and 8) myeloma.

The next two published works in Codman's "bone sarcoma" trilogy appeared in 1925, and they were two outstanding achievements in the study of bone sarcoma. The first was an article entitled, "The Nomenclature Used by the Registry of Bone Sarcoma," which appeared in the *American Journal of Roentgenology and Radium Therapy*.[351] This was a lengthy article that discussed the exact nomenclature, that had been developed by the Registry in consultation with the Clinical Pathological Association which included Dr. [William Carpenter] M[a]cCarty (1880-1964) of the Mayo Clinic, Dr. [Frederic Ewald] Sondern (1867-1966) of New York, Dr. [Armin Von] St. George (1892-1943) of New York, and Dr. [Elexious Thompson] Bell (né 1880) of Minneapolis. The nomenclature problem had been alluded to in the first article of the trilogy. Later that year Codman published a book entitled simply, **Bone Sarcoma**,[352] noting that it was reprinted, with additions, from the above mentioned journal article. The book began with a short dedication:

To
Future Sufferers From Bone Sarcoma
may they be fortunate enough to fall
into the hands of roentgenologists,
pathologists and surgeons who have
the courage to accept the invitation
of the American College of Surgeons
to register their cases.

The book is a small one, both in number of pages (93) and size. Its content is almost exactly the same as the article which was published in the *American Journal of Roentgenology and Radium Therapy*. It again

---

351*Amer. J. Roentgenology Radium Ther*, 13(2): 105-126, February 1925.

352Codman EA. *Bone Sarcoma*, (New York: Paul B. Hoeber, 1925).

discussed the nomenclature described above in the early article but in much more detail.

The book began with a discussion of metastatic tumors, noting that the prognosis in these cases was universally unfavorable. He described the location in bone and noted that histologically they were usually similar to the original tumor.

Under periosteal fibrosarcoma Codman noted that they were tumors lying next to bone but not invading it and were indistinguishable histologically from fibrosarcomas of the fascia. He stated that they formed no osteoid tissue which separated them from osteogenic sarcomas.

Codman devoted the largest part of the nomenclature section to his discussion of osteogenic tumors, notably osteogenic sarcoma. He described several subtypes of this tumor including medullary, subperiosteal, periosteal and telangiectatic. Among these subtypes he discussed their radiographic characteristics, their histologic characteristics, and the varying prognoses. He stated that telangiectatic sarcoma had clinically the poorest prognosis, a statement which is still true today. Codman's description of inflammatory conditions reflects the era in which he lived. He subdivided inflammatory conditions into traumatic, syphilitic, and infectious, and included tubercular among the infectious. Syphilitic and tubercular bone infections are very rare today in the United States.

Codman discussed giant-cell tumors at some length. At this time it was felt that there were both benign and malignant giant-cell tumors. Codman demurred that he had never seen a case of a malignant giant-cell tumor of its own that caused metastasis. He felt that all giant-cell tumors were actually benign and that the malignant variety was probably an osteogenic sarcoma, as most of those actually formed bone. Some of these same arguments are still being made by pathologists today, although giant-cell tumor is <u>almost</u> always believed to be benign.

Codman further discussed Ewing's sarcoma, a malignant round cell sarcoma of bone which usually occurs in the mid-substance, or diaphysis, of the bone. Codman described all of this exactly as we do today. He also noted that these tumors were sensitive to radiation treatment which was not true of the osteogenic sarcomas to any degree. For decades after this paper, until just recently, radiation treatment of Ewing's sarcoma was among the mainstays of treatment for this tumor that usually occurs in adolescence.

The last group of tumors discussed by Codman was myelomas, which he noted were almost always multiple and, in a later article, he stated that he had never seen a solitary tumor from myeloma.[353]

Bone Sarcoma was essentially the first book written in this country that discussed bone tumors exclusively and it remains an important work of the early orthopaedic literature. Although not nearly as well-known as his later book on the shoulder, it was, in every way, as important to the advancement of orthopaedic science. It was perhaps equally important as an example of using the End Result Idea to study a disease in detail.

A few years later, in 1927, another book appeared on bone sarcomas. This book, ***Bone Sarcoma: The Primary Malignant Tumors of Bone and the Giant-Cell Tumor***, written by Anatole Kolodny, M.D., Ph.D. (né 1892), summarized additional information from the Registry of Bone Sarcoma. The dedication read:

> *Respectfully Dedicated*
> *to*
> *the organizer of the registry of*
> *bone sarcoma of the American college of surgeons*
> *and the first registrar*
> ERNEST AMORY CODMAN, M.D.
> *Whose tireless work and*
> *idealism has inspired a generation of students*
> *in their investigation of bone tumors.*[354]

Kolodny's book was only an extension of Codman's work. He added little new information that was not already presented by

---

353Current nomenclature describes myeloma as either multiple myeloma or plasmacytoma, in cases in which it is solitary.

354Kolodny A. *Bone Sarcoma: The Primary Malignant Tumors of Bone and the Giant-Cell Tumor*, Chicago: Surgical Publishing Company of Chicago, 1927. Dedication page.

Codman, but simply summarized the additional cases which the Registry had received in the past two years.

In 1925 Codman and the Massachusetts General Hospital (MGH) reconciled somewhat. The passage of 10 years since the meeting at the Boston Medical Library, and 11 since he had resigned from the MGH, and his pioneering work on a less controversial topic, bone sarcoma, had again made him acceptable to his mother institution. The MGH gave him an office from which he could see patients and conduct his clinical research into bone sarcoma.

In 1926 Codman published his last paper which dealt with the Registry of Bone Sarcoma, summarizing the first five years of the Committee of the American College of Surgeons. At the end of five years, the Registry of Bone Sarcoma had been able to collect only 17 cases of primary malignant bone tumors that had been considered cured, four of Ewing's sarcoma, and 13 of osteogenic sarcoma. He listed the important contributions that had been made by the Registry of Bone Sarcoma as follows:

> **Five years have passed since the first circular letter went out and some of our by-products may be listed as follows:**
>
> 1. **Many contributions to the medical literature on bone tumors.**
>
> 2. **A more or less acceptable standard classification, presented and discussed in the form of a small book. (Reprinted in Bull. Am. Col. of Surg., 10(1A): 1926)**
>
> 3. **The impersonal proof of Dr. Bloodgood's contention that giant cell tumor is benign.**
>
> 4. **The impersonal proof that cases of giant cell tumor may be cured by radiotherapy.**
>
> 5. **The diffusion of Dr. Mallory's contention that benign giant cell tumor is not a neoplasm but a faulty repair phenomenon.**

6. The impersonal proof that many of the cures from combined treatment by surgery, mixed toxins, and radium claimed by Dr. Coley are authentic.

7. The principle of co-operative education (concerning rare diseases) among laboratories (the founding of other Registries).

8. The possession by the American College of Surgeons of collections of data on 100 standard benign giant cell tumors, 100 standard osteogenic sarcomata of the femur, 100 standard osteogenic sarcomata of other bones, 50 standard cases of Ewing's tumor. (These data are neatly packed in trunk-like boxes available for study by investigators or by pathologists or surgeons who see few bone tumor cases but who occasionally must decide questions of life and limb.)[355]

9. A principle suggested for the new Museum of the College (and for other museums) of accumulation of data on accepted standard clinical entities, in available form for intensive research and educational study.

10. The idea that the Museum might become a sort of patent office of new clinical entities. A practical example of this idea by submitting a collection of over 50 cases of Ewing's tumor.

11. The suggestion that the College should devote its energies to the standardization of series of surgical cases,

---

[355]After Codman's death, the Registry of Bone Sarcoma was kept by the American College of Surgeons for a few years but fell into disuse, as surgeons stopped registering their cases. In 1953, the American College of Surgeons donated the collection to the Armed Forces Institute of Pathology (AFIP) in Washington, DC, where the collection still resides to this day. At that time it consisted of the records and specimens of 2,374 cases. The collection became a part of the Registry of Musculo-Skeletal Pathology, but retained its name so as "to preserve the identity of the first such Registry created, and to honor Dr. Codman who first conceived the idea of a Registry and follow-ups as an essential feature of medical investigation." [from Henry RS. *The Armed Forces Institute of Pathology: Its First Century 1862-1962.* (Washington: United States Government Printing Office, 1964), p. 325]

asking from hospitals duplicate records of one series after another. (For instance, a check on the standardization of hospitals might be made in epitome on the manner in which the cases of bone sarcoma are registered since such registration tests not only the apparatus of roentgenologist, pathologist, and surgeon, but the education, cerebration, and practical efficiency of the staff and perhaps even their consciences.)[356]

He continued by listing 25 criteria by which a doctor could make the diagnosis of osteogenic sarcoma. These criteria included both radiologic and pathologic criteria and were separated into five subcategories:

History:
1. Onset with pain without fracture or tumor

2. Duration of months but not weeks or years.

3. Usually occurred in healthy individuals.

4. Onset less than fifty years of age except in cases arising in Paget's disease.

5. Steady enlargement month by month.

Examination:
1. Immobility of the soft tissues overlying the tumor.

2. Occurring primarily in the femur, tibia and other long bones.

3. No local signs of inflammation.

4. Neighboring joints not affected.

356SGO, 42: 381, 1926.

5. Size and shape usually large and not pedunculated.

Radiographic:
1. Central and subperiosteal involvement.

2. Old shaft present and not expanded.

3. Poorly marginated with an invasive character.

4. Both osteolytic and osteoblastic components.

5. No radiographic invasion of the contiguous soft tissues.

Histologic:
1. Numerous mitoses present.

2. Pleomorphism of the cells.

3. Presence of giant cells.

4. Incomplete differentiation of tissues.

5. Presence of tumor vessels.

General:
1. Nature of the pathologic examination.

2. Quality of the clinical date available.

3. Unanimity of varying specialists.

4. Classification by the Registry.

5. The ultimate result.[357]

There is very little in the above, if anything, which is not still true in 1998.

357*Ibid.* p. 384.

Interestingly, Codman also describes a triangular extension of bone which occurs in Ewing's sarcoma.[358] (Figure 13A-B) Today, we would actually expect this triangular expansion to occur far more often in an osteosarcoma, and it now carries the eponym of Codman's Triangle.[359] (Figure 14) The last half of his final article on the Registry of Bone Sarcoma listed the 13 cases of five-year cures of osteogenic sarcoma, giving details of each case.

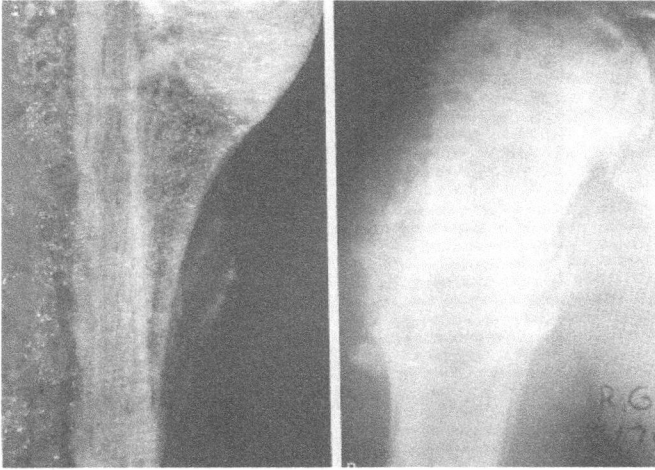

Figure 13A-B—A photograph of a specimen of Codman's Triangle, showing the periosteal elevation on the medial surface of the proximal humerus, with accompanying radiograph. (Courtesy John M. Harrelson, M.D.)

358*Ibid.* pp. 386-287.

359See Appendix I which lists Codman's Eponymic contributions to the medical literature for a fuller description of Codman's Triangle.

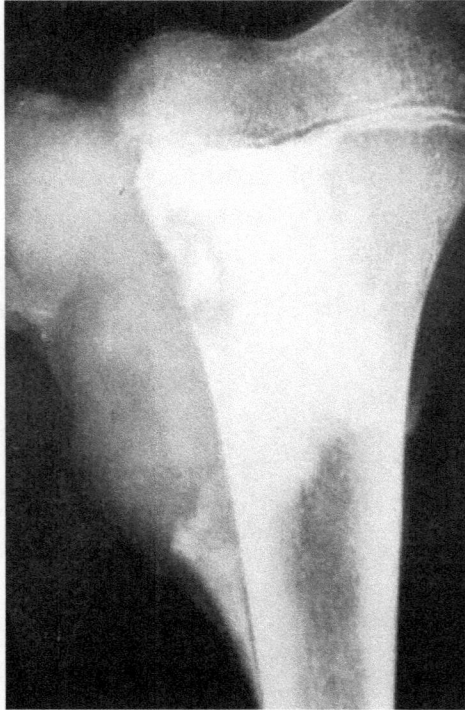

Figure 14—Radiograph of a specimen of osteosarcoma of the proximal tibia, showing the radiographic appearance of Codman's Triangle. (Courtesy John M. Harrelson, M.D.)

Although the 1926 paper was the last that Codman published summarizing the results of the Registry of Bone Sarcoma in detail, it was not his last publication in the medical literature on bone sarcoma and bone tumors. In 1931 he published the paper which would again bring him eponymic fame, "Epiphyseal Chondromatous Giant Cell Tumors of the Upper End of the Humerus."[360] Although he used this unwieldy name to describe the tumors, we now know them as chondroblastomas, though they are often referred to as "Codman's Tumors."[361]

360SGO, 52 (2A): 543-545, 15 February 1931.

361See Appendix I which lists Codman's Eponymic contributions to the medical literature for a fuller description of Codman's Tumor.

Despite the eponym he would eventually earn (See Appendix I), Codman stated in his article that he had never treated a case of this type of tumor himself. The article described nine tumors that he had been able to find from all the cases sent to the Registry which, by 1931, totaled over 1,000. He began the article by giving detailed case summaries of the nine cases. He then described the X-ray characteristics noting that the tumors were often found at the upper end of the humerus but were checked by the epiphyseal line. Currently we know that chondroblastoma is one of the rare tumors of bone which occurs in the epiphyses rather than the metaphyses or diaphyses. Codman described the histologic appearance as "distinguished by the presence of peculiar epitheloid cells which merge into a low grade type of cartilage cell on the one hand and into the cells of the tumor on the other."[362]

Codman ended the article by prophetically discussing the difficulty with the name he had used for these tumors.

> **With regard to the name by which to designate this type of tumor, I have used the adjective epiphyseal because I believe that these tumors are characteristic of the period of life when the epiphyses are uniting and that their peculiar cells arise from the epiphyseal cartilage. I have used the adjective chondromatous as descriptive of their histology. I believe that they are essentially benign giant cell tumors and thus that part of their name is justified. Yet I am not satisfied with such a long cumbersome name. Ewing speaks of them as calcifying giant cell tumors but that does not seem to me descriptive enough. We must find a name which will not tie the tongue but it should associate adolescence with this puzzling type of lesion.**[363]

362*Ibid.*, p. 546.

363*Ibid.*, p. 548.

The nomenclature problem would later be solved by simply describing it as Codman's Tumor (Figure 15).

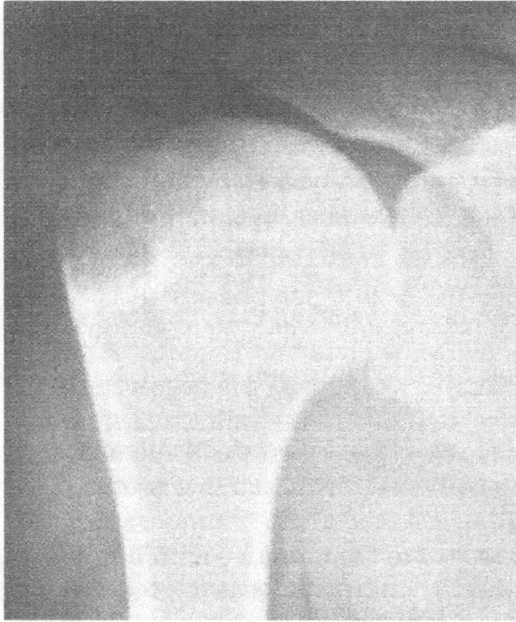

Figure 15—Codman's Tumor—a radiograph of a chondroblastoma of the proximal humerus, showing the lytic lesion on the lateral aspect surrounded by a sclerotic border. (Courtesy Julia R. Crim, M.D.)

Between 1927 and 1934, Codman put aside his work on bone sarcoma, and devoted himself to writing his book on shoulder problems. But he did not abandon bone sarcomas, nor their importance to the End Result Idea, and he returned to them when his shoulder book was finished. In 1934 Codman was asked to chair a symposium on the treatment of bone sarcoma, held at the New York Memorial Hospital, and the *American Journal of Surgery* published the results of that symposium in the January 1935 issue.[364] Papers were given at this symposium by Dr. Henry W[illiam] Meyerding (1884-1969), Dr. Joseph C. Bloodgood, Dr. Bradley L[ancaster] Coley (1892-1961), Dr. William

---

[364]Codman EA. Symposium on the Treatment of Primary Malignant Bone Tumors, *American Journal of Surgery*, 27: 3-6, January 1935.

B[radley] Coley (1862-1936), Dr. James Ewing, Dr. Channing C[hamberlin] Simmons (1877-1953), and Dr. Bowman C[orning] Crowell (1879-1951). Codman wrote the conclusion that appeared in the journal, which summarized his opinions of the various papers presented. As always, Codman was blunt, criticizing when he deemed it necessary, but he could also be laudatory, as he was when describing Simmons' paper, "Should the general surgeon or roentgenologist wish to read one paper which gives a clear, succinct statement of our present-day knowledge of the diagnosis of bone tumors, he will find what he desires in Dr. Simmons' paper."[365]

Several other statements in the papers that were presented are especially prescient and reflect current medical opinion concerning bone tumors. Bloodgood noted that preoperative radiation seemed to help in the treatment of these tumors, and this is now often used as adjunctive preoperative radiotherapy. He further discussed William Coley's conclusions that in cases of Ewing's sarcoma the use of Coley's toxins was definitely recommended. Chemotherapy remains a mainstay of the treatment of Ewing's sarcoma into the 1990s, though not with Coley's toxins, which are no longer used medically. [366]

William Coley also discussed biopsy, "It should be performed only by the surgeon who is to have the subsequent care of the patient, and who is prepared to carry out the best method of treatment as determined by the biopsy."[367] This is exactly what is recommended today by the Musculoskeletal Tumor Society, whose policy is that the treatment of bone sarcoma begins with a biopsy performed by the eventual treating surgeon in all cases, when possible.

Finally, Simmons advanced what Codman described as "the only important new suggestion which was presented at the Conference ..."[368] This was an observation of the increased alkaline phosphatase

---

365*Ibid.*, p. 5

366Coley's toxins was an early form of immunotherapy. In the 1890's, Coley observed 38 cases of malignant tumors which had spontaneously resolved after the patient came down with erysipelas, caused by the bacterium, *Streptococcus erysipelas*. Coley began using the toxins produced from *Strep. erysipelas* in an attempt to induce regression of tumors. To this mix, he later added toxins produced by the bacterium now called *Serratia marcescens*, then called *Bacillus prodigiosus*.

367*Ibid.*

368*Ibid.*, p. 6.

level of the blood in cases of bone sarcoma. Clinically, we now know this to be completely accurate, as in cases of osteosarcoma, and any sarcoma in which bone is formed, the alkaline phosphatase level in the blood can be exceptionally high.

In June 1936 Codman received a letter from Drs. Charles M. Duke and Bowman Crowell of the American College of Surgeons, in which they asked Codman to give a talk at a cancer symposium to be held in Philadelphia in late October. Codman originally suggested speaking on the topic of, "The Open Registry of Bone Sarcoma; Its Aims and Its Progress." However, after several letters had gone back and forth between the doctors, Codman eventually spoke instead on "The Treatment of Giant Cell Tumors Near the Knee Joint."[369] This was probably a disappointment to Codman, as the first topic would have given him more chance to expound again on the Registry of Bone Sarcoma and its use for promoting the End Result Idea.

Codman wrote one final journal article concerning tumors: "Treatment of Giant Cell Tumors About the Knee," which summarized his talk in Philadelphia.[370] In this article he discussed 153 of these cases that had been reported to the Registry of Bone Sarcoma and gave further details of the 91 surviving cases, separating them into those that had amputations (44 cases) and those which had not (47 cases). He further gave his own specific recommendations as to treatment which involved an unusual periosteal flap that he imbricated over the tumor cavity after it had been surgically evacuated. Codman thought that there were five general principles that could be deduced from his study of giant cell tumors about the knee:

General Principles Deduced from This Study
1. **The expansion and progress of these tumors is due to their pulsation, not to the malignant quality of their cells. Therefore, we should pay scrupulous attention to stopping their blood supply.**

369CA 1/1.

370SGO, <u>64 (2A)</u>: 485-486, February 1937.

2. The persistence of a large cavity in the bone is one main reason for the inadequacy of the modes of treatment in vogue. Therefore, we should collapse the bony wall of the cavity and by using a flap of periosteum we may make the defect outside instead of inside the cortex.

3. We should bear in mind Wolff's law: that regeneration of bone tends to occur in lines of stress and absorption tends to take place where there is no stress. Therefore, we should place periosteum where new bone will be formed on the concave side of the defect, from which the tumor has been removed.

4. After operation we should support the limb, not only to prevent fracture, but in a manner that will assure stress in the normal line of weight bearing.

5. We should not jeopardize the normal repair process by the use of chemical or electrical cautery or by radiation.[371]

By this time, near the end of his life, Codman had become the country's foremost expert on bone sarcoma. On 10 July 1939 Dr. Joseph [Seaton] Barr (1901-1964) of the American Academy of Orthopedic Surgeons (AAOS) asked Codman to make a presentation at the AAOS Annual Meeting in Boston in January 1940. He accepted and later gave his presentation with Drs. Channing Simmons and Clifford C[arlton] Franseen (1903-1979), at the Hotel Statler on 24 January 1940. At the meeting, Codman was given a gold medal by the American Academy of Orthopedic Surgery in recognition of his work on bone sarcoma.[372]

Codman's recognition by the American Academy of Orthopaedic Surgery (AAOS) came near the end of his life and was quite ironic. No

---

371*Ibid.*, p. 487.

372The Gold Medal of the AAOS was given to Codman, Simmons, and Franseen titularly for the top presentation at the Annual Meeting. However, it appears, since the presentation was requested, that this was a planned tribute by the Academy to Codman for his years of work on bone sarcoma. Simmons and Franseen were also given gold medals for the presentation, but they must have somewhat "ridden on Codman's coattails." Simmons was a Boston surgeon who followed Codman as a top expert on bone sarcoma. Little is known about Franseen but he did not contribute significantly to the literature on bone sarcoma.

mention was made of the End Result Idea, the great passion of his professional career. It is especially strange that the AAOS made no mention of his work on the shoulder, although the award was given to him more than five years after the publication of his book on that topic, perhaps because the book (see Chapter Twelve) contained so much controversial biographical material. Finally, although Codman spent much of his career studying orthopaedic problems, especially the shoulder and bone sarcoma, he never joined the American Academy of Orthopaedic Surgery. In fact, the only orthopaedic organization to which Codman ever belonged was the Boston Orthopaedic Club, although he is now a posthumous emeritus member of the American Shoulder and Elbow Surgeons.

This belated, somewhat backhanded recognition of Codman's work also merits comparison to the most famous scientist of the 20th century, Albert Einstein. Einstein is best known for his theory of relativity, of which there are two, the special theory and the general theory. He published his paper on the special theory of relativity in 1905 and on the general theory of relativity in 1915. But strange as it may seem to us now, these theories were highly controversial for that time, and some physicists did not believe them to be true at all. Unlike Codman, Einstein did not antagonize his peers, but like Codman's End Result Idea, his ideas on relativity were only accepted and appreciated by the elite physicists of the 1910s. Finally, Einstein also received recognition for his work belatedly, winning the Nobel Prize for Physics only in 1921. And then, as with Codman's AAOS Gold Medal, the Nobel Prize was given not for his greatest work, relativity, but for his work on the photoelectric effect and Brownian motion, topics which he had published in 1905, the same year as his seminal paper on the special theory of relativity. While the photoelectric effect and Brownian motion were two important discoveries, they were dwarfed by Einstein's work on relativity, as Codman's work on bone sarcoma was surpassed by his work on the shoulder and the End Result Idea.[373]

373This information on Einstein can be found in the many biographies of the great scientist. The earliest encyclopaedic one is probably *Einstein: The Life and Times*, by Ronald W. Clark (New York: World Publishing, 1971). A good, more recent one, is *Albert Einstein: A Biography* by Albrecht Fölsing (New York: Penguin Books USA, 1998).

Through 1927, Codman had made three pioneering contributions to medicine: the End Result Idea, the Registry of Bone Sarcoma, and his study of the shoulder. Since 1912, he had published little on the shoulder, first devoting himself to the Codman Hospital and the End Result Idea, and then to his work on bone sarcoma. He turned 58 years old in 1927 and, with the professional rapprochement that had begun around 1915, his medical career was surely slowing down somewhat. It probably seemed time for him to begin summarizing his life's work, yet he was not ready to abandon his attempts to establish the End Result Idea as a way to reform medicine. In 1927, he began work on the book for which he is best remembered today by the orthopaedic community, *The Shoulder*. But the book, while far ahead of its time in its orthopaedic contributions, was more than a simple book about one joint in the human body. It also reviewed the life and professional career of a man who had become a thorn in the side of the medical community, while all the time believing that he was working for the good of that community. The book, in which Codman discussed in full the End Result Idea and his reasons for espousing its use, would push that thorn in only deeper.

CHAPTER 11

THE BOOK ON THE SHOULDER

If one but tell a thing well, it moves on with undying voice, and over the fruitful earth and across the sea goes the bright gleam of noble deeds ever unquenchable.

Pindar, *Isthmian Odes*, IV, line 67 [*ca* 450 B.C.]

In approximately 1928 Ernest Amory Codman sat down to tell the world about his knowledge of *The Shoulder*. It was to be a summary of all that he had learned about this joint during his many years of studying it.

Fully entitled *The Shoulder: Rupture of the Supraspinatus Tendon and Other Lesions In or About the Subacromial Bursa,* the book was originally published in 1934. It was printed by the Thomas Todd Company of Boston at Codman's urging, and was, in fact, essentially a vanity publication, financed by Codman himself. Thomas Todd Company of 14 Beacon Street in Boston had printed Codman's earlier book, *A Study in Hospital Efficiency*. He also used this firm to print the flyers he sent to out to doctors, to publicize both his own hospital and the Registry on Bone Sarcoma. In a letter from Thomas Todd to Codman dated 10 July 1934, the cost of 1,000 copies of the book to Codman was given as $1,981.20.[374] Codman did not pay the Thomas Todd Company until July 1935 at which time he sent them a check for

$500 and noted that he now owed them $1,500. By then, late in his life and not doing well financially, Codman did not have the money to pay for the remainder of the printing of the book and asked the publisher to go to his bank and ask them for the money as a loan, applying it against other loans that he had. The Thomas Todd Company elected not to do this, stating that there was not a pressing demand for the money and they would allow Codman to pay as he could.[375]

Codman advertised the book with a circular announcing the publication as follows:

A Book on Diseases and Injuries of the Shoulder
Rupture of the Supraspinatus Tendon and Other Lesions In and About the Subacromial Bursa

by E.A. Codman, M.D.

In a circular letter, three years ago, to the Fellows of the American College of Surgeons, announcing that this book was to be written and asking for subscriptions, it was stated: "The price of copies of the first edition will be five dollars. The first printing will be limited to 500 more copies than the total number of affirmative answers ..." There were 500 such answers and accordingly 1,000 copies have been printed. These copies will be for sale exclusively to Fellows of the College, and at the above price.

Since the cost of this edition has been $9,376.19[376], without including any estimate for the author's work or that of his assistants, the next printing must command a higher price, namely, $10.00, even for hospitals and libraries.

375*Ibid.*

376As mentioned above, Thomas Todd listed the cost as $1,981.20 for 1,000 copies in a letter to Codman. It is unclear why the numbers are so different although I suspect Codman is quoting the cost for about 5,000 copies.

This limited first edition should suffice to attain some of the main purposes of the book, if each subscriber would help as follows:

1. Read the preface and epilogue attentively, and as much of the shoulder part as may be of interest.

2. Write frankly on the pages provided for this purpose in the Introduction, whatever criticisms you may have of the original statements or suggestions made in the book, especially those on page 21 of the epilogue.

3. Hand the book to some other Fellow of the College and ask him to hand it on to others, until all the members in your vicinity have seen it.

4. Then give it to your hospital library and interest some young surgeon on your staff to study it in connection with all available clinical and autopsy material at your clinic, in case the author's suggestions as to a joint investigation of shoulder injuries is adopted next October.

In this way copies of the book would be distributed to most of the larger hospitals in the United States, and every Fellow of the College would be given an opportunity to form his opinions as to the author's suggestions and to express these opinions to the officers of the organization before the meeting in October, 1934.

If the Regents accepted the suggestions in the epilogue, the following results might be attained:

1. Rupture of the supraspinatus and its symptoms would become known to the members of the staff of each hospital and to a constantly widening circle of the practitioners who use each hospital.

2. Eventually, general practitioners everywhere would know the name of the surgeon in a nearby hospital who would be given intensive study to lesions of the shoulder, and yet was not a "specialist."

3. Patients with sore shoulders, everywhere, might receive more intelligent treatment than they do now.

4. The cost to industry of injured shoulders might be greatly lessened. One neglected case of ruptured supraspinatus may now cost the community over $3,000.00; if each of the 1,000 hospitals to which you give the book, succeeds in preventing the neglect of only one case, industry might be saved over $3,000,000.00.[377]

It is interesting to note that Codman ended the circular with a mention of how treating shoulders better would benefit medical care in general. Although a bit oblique, it was obvious he was still interested in the End Result Idea, and he considered how work on shoulder injuries could help him implement that Idea.

The book begins with a Preface that many people feel is the most valuable part of the book. To many readers it is certainly the most interesting part. Codman, himself, defended it right from the start, noting that, "No one is obliged to read a preface, but in it the author should introduce himself to the reader and give him a glimpse of his own personality, amusements and intellectual processes."[378]

Codman definitely gives the reader a glimpse of his own intellectual processes in his preface. In fact the preface is labeled "An Autobiographic Preface," and it definitely is. Within the preface, on page vi he includes a beautifully done chart of his life. Every year from 1869 to 1933 is labeled, telling exactly what happened during that year in one of fifteen categories: 1) inheritances, 2) environment, 3) opportunities, 4) education, 5) religion, 6) philosophy, 7) marital, 8) nephews/nieces and grand ones, 9) diversions, 10) dogs, 11) travel, 12) ambitions, 13) honors, 14) advertisements[379] and 15) income.[380] The

---

377CA 5/100.

378Preface, p. v.

379By advertisements Codman meant his published literature. Codman attempted to list herein his *curriculum vitæ* in terms of journal articles. However, he missed a number of articles. He lists sixty journal articles and four books which he had published previously to *The Shoulder*. My research has turned up just under one hundred journal articles, two book chapters and the same four books as well as *The Shoulder*.

380The chart was drawn by Charles D. Vaillant.

reader who does not wish to read an entire biography of the man by simply reading the preface and especially studying the chart in detail.

In the pages after the chart Codman described his early discoveries of the subacromial bursa and his first presentations on that subject, followed by his early years in Bowditch's lab at the Massachusetts General Hospital, where he did his pioneering work on X-rays. He discusses his dissatisfaction with the hospital and his own reasons for leaving it on page xv.

> I determined that, as any increased opportunity at the M.G.H. was most unlikely since the tradition of a seniority system was so firmly fixed, I would start a small hospital where I would be my own master and could work out my own ideas. I especially wished to make it an example of the End Result Idea.[381]

Codman then discusses the End Result Idea, his meeting at the Boston Medical Library, and his resignation from the Massachusetts General Hospital, and subsequent request to be appointed Chief of Service, "Naturally, my letter was ignored, and I was not appointed Surgeon-in-Chief. However, it was not too long before the seniority system was dropped, and a portion of their budget became devoted to a Follow-up System."[382] The preface also contains, on page xvi, a reprint of the famous cartoon that was displayed at the Boston Medical Library Meeting. He commented on the cartoon in his book:

> I publish this cartoon now, because, having been condemned by a previous generation on its account, I hope that I may be judged by a future one to whom the subject will appear less serious. It depicts President Lowell standing on the Cambridge Bridge, wondering whether it would be possible for the professors of the Medical School to support themselves on their

---

381Preface, p. xv.

382Preface, p. xxi.

salaries, if they had no opportunity to practice among the rich people of the Back Bay (the residential portion of Boston). The Back Bay is represented as an ostrich with her head in a pile of sand, devouring humbugs and kicking out her golden eggs blindly to the professors, who show more interest in the golden eggs than they do in Medical Science. On the right is the Massachusetts General Hospital with its board of trustees deliberating as to whether, if they really used the End Result System, and let the Back Bay know how many mistakes were made on the hospital patients, she would be willing to give her golden eggs to support the hospital, and would still employ the members of their staff and thus save the expense of salaries. Across the river and over the hill are seen armies of medical students coming to Harvard because they have heard the End Result System will be installed in her affiliated hospitals.[383]

Codman further noted that a few of his contemporaries had credited him with moral courage for his forthright stands to reform medicine. However, he did not feel that this was true, stating that, "Whatever credit I may deserve for my tirade should not be for moral courage, but it seems to me that I deserve some credit for restraining myself as well as I have done having once started on the campaign."[384]

After a brief description of his time at Halifax and serving in the Army, Codman began to discuss his own work with bone sarcoma. In this section, he states explicitly what many have thought, that Codman was using the Registry of Bone Sarcoma as a test of his own End Result Idea:

[I] subtly drifted into the organization of the Registry of Bone Sarcoma, because one of my best patients had a bone tumor. My dream was that this one

---

383Preface, p. xvi

384Preface, pp. xxviii-xxix.

disease could be used as an example of the inadequacy of our present methods, and that some day the results would serve to demonstrate the value of the End Result System in hospital organizations.[385]

And he finally ended his discussion of bone sarcoma with, "My chief interest in all this work was to show, in epitome, an example of the End Result Idea.[386]

Near the end of the Preface, Codman begins to wax somewhat philosophic and these rather incoherent ramblings, probably describe him as well as anything in the book. He mentioned the fact that his ideas had neither reached fruition, nor achieved him fame or riches, but that he felt satisfied as long as he had made contributions that may someday better the world of medicine for his children and his children's children. He also described his own passion for hunting and fishing, and defended this hobby on the grounds that perhaps he had had somewhat less professional success as a surgeon due to his time in the woods, but he did not regret it.[387]

Codman was not yet ready to start the clinical part of his book. He next included what he called an "introduction" in which he invited the reader to give his opinion of it:

This book is confessably 'somewhat unusual' as it was heralded to be, three years ago, in my circular letters to the members of the American College of Surgeons. For example the preface is illustrated, the epilogue offers resolutions, the index is a chart of differential diagnoses, and every chapter in the central portion presents original ideas which may, or may not, be of value. The introduction should be in keeping, and it shall be, for I invite each reader to write his own introduction and provide for him several blank pages on which to do so in ink. If his opinions on the

---

385Preface, p. xxxii

386Preface, p. xxxv

387Preface, pp. xxxviii-xl.

frequency and importance of rupture of the supraspinatus or on professional advertising differ from mine, let him record them now, so that in ten years he may look back and see which of us was right. Let him attack my views as sharply as he likes, but let him not in the intervening years excise and burn the pages bearing his handwriting! I am on record as long as copies of the book exist; let him be fair and commit himself also.[388]

Codman knew that his book, especially the Preface, would be controversial, and he did not shy from this. "After indulging in a luxurious preface and speaking frankly of various taboos mentioned by doctors only in hushed voices—incomes, results, motives, religion, advertisements, dependence on bankers, personal poverty—I must have made plenty of enemies! Let *them* write introductions. An introduction from an enemy who has read the book should be more enlightening than from a friend who only dozed through it."[389]

Codman was still not ready to get into the main subject of the book—the shoulder. Next came several pages of acknowledgments. Here, despite his many diatribes against them, he stated, "In spite of my jibes, I take great pride in having been a product of the Harvard Medical School and of the Massachusetts General Hospital, and in being a member of the American College of Surgeons, which I have seen arise and grow in strength."[390] At the end of these Acknowledgments he thanks a younger surgeon who was promoting some of Codman's ideas about shoulder problems, stating, "A dog may bark up a tree a long time before anyone comes to see what is up in the branches. For twenty years I bayed, though not continuously, about the frequency and importance of rupture of the supraspinatus, and I owe a debt to Dr. Philip L [*sic*] Wilson, the first prominent surgeon to take time enough to study the evidence that there was something at which

---

388Preface, p. xliii

389Preface, p. xliii

390Preface, p. xlix.

to bay."[391] Philip Duncan Wilson (1886-1969) published a paper in 1931 on rotator cuff injuries and gave credit to Codman as his inspiration in that article.[392]

Still he did not begin the medical text, but instead included next a beautiful two-page illustration of a rupture of the supraspinatus tendon. He described in detail the pathology of this lesion, stating near the end, "One can readily imagine the pain which this patient endured during the first few years after his injury form the mere mechanical irritation from the tuberosity striking on the edge of the acromion during efforts at elevation of the arm."[393] This described almost perfectly what is now called "impingement."

And then Codman began his book on the shoulder. It was the first book in orthopedics ever written in English[394] solely about the shoulder, and it is doubtful that his effort has been surpassed to this day. The first chapter is a description of the "anatomy of the human shoulder". Thirty-two pages long, the chapter deals with all aspects of the anatomy, including the bones, ligaments, tendons, muscles and bursae. In this chapter he includes numerous allusions to the anatomy of other animals, using comparative anatomy to its utmost.

As always, Codman was well ahead of his time. In discussing the coracoacromial ligament, he states, "It is wholly a scapular ligament, passing between the two processes from which it takes its name which are parts of one bone. ... Its function appears to be largely to restrain the head of the humerus from gaining a fulcrum on this joint or on the under side of the end of the clavicle. It is more elastic than bone but quite firm. Evidently the coracoacromial ligament has an important duty and should not be thoughtlessly divided at any operation." For

---

391Preface, p. 1

392Wilson PD, Complete rupture of the supraspinatus tendon. *J Am Med Assoc*, 96: 433-438, 1931.

393Preface, p. liii

394It is usually described as the first book ever written on the shoulder, language notwithstanding. However, during the course of my research for this book, I came across a French book entitled *L'Épaule*, or "*The Shoulder*," written by Antoine Basset and Jacques Mialaret. It was also published in 1934, so which book came first is arguable. Both were reveiwed in the *Journal of Bone and Joint Surgery*, Codman's in Volume 16, No. 3 in July 1934, and the Basset/Mialaret book in Volume 17, No. 1 in January 1935. But because of the era and the delay in posting a book from France across the Atlantic, it is likely that they were published almost concurrently.

years, division of the coracoacromial ligament has been advocated by surgeons as a method of treating problems of the rotator cuff. But some recent work in the early 1990s supports Codman's thoughts here, and recommends that the coracoacromial ligament shoulder not be needlessly divided.

The last nine pages of the first chapter are a detailed description of the bursae about the shoulder, especially the subacromial bursa. Codman attributed great importance to these bursae and considered most of the inflammatory problems around the shoulder to be bursitis, and not tendinitis, as was often thought at that time. Today both are considered important sources of pain in the shoulder, but it is not clear that the pathology is inflammatory in nature.

Chapter Two is a 33-page description of the "Normal Motions of The Shoulder Joint," although it is essentially a chapter on the biomechanics of the shoulder. Of the many impressive chapters in the book, this may be the finest. Codman took his study of comparative anatomy, which he started in the first chapter, and extended it herein to comparative biomechanics, discussing the motions of the shoulder in other animals, mostly the horse, and comparing it to the motion of the human shoulder.

He noted the great difficulty with the nomenclature of motion about the shoulder, a problem that still exists to this day. For two full pages he discussed what he termed a curious paradox in which one can prove that the completely elevated arm is either in extreme external rotation or extreme internal rotation, calling it the pivotal paradox. Today, this is known as Codman's Paradox, or occasionally, Codman's Pivotal Paradox (Figure 16).

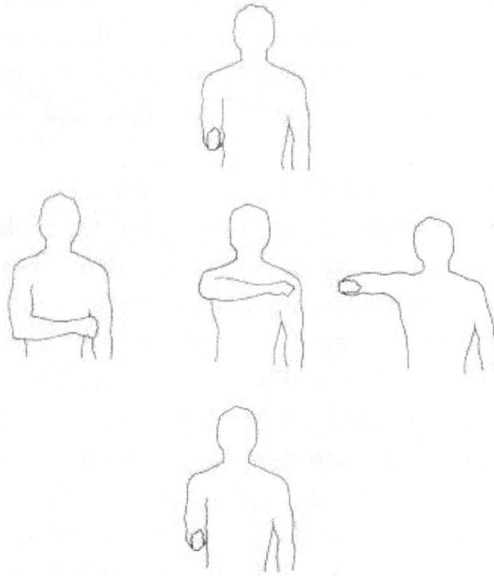

Figure 16—A diagram demonstrating Codman's Paradox, the conundrum
that the overhead elevated arm can be proved to be in either maximal
internal rotation or external rotation. On the top left, the subject internally
rotates his arm. In the two drawings below that, the arm is forward flexed
180° from that position. On the top right, the subject externally rotates his
arm. In the two drawings below that, the arm is abducted 180° from that
position. The two bottom drawings show that the arm reaches the same final
position—Codman's Paradox. (Courtesy Bill Mallon, M.D. Collection)

Some of his observations conveyed information not previously
known about the shoulder, and described here for the first time,
notably, "In other words, complete elevation of the arm from the
anatomic position in a sagittal plane is not possible; in order to arrive
at complete elevation the humerus must rotate on its long axis
externally at the start of this motion or internally at the latter part."[395]

---

[395]Shoulder, p. 45. All future footnote references to "Shoulder" refer to Codman's book *The Shoulder: Rupture of the Supraspinatus Tendon and Other Lesions In or About the Subacromial Bursa.*

Today external rotation is considered important because it is necessary to allow full overhead elevation of the shoulder.

In Chapter Three Codman discussed, "The Pathology of the Subacromial Bursa and of the Supraspinatus Tendon." The information in this chapter was based on his own pathologic studies in which he mentioned that he was certain that he had opened over 500 shoulders, perhaps as many as 1,000. Early in the chapter he listed ten pathologic changes that can occur in the subacromial bursa:

> **A.Changes within Bursa**
> **1. Acromial edge**
> **2. Calcified particles**
> **3. Defects in base**
> **4. Villus**
> **5. Band**
> **6. Inflamed fold**
> **7. Adhesion**
> **8. Fluid**
> **9. Straps**
> **10. A deep red, more or less circular zone.**[396]

He also noted that changes could occur within the substance of the "musculo-tendinous" cuff (rotator cuff) itself. He described five pathologic changes which occurred within the rotator cuff.

> **B. Changes Occurring in the Musculo-Tendinous Cuff Itself**
> **1. Degeneration of fibres**
> **2. Calcified bodies**
> **3. Rupture of fibres**
> **4. Rice bodies**
> **5. Eburnation**[397]

396Shoulder, pp. 68-73.

397Shoulder, pp. 74-90.

Codman devoted 10 pages to discussing calcific tendinitis and the pathology of the calcareous deposits therein. Well into the chapter, he discussed the clinical consequences a ruptured supraspinatus tendon, or a rotator cuff tear. Codman described four possible pathologic types of rotator cuff tears:

> Referring again to Fig. 9, it will be seen that stress on the supraspinatus tendon in the direction of its normal pull may result in four different forms of break in continuity:
>
> a. The tuberosity, facet and all may be pulled away. This may occur without making a communication between the base of the bursa and the joint.
>
> b. Evulsion may occur at the point of insertion and the superficial part of the facet be carried inward by the retracted tendon.
>
> c. True rupture of the tendon leaving a stub on the tuberosity usually occurs at the narrowest place shown in Fig. 6, leaving the broad, semi-cartilaginous fibro-cartilage still attached to the bone as a stub. This amount is barely sufficient to permit a good hold with at stitch.
>
> d. A fourth condition of great clinical importance consists of those cases in which a portion of the tendon is torn to a degree insufficient to tear the base of the bursa itself, so that a film of tissue is left between the joint and the bursa. I allude to these cases as "partial" ruptures or "rim rents." Repair takes place to a certain degree from the thickening of the film of the bursal base.[398]

Referring to the fourth type, Codman believed that, "… this fourth division accounts for many of the industrial shoulder injuries which recover after a few weeks or months, and which I have in the past

---

[398]Shoulder, pp. 87-89

classified as relatively trivial cases of traumatic subacromial bursitis."[399]

He continued with what is probably the most detailed pathologic description of rotator cuff pathology that has yet been published by a single author. He mentioned further changes that occur in the greater tuberosity as follows:

C. Changes in the Greater Tuberosity
1. Excrescences
2. Caverns
3. Eburnation
4. Bursal osteitis
5. Recession
6. Trabecular atrophy[400]

And changes which occur within the glenohumeral joint itself:

D. Changes Within the Joint Itself
1. Changes in biceps tendon
2. Rupture on joint side of tendon
3. Eburnation of sulcus
4. Raised articular edge
5. Adhesions of the extensions of the joint
6. Fluid[401]

Finally, he described the five pathologic processes that he had found when a rotator cuff tear existed and there was communication between the glenohumeral joint and the subacromial bursa:

1. Fibro-synovial edge
2. Erosion of articular cartilage
3. Stub of tendon
4. Recession of tuberosity

399Shoulder, p. 90.

400Shoulder, pp. 91-93.

401Shoulder, pp. 93-94.

5. Fluid in axillary pouch[402]

The chapter ended with multiple histologic slides of the pathology of the subacromial bursa and the rotator cuff.

Chapter Four is entitled, "Arthritis, Periarthritis, and Bursitis of the Shoulder Joint." This chapter discussed what we today call rotator cuff tendinitis in most cases, or possibly the "impingement syndrome." Prior to Codman's era, these cases were usually described as periarthritis, which was basically a wastebasket diagnosis to describe pain about the shoulder when no true arthritis was present. Codman delineated his feelings as to the etiology of the problem herein, "My present view might be expressed as follows: The starting point of most lesions of the shoulder centers in the tendon of the supraspinatus. Thence it involves the bursa and the adjoining tendons of the other short rotators, but the inflammation of the bursa give the most pronounced and often the only painful symptoms."[403]

He then described three types of subacromial bursitis as: Type 1) acute subacromial bursitis, Type 2) chronic adherent subacromial bursitis, and Type 3) chronic non-adherent bursitis. The chronic adherent type would currently be classified as adhesive capsulitis. All three of the types were described in his many earlier articles on the shoulder *circa* 1906 through 1908.

In Chapter Five Codman gave a beautifully complete discussion, almost 60 pages long, of "Rupture of the Supraspinatus Tendon," or rotator cuff tears. Much of the content of this chapter is simply reproduced from his earlier journal articles, in which he described this entity as the fourth type of sub-acromial bursitis. It is an awe-inspiring chapter anticipating much of what we know about the rotator cuff today. Codman knew of, and described, possible treatments for incomplete ruptures, and two relatively unusual shoulder lesions now described as rotator interval lesion and rim rents. The exact treatment of these in the 1990s is still highly controversial, and people who have not read Codman likely think that these problems were not even described until the 1980s.

402Shoulder, p. 95.

403Shoulder, p. 119

Little has changed in our classification of sub-acromial bursitis. Today we talk of three stages of the diseases—Stage 1) inflammation and edema, Stage 2) fibrosis and tendinitis, and Stage 3) bone spurs and rotator cuff tears.[404] We consider as a separate entity adhesive capsulitis, which would correspond to Codman's chronic adherent subacromial bursitis. Stage 1 is equivalent to Codman's Type 1; Stage 2 is equivalent to Codman's Type 3, and Stage 3 is Codman's fourth type, described in the book only as a rotator cuff tear.

In this chapter, Codman reproduced an X-ray of the shoulder with air entering both the joint and the bursa, after the shoulder has been dissected out. This could be considered the first known air arthrogram, or *pneumoarthrogram*, of the shoulder.

Further anticipating work in the 1980s and 1990s, Codman included a chart on page 137 that listed all of his rotator cuff cases and the age of the patient. This produced a bell curve in which one can relate the most common age of occurrence to one of four diagnoses: 1) complete rupture of the rotator cuff, 2) partial rupture of the rotator cuff, 3) calcific tendinitis, and 4) rotator cuff tendinitis. Recently, Dr. Frederick Matsen of Seattle has produced similar work on shoulder pathology, relating the age of the patient and his functional limitations to the most frequent diagnoses. Matsen's work is very helpful to clinicians, and much better organized than was Codman's, but Codman had the idea over 60 years ago.

Codman went into great detail in this chapter about physical examination and how to make the clinical diagnosis of a rotator cuff tear, a discussion which appears for the first time in the orthopaedic literature. He described such things now known to be common with rotator cuff pathology such as pain at night, loss of power upon elevation of the arm, normal X-rays (usually), age over 40, and an abnormal scapulohumeral rhythm. Codman also described a physical finding in which the pain disappears after a certain arc of elevation of the shoulder, a finding presently known as the "painful arc syndrome." He further stated that a faulty scapulohumeral rhythm is a *sine qua non* for the diagnosis.

404Neer CS II. Impingement lesions. *Clin Orthop*, <u>173</u>: 70, 1983.

It is almost shocking how well he understood the shoulder in 1934, and likely earlier.[405] The end of this chapter discussed the fact that rotator cuff tears often occurred in industrial or worker's compensation injuries and caused prolonged disability, usually at extreme costs to society and the patients who were out of work. Codman estimated (using 1934 dollar values), that 100 cases of complete rupture of the rotator cost society $300,000 both in medical costs as well as lost wages to the patients. He stated that "... complete rupture of the supraspinatus tendon is the most common cause of prolonged disability from industrial accidents to the shoulder."[406] Further anticipating the socio-psychological problems attendant on worker's compensation cases, he noted, "The actual physical deterioration from worry is still further aggravated by the doubt that is thrown on their veracity by the physicians employed by the insurer. Usually by the time they are sent to me some months later, their attitude of mind is defensive, and they at once begin to express their disgust with being told that they ought to go to work and think less about the pain."[407]

In Chapter Six, Codman discussed "Calcified Deposits in the Supraspinatus Tendon." It opened with Codman's description of what he believed was the first time an operation was performed on this condition. The operation occurred in 1902 when he and Dr. Harrington incised and drained what they thought was an abscess of the subacromial bursa, only to find sterile calcific deposits. Codman also stated that he thought the usual term in use for this condition, calcified subdeltoid bursitis, was a poor one. He noted that the calcified deposits were rarely in the bursa but were actually in the substance of the tendon of the supraspinatus or of the tendons of the other short rotators.

405I am primarily a shoulder surgeon in my own orthopedic practice. The more I read Codman's work, and especially his book on the shoulder, the more amazed I become by his knowledge of the shoulder. Much of what I learned about the shoulder in the 1980s I assumed to be knowledge which had been discovered only in the 1960s through the 1980s, often primarily through the efforts of Dr. Charles F. Neer of New York. Neer is usually considered the greatest shoulder surgeon of modern times, but this does somewhat of a disservice to Codman. Working 60 to 70 years before Neer, he seemed to be able to explain many of the things that Neer did later. This is not to demean Charles Neer, who expanded on Codman's work and often organized and categorized it better, but simply emphasizes how Codman was so far ahead of his time.

406Shoulder, p. 158

407Shoulder, p. 153.

Based on his own microscopic and pathologic study of rotator cuff tendons, Codman disputed the prevailing dogma that calcified deposits often resorbed, allowing the shoulder to heal on its own. He reported that this resorption must be accompanied by some atrophy of the tendon and he did not feel the complete and normal repair could take place.[408]

In this chapter he gave a brilliant description of normal and abnormal scapulohumeral mechanics:

> ### Loss of Scapulo-humeral Rhythm
>
> Normally when one raises the arm to a position pointing straight toward the ceiling, much of the motion is performed by rotation and elevation of the scapula on the chest wall, while the remainder is performed by the true joint. (See Fig. 25.) The two motions go on pari passu, so that as one watches from behind it is impossible to a say that either motion proceeds faster than the other. In nearly all affections of the joint or bursa, this even distribution of motion is destroyed, because the sensitive point, unwilling to move, sends it reflex telegram to the short rotators to lock the joint in a fixed position and to hold it there by spastic tension. This phenomenon is one of the most important for the student of shoulder conditions to learn, and its behavior in these cases of calcified deposit is very characteristic.[409]

All orthopaedic surgeons who operate on the shoulder will eventually realize that patients with rotator cuff tears, or rotator cuff tendinitis rarely isolate their pain directly to the top of the shoulder but often a few inches further down the upper arm. Codman, as he always seemed to, understood this situation as well: "The location of pain in the region of the lower fibers of the deltoid six inches or so below the real lesion, is a curious but very constant phenomenon in these cases,

---

408Shoulder, p. 185.

409Shoulder, pp. 188-189

in all stages of their course. The complaint of pain in this region is almost diagnostic without other symptoms. I am uncertain whether it is to be explained as reflex pain or directly due to spasm of the lower deltoid fibers."[410]

Within this chapter, Codman described what he called stooping exercises, which he described in some of his papers from the early 1900s. These are often called pendulum exercises, in which the patient leans forward from the waist and lets his arm hang down so that the shoulder is effectively elevated 90° in relation to the torso. From this position the patient may make small pendulum circles of the shoulder and is usually able to do so painlessly, even in the case of very painful shoulders. This exercise is now frequently described as "Codman's Exercises," or "Codman's Pendulum Exercises." (Figure 17)

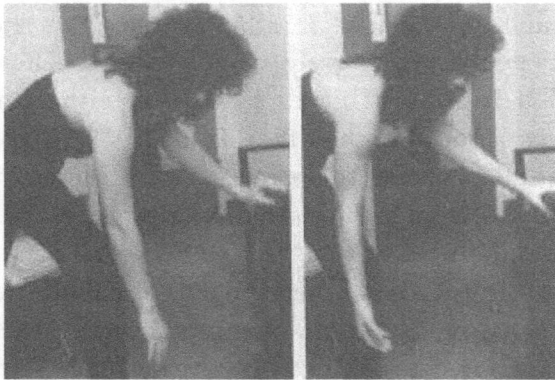

Figure 17—A demonstration of Codman's Exercises, also called Codman's Pendulum Exercises. While leaning forward from the waist, the arm may be elevated to 90° without the influence of gravity opposing the shoulder muscles. (Courtesy Louis U. Bigliani, M.D.)

In each chapter of the book, including this one, Codman usually summarized his own results, again emphasizing the End Result Idea. In his chapter on calcific tendinitis, Codman noted that all the patients who had been operated upon had no further trouble with the shoulder

---

410Shoulder, p. 191

upon which the surgery was performed, but 10 of the 20 later developed similar problems in the opposite shoulder.

Codman discussed "Tendinitis of the Short Rotators" in Chapter Seven. This chapter, however, dealt only with what he termed adherent subacromial bursitis (now called adhesive capsulitis) and he coined the term here "frozen shoulder," the lay term by which it is often known to this day. He noted, however, that he did not feel that this was really a true bursitis but rather a tendinitis, with only secondary involvement of the bursa. He also noted that the most common diagnosis made in these cases, before referral to him, was either periarthritis or neuritis. He described the difference between generalized arthritis and frozen shoulder as follows, "The great clinical differences are that they are not a part of a generalized arthritis and that they run a self-limited course and clear up entirely without leaving the joint deformed or otherwise permanently damaged."[411]

In his earlier articles, Codman described his treatment of adherent subacromial bursitis as manipulation under ether (anesthetic) or even open lysis of adhesions. In the book, however, he differed from his earlier opinions. He now recommended rest in bed with the arm in elevation and felt that this treatment would frequently heal the problem, "I am confident that I can shorten the convalescence of any case by the elevation treatment outlined above, but in most cases I do not advise it, and the mere assurance that they will recover in time seems to be of wonderful therapeutic value."[412]

In the chapter on "Operative Treatment of Shoulder Lesions" (Chapter Eight), Codman discussed two basic operations about the shoulder: 1) the technique for removal of calcific deposits, and 2) the repair of rotator cuff tears. He also gave a long description concerning the use of a large incision known as the sabre-cut incision about the shoulder joint but eventually condemned that incision for routine use.

He began his description of removal of calcific deposits by stating, "I prefer to do this operation under local anesthesia in suitable cases, because it is easier for the patients."[413] His description of the removal

---

411Shoulder, pp. 216-217.

412Shoulder, p. 223.

413Shoulder, p. 226. To my knowledge this is never attempted today by anyone in this country, and I am

of the deposits is that after a nick is made in the tendon, "there emerges a ribbon of whitish material just as one sees as a tube of zinc oxide ointment is squeezed."[414] This is very similar to the now oft-used analogy of "toothpaste being squeezed from its tube."

When it came to the shoulder, there was very little which escaped his study. Consider this description: "In ladies it is well to have the patient try on a low-necked dress and to make the incision at a point where the scar would be concealed by the shoulder strap."[415] In his description of the sabre-cut incision, which he stated he seldom used, he again showed his understanding of the psychology of personal injury or worker's compensation cases, using this as one of the reasons which kept him from using this incision. "A third reason is less technical and more in the domain of human nature. In Industrial Surgery there is not a frank understanding between surgeon and patient as in their ordinary profession relation. The patient is apt to have the element of compensation too strongly in mind, as compared to a coöperative tendency to make the best of the surgeon's attempt to better an injured limb, although both know it may never again be 'as good as new.' The extent of the sabre-cut incision exaggerates in the patient's mind the degree of the injury and the scar would certainly be impressive to a commission or jury."[416]

His description of rotator cuff repair began with him listing the common difficulties that occur during the surgery and discussing each one of them:

Special Points and Special Difficulties

I have found in the old cases on which I have operated, it is seldom easy, often difficult and sometimes impossible to repair the tendon. It seems best to list the difficulties and then to discuss each.

1. Position on table.
2. Mobilizing the tendon.

---

not certain patients would tolerate it very well.

414Shoulder, p. 233.

415Shoulder, p. 235.

416Shoulder, p. 252.

3. The long head of the biceps.
4. Drilling the tuberosity or removing it.
5. Suturing the rent.
6. Formation of a new sulcus.
7. Frictionless surface.
8. Material of suture.
9. Shape of needles.
10. Closure of bursa. Disposal of fluid.
11. Postoperative treatment.[417]

He further discussed what to do if there was insufficient tissue to repair the tendon, mentioning his own method and that of Philip Wilson. Both involved making drill holes in the greater tuberosity, passing either large sutures or fascia lata through the tuberosity over the top of the humeral head, and then sewing the remnant of the rotator cuff to either the fascia lata or the sutures.

Codman's postoperative treatment again showed him to be a surgeon of the '90s and not the '30s. Early motion is a mainstay of current treatment of rotator cuff surgery and Codman espoused the use of this principle himself, "I find that my tendency has been, as the years go by, to allow more motion and to allow it sooner. It is possible to lay down more definite directions, but I may say that by the end of the first week I expect the patient to be able to bend his body at the hips to a right angle, and to let both the injured and well arm fall in a relaxed position at right angles to his body."[418]

Codman described his non-operative treatment for supraspinatus rupture using both his stooping exercises (Codman's Pendulum Exercises) and his abduction splint mentioned in Chapter Four, that fixed the shoulder in elevation to relax the tendon, improve the blood supply, and approximate the torn ends.[419] He ended this chapter with a table listing all 144 cases of his surgical repair of the rotator cuff during his career. It was another example of his use of End Results — he continued to publish his own, even his others did not.

417Shoulder, pp. 238-239

418Shoulder, p. 249.

419Shoulder, p. 253.

Chapter Nine, the next chapter, was somewhat unusual in the context of the book, as it did not deal directly with rotator cuff pathology, but rather discussed dislocations and fractures of the shoulder joint, and was entitled, "The Role of the Supraspinatus in Dislocations and Fractures of the Shoulder Joint." However, he hardly discussed the treatment of shoulder dislocations, but rather described the biomechanics of how they occur, noting that the humeral shaft acts as a lever and the acromion as a fulcrum to force the humeral head out of the glenoid fossa. He also correctly noted that dislocations tend to predominate in a younger age group, and fractures tend to predominate in the older age group, information still considered correct today.

In his discussion of treatment of shoulder dislocations, however, he further anticipated modern orthopaedic attitudes when he stated, "The writer believes that at present there is too great a tendency to confine the arm after reduction. It would seem more logical to let the patient use his arm a little—even to urge him to do so, in order that *débris* and blood clot may work out of the joint capsule into the areolar tissue, where they would be readily absorbed. If the capsule were emptied of the blood clot, it would seem that it would be more likely to have its edges fuse together again without leaving any distortion or undue irregularity. On the other hand, I believe that motion should not be forced for fear of tearing edges which are beginning to unite. For those who think this policy too radical, it would be safer to treat most cases in the sling position than in the abducted one, unless the surgeon were very well versed in the study of the shoulder joint. I think stooping exercises should be begun at once and continued daily in any case. We should use fixation only for comfort, and this means very little, for one may be sure that if there is severe pain after reduction some complication exists."[420] It was another example of Codman advocating the modern principle of early motion after shoulder surgery.

In Chapter Ten, "Fractures in Relation to the Subacromial Bursa," Codman elaborated further on fractures about the shoulder. He

420Shoulder, p. 283

included a figure showing the various types of fractures that can occur about the proximal humerus. He described this in detail.

> **Reference to Fig. 60 shows that the epiphyseal line is retained in adult life as a thin wedge-shaped subdivision, marking off the tuberosities and the anatomic head from the diaphysis. The lines of cleavage of most fractures in this region follow near these old lines of epiphyseal union, and the head of the bone tends to become divided into four main fragments, or various combinations of these four fragments.**

> **The tuberosities break off from the shaft at or near the transverse epiphyseal line, and the two tuberosities are also frequently partially separated by a line of fracture down the biciptial groove, this line representing very nearly their former vertical epiphyseal union. The fragments of the tuberosities usually remain in continuity with the tendinous insertions of the short rotators which are attached to them. The articular head forms the third unit and the shaft the fourth.**[421]

He continued, "Bearing in mind the four fragments which usually occur in the severe fractures, we may form subordinate types according to whether any two or three fragments remain united. Usually the four fragments are only partially separated, and either because held by periosteum and the musculo-tendinous cuff, or because prompt reduction has taken place, lie in mutually normal relations, even if as a group they are not in line with the shaft."[422] (Figure 18)

421Shoulder, p. 314-315

422Shoulder, p. 322.

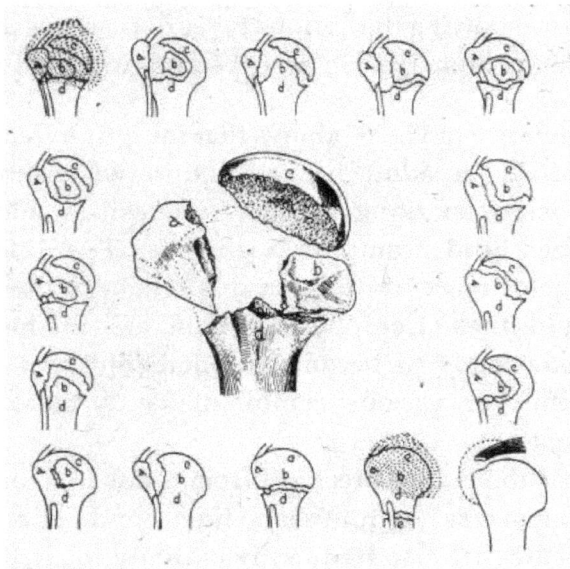

Figure 18—Codman's four-part classification of fractures of the proximal humerus. (from p. 319 of his book *The Shoulder*) (Courtesy Bill Mallon, M.D. Collection)

This was a landmark description. From mid-1950s through the early 1990s the gold standard for classification of fractures about the shoulder has been the Neer four-part classification. Neer's two articles on this problem are considered classics of the orthopaedic literature.[423] They are far more organized and complete than Codman's description in his chapter, but Neer obviously used much of what Codman had to say in terms of the description of the fracture patterns that occurred around the humeral head. Codman described, exactly as did Neer, the four major parts that can occur in any fracture of the proximal humerus and humeral head.

In his classic article on the classification of proximal humerus fractures, Neer quoted Codman early on, "As Codman observed, fractures at the humeral neck separate one, two, or three of the four major segments from the rest: the segments are the head, the lesser

---

423Neer CS. Displaced proximal humeral fractures. Part I: classification and evaluation. *J Bone Joint Surg* 52-A (6): 1077-1089, 1970, and Neer CS. Displaced proximal humeral fractures. Part II: treatment of three-part and four-part displacement. *J Bone Joint Surg, 52-A (6):* 1090-1103, 1970.

tuberosity, the greater tuberosity, and the shaft."[424] And as Neer did later, Codman realized that a fracture of the proximal humerus was a difficult problem, but much less so than a fracture-dislocation:

The really important question is whether there has been escape of the articular head out of the capsule. So long as the articular head remains attached to a tuberosity, it cannot displace permanently, and so long as it remains between the tuberosities and the glenoid we may hope for a good result; but if it has escaped from the capsule there should be no delay in deciding between operation and a stiff shoulder.[425]

Codman was optimistic about the results of proximal humerus fractures, however, when they were not accompanied by a concurrent dislocation. He stated, "There is one very striking thing about fractures of the humerus, and that is that most cases eventually recover pretty good use of their shoulders *in spite of* any kind of treatment. Only those in which the displacement is very great or in which the treatment is neglected very grossly (perhaps by the patient) result in ankylosis."[426]

Chapter Eleven is the only chapter in the book not written by Codman. Entitled "Brachial Plexus Paralysis," it was written by one of his neighbors, Dr. J[ames] H[erbert] Stevens (1871-1932) who had, for a long time, made a hobby of studying the brachial plexus. Stevens had written a manuscript on the brachial plexus, and although he died in 1932, shortly before the publication of the book, Codman copied his manuscript and used it for this chapter, giving full credit to Stevens.

Codman recounted his own description of brachial plexus problems in Chapter Twelve, entitled, "Lesions of the Brachial Plexus Complicated by Rupture of the Supraspinatus Tendon." In this chapter Codman made several cogent points.

424Neer CS. Displaced proximal humeral fractures. Part I: Classification and evaluation. *J Bone Joint Surg*, 52A(6): 1077, September 1970.

425Shoulder, p. 322-323.

426Shoulder, p. 331.

The most important point I have in mind to accent in this chapter is that one should never be misled by the fact that the patient's deltoid is paralyzed, into thinking that the supraspinatus is undamaged. As a matter of fact, the combination of these two injuries is not infrequent, and the supraspinatus injury remains undetected because the deltoid paralysis seems to be accountable for the fact that the patient cannot raise his arm.[427]

It is now known that the most common long-term injury in a dislocation occurring in an older age group is a tear of the rotator cuff, but Codman knew this sixty years ago, "Taking all these considerations into account, I should lay it down as a dictum that if, following such injuries, one finds the deltoid paralyzed and the patient is unable to slowly raise his arm with the supraspinatus alone, the probability of a diagnosis of a ruptured supraspinatus tendon is so likely that exploration of the bursa should be done, unless there is a coincident paralysis of the rhomboids or the clavicular portion of the pectoralis major."[428]

Codman ended most of the chapters in his book with a short bibliography listing the important references on the subject. His chapter on brachial plexus lesions complicated by rotator cuff tears, however, was obviously original material and he finished it with the following statement, under references, "I know of no writings on the subject considered in this chapter."[429]

When reading the title of Chapter Thirteen, one might think it was mostly of historical interest, as several of the terms in it are not often used today in relation to the shoulder: "hysteria, neurasthenia, neurosis, traumatic neuritis, malingering." However, the chapter is remarkably current and, again, one finds that Codman discussed

---

427Shoulder, p. 382.

428Shoulder, p. 384)

429Shoulder, p. 399

worker's compensation cases and their relationship to patients' symptoms and mental status. He described this as follows:

> It would seem to me that a twenty-five per cent allowance for exaggeration might be fairly given to any normal patient when there are Medico-Legal questions involved. Furthermore, it is also true that the longer a patient is laid up as the result of an injury, the more his mental state is involved in relation to the physical side. His mind becomes riveted on the injured part; he notices every little point of soreness, and marks it deeper and deeper on his mentality in order to use it to strengthen his case. He goes to bed thinking of his troubles and thinks of them when he wakes—perhaps he dreams of them. Often in industrial cases, he is insufficiently fed; his general condition deteriorates; he talks to every one who will listen, and described the details of the accident, the character of his suffering, and his feeling that injustice has been done him. From a life in which his whole mind has been filled by his occupation, he is thrown into idleness and has nothing to do but dwell on his misfortunes. Such a man is not abnormal, in my opinion, and cannot be considered hysterical or malingering, until he passes from the twenty-five per cent class into the fifty or seventy-five per cent class. One of the strongest arguments against our Workman's Compensation Laws is, that they so often result in producing this state of mind.[430]

He ended this chapter by again implying that all the work here was original: "I know of no article which relate to hysterical manifestations in lesions of the shoulder."[431]

430Shoulder, pp. 400-401.

431Shoulder, p. 410

It is certainly important when the absolute world's expert on one problem writes the definitive treatise on it. It is even more important, and quite rare, when the two recognized experts write a definitive treatise on two topics concurrently. In Chapter Fourteen of his book, Codman, who was in this case both experts, wrote on "Tumors in the Region of the Subacromial Bursa." Codman was the world's foremost authority on the subacromial bursa and he was also the world's foremost authority on bone tumors, the two topics of this chapter.

In this chapter he gave a useful table listing all the cases from the Registry of Bone Sarcoma that occurred in either the humerus, clavicle or scapula and classified them according to their pathologic diagnosis, such as osteogenic sarcoma, Ewing's sarcoma, multiple myeloma, etc. There were 144 cases involving the humerus, clavicle and scapula of the 1,335 cases that had been submitted to the Registry of Bone Sarcoma by 1934. Codman also included a reprint of his article entitled "Epiphyseal Chondromatous Giant Cell Tumors of the Upper End of the Humerus."[432] In addition, he emphasized what is probably the most important point to be remembered, even today: "The details of this chapter need not be remembered by the average physician if he will only bear in mind his obligation to see that every patient complaining of pain or swelling about the shoulder is promptly referred to a röntgenologist."[433]

The medical chapters of the book end with Chapter Fifteen, "Rare Lesions of the Shoulder." It is an interesting chapter, and reflected Codman's complete devotion to full analysis of problems about the shoulder. However, out of the 1,151 shoulder cases that formed the basis for his book, he covered only 42 of these in this chapter. Many are of mostly historical interest only, such as syphilis, cervical Pott's disease (tuberculosis of the cervical spine), and lead palsy.

Codman ended the medical section of the book with a two-page chart that could help any physician make the diagnosis in problems about the shoulder. The chart is essentially a spreadsheet listing 51 clinical entities or diagnoses along the top, and 36 diagnostic points

---

432SGO, 52 (2A): pp. 543-548, 15 February 1931.

433Shoulder, p. 424.

down the left side. Each of the squares of the spreadsheet, combining rows and columns, contain one of six symbols relating a specific diagnostic point to a degree of importance in making the diagnosis of that clinical entity. The symbols range from positive importance in making the diagnosis to no importance in making the diagnosis.

After 513 pages of discussion of the medical problems of the shoulder, he concluded his life's work on the shoulder. But Codman, as he usually did, still had more to say. He ended the book with an Epilogue of 29 pages in which he pontificated a bit on the shoulder, End Results, and life in general. First, he summarized his own claims as to the importance of the rupture of the supraspinatus as follows:

My Claims in Regard to Complete Rupture of the Supraspinatus Tendon

1. The lesion exists, is not uncommon, causes prolonged disability, has a clear symptom complex, and may be relieved by a minor surgical operation, if it is promptly done.

2. Since it occurs at a time of life when general mental and physical degeneration readily ensues from enforced idleness, most patients never do heavy labor again, even after their compensation ceases. Thus the economic loss is great.

3. In Massachusetts, the cost in compensation for this disability in an individual case is as great as from any major injury. To the man incapacitated it is a major injury. One hundred such neglected cases cost us more than the entire gross income of the average doctor during his lifetime.

4. Since the lesion is important to the employee and to his family, to the physician, to the hospital, to his employer, to the insurer, to the industry, and to the consumer, the above facts should be advertised to all, because the relief of the patients, as well as a great saving, largely depend on its prompt recognition.

5. Hitherto, for twenty-three years the burden of advertising it by the usual professional methods has been assumed chiefly by me, at an expense greater than all my earnings from treating such cases.

6. My advertising has been ineffective, for I have not yet had a patient referred to me immediately after his injury. Moreover, the operation which I recommend is as yet rarely done in any hospital in the world; in fact, the lesion, frequent as it is, is still unknown, much less recognized in many of them.[434]

The epilogue is actually difficult to follow. The thrust of it, however, is that to some degree Codman felt his life to be a failure. He admitted that he had not done well financially despite his efforts to advertise his services as a shoulder surgeon and an expert on bone sarcoma. With text shaped like two pyramids he described his own ambitions in life in 1928, when he started writing the book, and in 1933, when had he finished the book. They were as follows:

Later (1928), when I laid out my plan to use this lesion as an illustration of the End Result Idea, it was at a time of plenty as shown by the chart in the preface. At that time my mind projected my ambitions in somewhat the following order:

1. To hasten better medical service to the public through improved hospital organization.

2. To illustrate to all hospitals some of the advantages of the End Result Idea.

3. To make the life of a doctor count more to himself and to his patients.

4. To enable great medical societies to be of more service.

5. To render our medical journalism more effective.

6. To make our medical education more logical.

434Epilogue, pp. 7-8. All future footnote references to "Epilogue" refer to the Epilogue at the end of Codman's book on the shoulder.

7. To contribute to the advance of medical science.

8. To influence the H.M.S.[435] to seize the E.R.I.[436]

9. To help people with sore shoulders.

10. To obtain more such cases to treat.

11. To lay up money for my heirs.

12. To get some just to spend.

13. To enjoy my life.

14. Ego.

1. Ego.

2. To enjoy my life.

3. To get some just to spend.

4. To lay up money for my heirs.

5. To obtain more such cases.

6. To help people with sore shoulders.

7. To influence the H.M.S. to seize the E.R.I.

8. To contribute to the advance of medical science.

9. To make our medical education more logical.

10. To render our medical journalism more effective.

11. To enable great medical societies to be of more service.

12. To make the life of a doctor count more to himself and his patients.

13. To illustrate to all hospitals some of the advantages of the End Result Idea.

14. To hasten better medical service to the public through improved hospital organization.[437]

It was obvious he had changed his priorities and by 1933, as we will see in the final chapter, money, or his lack of it, was a major priority in his life. He described the financial straits that came to him in his last decade, "Now, 1933, my Ego sees in large letters chiefly the narrow portion; to enjoy life, I need money, and I have none to spend. My fixed

---

435Harvard Medical School.

436End Result Idea.

437Epilogue, pp. 13-14.

expenses so nearly equal my income that my heirs would receive nothing, should I die."[438]

Codman knew that his Preface and Epilogue would anger some people and stated that he expected some doctors to say "Leave out your outrageous egotistical preface, your insulting epilogue and your commonplace cartoon ..."[439] He also expected other doctors to make the following comment concerning the book, "Your own moderate success shows that you can be a humbug, when it is necessary for your personal comfort. Be moderate in your old age. Your friends and relatives will be glad to have you retire, and go fishing, and so will your fellow members, if you will stop writing. The shoulder part of your book is all right; why not leave out this End Result Stuff?" [440]

But Codman would have none of that. He stated that the purpose for writing the book was not necessarily to educate the orthopaedic world about the shoulder, but rather to educate the medical world about the End Result Idea.

> **I designed the balloon to advertise the End Result Idea, and I was planning to pay for the trip as a luxury, provided the whole affair was built on my specifications. I did not submit the manuscript to a publisher, for I felt there was little chance of one accepting it with the "sales value" destroyed by two cartoons, a preface and an epilogue, which ridiculed our most sacred medical institutions.** [441]

In the Epilogue, Codman lamented somewhat that he had not received more recognition and financial gain for his efforts. But at the end of the book, in the last two paragraphs, he asked that Argentina not cry for him:

438Epilgoue, p. 14.

439Epilogue, p. 15

440Epilogue, pp. 15-16.

441Epilogue, p. 16.

However, if my work or my writings succeed in bringing about the establishment of an End Result System of Organization in our hospitals, even a few years earlier than it would otherwise have arrived, I shall have left to the children of my great nieces and nephews, more than a money value, although they will share it with all the other heirs of the world.

Most people desire to leave money to their heirs chiefly to protect them against sickness and injury. If our children's children have health, and are assured of the maximum benefits of medical science when sickness or injury does overtake them, they should enjoy looking out for themselves, and providing better conditions still, for their own third and fourth generations.[442]

And thus it ended. However, in a larger sense, it still goes on today, as no better book on the shoulder has been written, and the book is frequently used as a reference by orthopaedists, especially those with an interest in shoulder surgery. And that statement deals only with the medical portion of the book, omitting entirely the book's importance because of the autobiographical preface and epilogue that both discuss Codman's philosophy and life, including his feelings about the End Result Idea. Carter Rowe described the book's impact thusly: "One has only to read a portion of his book to appreciate the uniqueness of Ernest Amory Codman. The reader will quickly realize that he has been introduced to a man of intellect, courage, conviction, controversy, and irrepressible honesty, in fact, at times too much honesty for his own good."[443]

Plaudits were quick to appear. The following notes appeared in a book review in the *Journal of Bone and Joint Surgery*:

442Epilogue, p. 29.

443Rowe CR. Codman - His Influence on the Development of Surgery of the Shoulder, In: *Shoulder Surgery*, I. Bayley, L. Kessel, eds. Berlin: Springer-Verlag, 1982, p.1.

A notable book, this of Codman's and an important one ... No one else has done as much as he in this field and the data here given must be accepted as authoritative ... This volume is destined to take a place with such works as that of Poland on epiphysis, Poirier and Cuneo on bursae, Dwight on anomalies of bones of the hand and foot, - to become one of the books on special subjects with which one must perforce be familiar in order to qualify for discussion of the subject in hand ... the only real word is that of tribute to an unusual record of research.

The establishment of the Registry of Bone Sarcoma and the long, dogged fight for evaluation of our work in surgery in terms of end-result study are the things for which Codman will be remembered as one of the outstanding personal influences of our time.

Every reformer, to be good, must have a smear of the fanatic about him, must be a bit intolerant, not only of opposition but of what seems to him half-hearted support.

"Leave all and follow me," was ever a hard commandment to follow. As the world goes, it is given to few of us to consecrate ourselves to that uplift in which we none the less believe."[444]

Another book review appeared in *Surgery, Gynecology & Obstetrics*[445] in early 1935. It was also a favorable one, although slightly less laudatory. Four years later, however, an entire book was written as a review of Codman's shoulder book, entitled, *Observations on "The Shoulder": A Book Review*, written by L[eeman] E. Snodgrass (1899-1976) of Philadelphia.

Snodgrass's book review/monograph was highly critical. However, he began it with a foreword in which he noted, "An enemy of Dr.

444Book Review of The Shoulder: Rupture of the Supraspinatus Tendon and Other Lesions in or About the Subacromial Bursa. In: *J Bone Joint Surg*: 16 (3): 745-746, July 1934.

445SGO, 69 (1): 130, January 1935.

Codman, if such there be, may look elsewhere than in these pages for aid, comfort or appeasement. Let no one read into these pages a non-existent, subtle attack on the personality or professional qualifications of a sterling character, whose entire life has been devoted to the improvement of American Surgery.[446]

From there, however, Snodgrass spent 80 pages criticizing Codman's shoulder book. He stated that there were some very good chapters in it, notably those discussing rotator cuff injuries and their treatment. However, he had three main complaints with the book: 1) he felt it was too long, 2) he did not like the Preface nor the Epilogue, and 3) he felt Codman was simply wrong in many of his statements in the anatomy and biomechanics section.[447]

On the contrary, Codman's best friend, Harvey Cushing, loved the book, and state so in two letters to Codman:

> **20 July [no year - probably 1934]**
> **Dear Amory:**
> **That's the best—far and away the best— monograph that has been published in terms of any surgical subject ...[448]**

Cushing then noted it should be called, "Codman's Disease of the Shoulder." In an earlier letter he elaborated further, surmising that the Preface and Epilogue might keep the book from receiving the acclaim it deserved:

> **May 14, 1934**
> **Dear Amory:**
> **... [middle paragraph] The central treatise on the shoulder of course constitutes one of the greatest monographs on any single subject of all times.**

446Snodgrass, LE. *Observations on "The Shoulder": A Book Review.* Philadelphia Westbrook Publishing, 1938, p. 5. I am indebted to Dr. Charles Rockwood of San Antonio for providing me with a copy of this rare book.

447I have not heard similar complaints from any other source and I stand by my earlier comments praising these chapters.

448CA 2/24.

Whether you have probably smothered it by introductory and concluding chapters I can't be sure. You have one who admires you and understands you as well as I do, I found these two accessory chapters to be so interesting that I may enough have entirely skipped the monograph itself, because many people in these days rarely read books through but only look at the beginning and end of them. However, I trust that this won't be what happens to your important monograph ...

With love to Katie and my affectionate regards to yourself, I am sincerely yours,

Harvey Cushing[449]

To a physician, *The Shoulder* is a stunning book, not simply for its comprehensive study of shoulder problems, but for its insight into the career and philosophy of one of the most important surgeons of the 20th century.. In it we have learned about the shoulder to a degree sufficient to make one knowledgeable in the 1990s, we have learned about bone sarcoma, we have learned about the End Result Idea, and, perhaps most importantly, we have learned about Ernest Amory Codman.

449CA 2/24.

CHAPTER 12
WHAT HE LIVED FOR

I went to the woods because I wished to live deliberately, to front only the essential facts of life, and see if I could not learn what it had to teach, and not, when I came to die, discover that I had not lived.

Henry David Thoreau, *Walden: Or Life in the Woods*, [1854]

Who was Ernest Amory Codman? Was he an irascible eccentric who dreamed only of a heroic, idealistic reform of American medicine, and cared nothing about the methods he used to achieve that—insulting and alienating many of his colleagues in the process? Did he begin the End Result Idea only because he saw in it a chance for self-promotion, to overcome the seniority system at the MGH? Or was he the ultimate altruist, attempting his reform only for the betterment of medicine, and demonstrating that altruism when he left his own hospital, his own wife and dogs, and sustained great financial and personal losses in the process, all to care for the victims of a horrible disaster in a nearby province? He was all of the above. His personal life is as complex and as interesting as his professional one had been. To understand what he was like personally, we must understand his hobbies of hunting and fishing, his love of his dogs, his marriage and his wife, Katy, or Katherine Putnam Bowditch Codman, and his philosophy and religion, or lack of both.

With all of his professional achievements, it is hard to fathom how Codman found time to hunt and fish as much as he did. And he loved those days he spent in the woods and on the lakes, noting,

> Since I have practiced surgery, my attention has been riveted on so managing my life that I could get 'days off' during the spring for trout fishing, in the fall for partridge and woodcock, that I have given little thought to morals and have substituted reasonable habits. If you are to know me, I may as well admit that I have averaged at least thirty days a year in hunting and fishing. I have tried these things in thirty-six States of the Union, and England, Scotland and Ireland: and Ontario, New Brunswick, Nova Scotia, Quebec, Cape Breton; Egypt and in Yucatan; and in the case of two New England states [Massachusetts and New Hampshire], in nearly every township ... Perhaps I have sacrificed my success as a distinguished surgeon to these pursuits. I have loved them better than teaching dozing medical students, the pride of amphitheater dexterity, or the hushed dignity of being insulted at the bedsides of important persons. On many a bright October day I have been glad that my talents as a teacher were not in demand. In the spring when I dig up the first worm in my garden, I say with Hambone: 'That old red worm he look up in my face and say, 'whar yo' fishing pole?" Then I get my reward for not being an overworked 'Chief of the Surgical Service.' In summer as I drift about on some out-of-way pond in my portable boat, watching the cotton wool in the clouds, and momentarily expecting a strike from 'a big one,' I am grateful that I am not in demand at the banker's bedside.[450]

450Preface, pp. xxxix-xl.

He was well-suited to a strenuous physical life in the outdoors. Although he had some minor ailments over the years—a duodenal ulcer and problems with his left knee—he was described as tall, almost 6'2" (1.88 m.), and stocky. He was solid, but photographs of him (see the many herein) never suggest that he was overweight. He was fair-skinned, and freckled, with a typical Celtic complexion, topped by light-brown, almost reddish hair, and blue eyes.

Codman occasionally hunted alone but usually did so in the company of friends, often either Bob Barlow, or Richard Cabot. One such person who remembered hunting with him while a young boy was Dr. William C. Quinby, Jr. Quinby accompanied Codman on many hunting trips along with his father, the Dr. William Quinby, Sr. In a recent reprint of Codman's book, *A Study in Hospital Efficiency*, Quinby reflected on grouse hunting with Codman.

> Dr. Codman and his setter, Luke, would pick us up by 7 AM in his aging Franklin sedan with its soft air-cooled engine and squeaky wooden frame. I shared the back seat with Luke and the gun cases. We usually hunted in Massachusetts Saturday mornings, but by afternoon would move into New Hampshire where hunting was possible on Sundays ...
>
> Our host generally managed the whole trip since he seemed to know everything. He had memorized the main roads, side roads, abandoned farms, old apple orchards, corn fields, alder runs, brook watersheds, country paths, stone walls, and the contour of the land. This detailed knowledge made it possible for him to set up a hunting plan for three shooters so designed that if the cover contained a bird, Dr. Codman often could predict which direction it would take when flushed ...
>
> Noontime usually found us eating box lunches in a field near the car. Dr. Codman always carried a large thermos of milk in the game pocket of his hunting coat. Sometimes during the morning or afternoon he

> would call a halt and lie down, manifesting abdominal
> pain.
> Saturday night might be passed at a farmhouse
> where Dr. Codman was welcomed like a long-lost son
> ...[451]

Quinby closed this delightful essay by noting that his father affectionately referred to Codman as "the last of the Puritans."[452] Perhaps it was somewhat a remnant of Codman's Brahmin heritage.

Codman kept a detailed record of his hobby of hunting and fishing in a diary which is still available to us.[453] It is an enlightening summary of his life in the woods, containing 123 pages detailing his hunting activities from 1889 to 1936. For each date there is an entry listing, among other things, with whom and where he hunted, how many shells were used, and how many birds were killed. He often included short summaries of the year and the season and, seemingly applying the End Result System to his hunting, he also often discussed how he could have shot better and how he could improve his hunting technique.

Codman described his first hunting experience, which occurred in 1888 when he shot his first partridge out of a tree in Medford, Massachusetts. The details of many of his trips, even overseas, are in here as well. The first ten years of the diary are more detailed, taking up a full 53 pages. The decade from 1910 to 1920, at which he was busiest professionally, with his own hospital and working on the End Result Idea, was covered only briefly, taking up six pages (106-111). This was probably due to his professional life keeping him too busy to hunt as much as he wished.

Reading the diary in detail is interesting, instructive and tells us a great deal about Amory Codman, and how important hunting and fishing was to him. He apparently loved shooting in both New Hampshire and Vermont, especially New Hampshire, and many of the

---

451SHE, pp. 2-4.

452*Ibid.*, p. 5

453CA 10/188. All of the many references to his hunting and fishing activities which follow can be found in the hunting diary in this location.

entries for the early years describe him hunting around Dublin, Hancock, East Washington, Antrim and Dearing in the Granite State. In the fall of 1892 he described hunting in New Hampshire in Hancock, Dublin, Loudon, Concord, Gilmanton, and Alton Bay. Most of the time he shot grouse, partridge, and woodcock.

In 1893 he described his western trip to North Dakota when he shot mostly ducks and a few birds. He gave details of shooting almost daily between 28 August and 30 September in North Dakota, especially around Dry Lake. On page 23 he summarized his western trip as follows:

Shells Used — 1,404
Days Shot — 25
Birds — 404
Average Shells Used Per Bird — 3.45

Few hunters can provide such a detailed study of the "End Results" of their hunting. His final comment on the North Dakota trip, however, was, "This is not a complete record as some days were left out—for more accurate account with the totals of kinds of ducks, see Bob Barlow's diary."[454]

In 1894 during his third-year in medical school, he took the previously described trip to Europe (see Chapter Two), during which he first became aware of the subacromial bursa, which spurred his own interest in the shoulder. But during that trip, he also found time to hunt in England, Scotland and Ireland, though there are few details in his journal about that. However, he also made a side trip to Egypt and in February 1894 he described seven days of shooting there, during which time he killed 13 ducks, as well as sandpipers, snipes and dove.

For the next few years, Codman hunted mostly in Northern New England and the Maritime Provinces of Canada. He was often accompanied by Bill Bigelow and Bob Barlow. But in an entry for November 1904, Codman mentioned hunting at Ponkapoag, a small neighborhood southwest of Boston on the border between Milton and Canton. This is the first known time that Codman ventured to

---

454CA 10/188.

Ponkapoag, but he must have liked it, for he and Katy eventually bought a retirement home in that small community which, in that era, must have been quite rural—perfect for Codman to get out to the woods and rivers. After 1916, they would live there in the summer and eventually in retirement as well.

His shooting at Ponkapoag was difficult, and he had some personal health problems which he described, "It has been the hardest work to get birds this year that I have ever known. We have had good luck in weather and the knee has been in better condition than ever before. On the whole I have shot better although the average of shells does not say so."[455] Again, he knew his own results—the End Result Idea in action. But it was not to improve for him. On 4 November 1905 he noted, "His worst shooting ever!" At the end of his entries for 1905 he stated, "... shot worse than for years! Elbow cause!!!"

Codman's often inserted a little bit of his own philosophy about hunting into the diary. Sample comments include, "It pays not to try to go for a whole day" and "the second half of a day is better than the first" and "two pairs of socks are better than one" and finally, "sodium bicarbonate is very useful by day and by night." These are more examples of his analytical mind, how he was always searching for ways to do things better.

Codman traveled to Europe in 1909 and briefly described his hunting near both Paris and Belgrade in the diary.[456] His trip to England and Scotland in the summer of 1910, during which he and Edward Martin became fast friends, and talked of establishing the American College of Surgeons, is described in the diary along with several of his hunting forays. He was back in the United States by October 1910, however, hunting in Massachusetts and Vermont from October 15 through the end of November.

In 1911 he made a trip to Minnesota with Katy and must have hunted there, although there are no details in the diary. In fact, presaging the fact that his diary would be less detailed for the next decade, at the end of his entry for 1911, it read, "Kept no record this

455CA 10/188.

456Strangely, although the chart on page vi of his preface lists his travels, no mention of this trip is made in that chart.

year. There are no further entries in the diary from 1912 until 1919. But he resumed keeping the diary in 1920, although he began to put less details of his hunting in it by then and often only summarized his season near the end of a year.

For the entry of 30 November 1923, he wrote, "This year I opened the season with Dr. Bowers at Harrisville with, I think, six birds. Then P. went home and [John] Homans and I joined Katie and Edith [Labus] at Chocorua at Hinshaw's old house. Later Quinby and M. Farley came up for a week each."[457] He also describes a southern trip he made in 1922 and 1923 as follows: "Left Boston with [Traylor] December 12 and A. N. Victor. Mr. Lampa about March 1. Shot quail in Delaware, North Carolina, South Carolina, and Georgia but not many anywhere. Best was in Delaware. At the Jones' in North Carolina, I shot a wild turkey with number H shot while I was shooting with old man Jones. On the Savannah River I did not have a single shot at a duck! After Katie found me in Florida we caught a lot of varied kind of fish, but on the whole had very poor luck according to local standards."[458]

Codman further described this trip in one of the few articles he had published in a non-medical journal.[459] Proving that he was no *prima donna* surgeon, Codman described his lodging, or lack of it, on this trip, "In 1922, I took a vagabond trailer trip to Florida, and J[oseph] L[ee] joined me at St. Augustine … In Florida, we sometimes slept in the trailer and sometimes on the ground … We stopped on the outskirts and, quite unrecognizable from soot and sand, at once rolled up our blankets beside the trailer, only to wake in the early morning and find that we had slept in the gutter beside the road, near the railroad station of a little village." He did note, however, that after Katy joined him, they lived in hotels, "like spendthrifts." [460] Joseph Lee (1862-1937) was one of his frequent fishing companions, and a well-known person in his own right. He was a pioneer in parks and recreations, and was the first President of the National Recreation Association.

457*Ibid.*

458*Ibid.*

459Codman EA. Fishing with J. L. *Recreation*, 31(9): 521-525, 582, December 1937.

460*Ibid.*

In the 1920s, he was older, getting closer to sixty and his health problems, especially with his knee, certainly had to limit him somewhat. However, he continued to hunt and to record his End Results. In 1933 he and Katy went to Ireland for a trip. There is a brief mention of the trip in the diary, but no real description of his hunting there, although one assumes that he did so. On 12 August 1933 he began day-by-day entries detailing shooting around New Hampshire and Massachusetts.

By the mid-1930s, the diary was close to finished. There are several blank pages and on page 140 he included a year-by-year summary of his life's shooting, describing the number of partridges, woodchucks, woodcocks, quail and snipes killed; the number of days shot, the number of shells used, and the average number of shells used per animal killed. But he resumed entries a few pages later, describing his efforts in 1935 and 1936, and then it ends—a summary of the hobby of a lifetime.

Hunting and fishing were obviously very important to Codman, and surely brought him relief from the pressures of his medical career. He commented on this in one his writings in 1911: "I know of no one else who has sense enough to go fishing and shooting as much [as I do]."[461] Strangely, fishing was rarely described in his journals or discussed in any of his writings in the Codman Archives; however, in an article he wrote, he did describe his frequent fishing forays with Joseph Lee.[462] In a well-known obituary of Codman, John Homans, (1877-1954) a fellow Boston surgeon and one of his hunting companions, summarized Codman's hobby as follows,

> **Very early in his boyhood, he took to hunting and fishing, sport which he pursued vigorously all his life, for which he always kept himself prepared, in which enabled him, in fact, to withdraw from, and forget at**

461Harvard College, Class of 1891. *Secretary's Report, No. V.* Cambridge: Privately printed, 1911, p. 48.
462*Ibid.*

intervals his exciting professional life. Few have made better use of an avocation.[463]

In addition to his descriptions of his hunting and fishing, Codman mentioned his dogs many times in his diary. As mentioned earlier, he and Katy had no children.[464] Codman once remarked to one of his hunting companions that his dogs were always, "like himself, a little queer."[465] It should be noted that Katy Codman obviously liked the dogs, too. There are several photographs in the Codman Archives of the Codmans together with their dogs out in the woods or on various hunting forays. Usually the Codmans had only one dog at a time, although for a few years, they had two, notably in 1922-1923 and 1926-1932. (Figure 19)

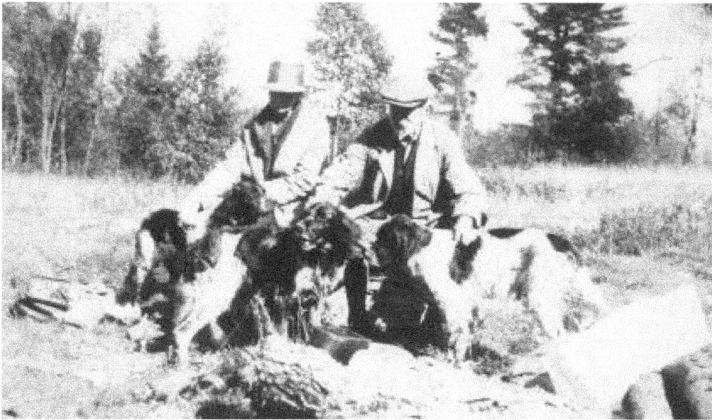

Figure 19—Katherine and Amory Codman with four of their hunting dogs. (Courtesy Francis A. Countway Library of Medicine, Rare Books and Special Collections Department)

463Homans, p. 299.

464It has been hypothesized that Codman sterilized himself with his early work on X-rays, although no real proof of this can be made. It is mentioned in Neuhauser's articles on him, and postulated by Richard Wolfe, former librarian at the Countway Library at Harvard, but there is no way to prove this.

465Homans, p. 299.

It is not known if Codman and Katy ever wanted children. There is no mention of children in the Codman Archives nor in the papers of Katherine Codman.[466] Codman obviously got on well with children, as he had many devoted nephews and nieces with whom he corresponded frequently and whose letters can be found in the Archives.

However, one could make a point that throughout his life, his dogs were his "children." He took them with him as often as he could, as evidenced by a letter from the Chicago Great Western Railroad Company dated 24 September 1913, giving him instructions as to how to bring his dog along with him on the train trip to Rochester, Minnesota.[467]

The dogs are known to have been setters and retrievers, although the exact breed of all of them cannot be determined. In the Preface, Codman listed most of his dogs and their life spans up through 1933, although he omitted several of them who are discussed further in his hunting diary.[468] The importance of dogs in Codman's life is exemplified by the first comment in his diary. It describes Dick, his first dog, noting that he bought him, a Gordon Setter, in November 1889 from Mrs. Outram Barys. Dick was quite a hunter in his own right. In the diary entry for 23 September 1894 he noted that Dick succeeded in getting one woodcock on his own. Sadly, only a few weeks later, Dick ran away and was never found.

In the Preface, Codman then mentioned having a dog named Dan.[469] He bought Dan in 1896 from his friend, Richard J. Cabot, but unfortunately the dog lived only a short time, apparently dying in 1897.[470] Codman's next "child" was Jacco, who was one of his most beloved hunting dogs but, again, only lived for four years with him.

466Katherine Codman's papers are kept in two boxes at the Schlesinger Library at Radcliffe College in Cambridge, Massachusetts.

467CA 6/115.

468Preface, p. vi.

469Preface, p. vi.

470In some cases it cannot be determined exactly if Codman's dogs died or were given away, although it is suspected in every case that, since Codman loved his dogs, he did not give them away.

He bought Jacco in October 1898, but his breed has not been recorded in any of Codman's papers.

Jacco was followed by Peter, who was with Codman from 1902 to 1911, and who is mentioned several times in the diary. He bought Peter from D. E. Russell of Keene, New Hampshire on 15 October 1902. While hunting with Peter on 28 October 1902 in the rain in Cordaville, Massachusetts, he mentioned, "Peter found wounded quail, probably of last week." [471] On 26 November 1902 he commented, "Peter found a bird with both wings broken."[472]

Rosie was the next hunting dog to accompany Codman, described by him several times in the diary. They had her from 1911 to 1913. She was followed by Prince, who was with him for as long as any dog, from 1913 to 1923. But Prince was not the hunting dog he had hoped for, and he had health problems as well. He wrote of Prince, "Prince was sick most of the season. Eczema and paralysis and fluid in the legs."[473]

Two other dogs not mentioned in Codman's chart in the preface, however, were described in the diary for this era. They were co-owned with other people, apparently sharing them as hunting dogs. He noted, "Sport owned with Cox in 1911. Tootsie owned with Bower in 1922 to 1923. Jenny's mother was Patsy, obtained from [Hurst] Springfield, New Hampshire through a friend of brother William." [474] Jenny was the dog that he got in 1922, while they still had Prince, and who was described numerous times in the diary. Jenny who lived until 1932, and Codman noted in his entry of 15 December 1925, "I have been out more than usual this year and am just as keen as ever. Jenny, now 4½, is the best partridge dog I ever had but absolutely the worst woodcock dog." [475] Two years later in an entry for 1927, he again discussed Jenny's ability, "Jenny is perfect on partridges and Luke had second season. He is good on woodchucks." [476]

471CA 10/188.

472*Ibid.*

473*Ibid.*

474*Ibid.*

475*Ibid.*

476*Ibid.*

In 1926, the Codmans added a second dog, the aforementioned Luke, an English Setter. The above is the only mention of Luke in the hunting diary, and it is not known how long he lived. After Jenny died, Amory and Katy Codman obtained a Chesapeake Bay Retriever named Spot, although the date is uncertain—it was likely after 1933, as he is not mentioned in the chart in the Preface. The 9 November 1936 entry commented on Spot, who obviously did not meet up to all of Codman's standards, "Bought Spot this summer for $100. He is good, full for form A-1. Does not back. Chews his bird, and about half retrieves. Nose not very good but showed when he does point few false points." In later entries concerning Spot, he again described his faults, "Spot is only slightly better", then described him further, "Spot improved a great deal but still breaks shot, does not back, seldom trails, and chews his birds. Nose poor but good on quail."[477] It is not known if Spot outlived his owner.

Dogs were obviously of great importance to the life of Amory Codman. One interesting note about this is that there is no record of Codman's family having dogs or pets when he was a child. But in adulthood, without children, they filled a void early in his marriage, they were his hunting and fishing partners later his life, and in his twilight years, they surely brought him companionship. They are mentioned more often in the diary than his wife, Katy, and the Codman Archives contains far more references to his dogs than it does to his wife.

———

Katherine Putnam Bowditch became the wife of Ernest Amory Codman on 16 November 1899 in Boston. She was born in 1871 in Geneseo, New York, and met Amory Codman while he worked in her uncle's laboratory. Katy Codman came from a renowned Massachusetts family and was a remarkable woman in her own right.

Like Codman's ancestors, the Bowditch family was of Puritan English descent. The first known ancestor was William Bowditch, who emigrated from England about 1639, and settled in Salem,

---

477*Ibid.*

Massachusetts. The first well-known descendant in the family was Nathaniel Bowditch (1773-1838), an astronomer and mathematician who also lived in Salem, Massachusetts. He developed the methods employed by sailors to sight the stars, using mathematical tables to find their position.

Nathaniel Bowditch had six sons and two daughters, the most famous of whom was Henry Ingersoll Bowditch (1808-1892), who was a physician and abolitionist who achieved fame in both fields. During the Civil War he assisted runaway slaves and was important in fostering anti-slavery feeling in the North. He became a major supporter of William Lloyd Garrison, who made violent denunciations of slavery. Henry Bowditch also published an important book, *Public Hygiene in America* (1877), which gave a history of preventive medicine and a summary of sanitary law in many parts of the world. He achieved renown as a crusader for the improvement of public health. His efforts to improve the health of the public were of a similar vein to Codman's, although his ideas were much better received.

Henry I. Bowditch's brother, Jonathan Ingersoll Bowditch, fathered two children who also made their mark on the world. One son, Henry Pickering Bowditch (1840-1911), became a well-known physiologist (1840-1911). He received his medical degree from Harvard in 1868 and then traveled to Europe where he studied in the world's top physiology laboratories in France, under Claude Bernard (1813-1878), Louis Antoine Ranvier (1835-1922), and Jean-Martin Charcot (1825-1893), as well as in Germany under Willy Kühne (1837-1900). He returned to Harvard in 1871 where he took up the position as Assistant Professor of Physiology and established the first physiology laboratory in the United States.

It was in this laboratory that Amory Codman eventually worked and made his early discoveries on X-rays from 1895 to 1900. While there, he also met Henry P. Bowditch's niece, Katherine, the daughter of his brother, Charles Pickering Bowditch (1842-1921), who was also an eminent scientist. Charles Bowditch was a very well-known archeologist, who was considered the greatest scholar of Mayan hieroglyphic writing of his era, did pioneering work in the field, and held a commanding position in the field of American archeology. His wife, and Katherine Bowditch's mother, was the former Cornelia Rockwell.

Codman and Katy Bowditch first met in late 1896. After a courtship of approximately two years, they became engaged in November 1898, and their wedding occurred about one year later in Chestnut Hill, Massachusetts, a Boston suburb, with the Minister Charles F. Dole presiding. It was attended by Harvey Cushing, who described it in a letter to his mother:

> **16 November 1899**
> **… Codman was married today and I do not know when I have seen a more simple and beautiful wedding or enjoyed one so much. His bride was a Miss Bowditch who lives up on a high wooded hill (Bowditch Hill yclept) in the centre of Jamaica Plain.**
> **…**

Codman and his wife moved into Codman's small home at 104 Mount Vernon Street in Boston, taking over the house that had originally belonged to his late brother, John. They remained there until 1904 when they bought a home at 227 Beacon Street in Boston, where they lived for the remainder of Amory's life. Katherine also lived there until her death in 1961. They would later buy a farmhouse with some land on Green Street in Ponkapoag, south of Boston, which served them as a summer home and eventually a retirement home for them both.[478]

As the wife of a prominent Boston surgeon, at least during the first two decades of his practice when Codman's career was still on the rise,

---

[478]The house at 227 Beacon Street still exists. It is an attractive Boston five-story "brownstone," built in 1879, although the exterior is of cinder-block material now painted a tan color, set off by deep mahogany-colored front doors with etched glass inserts. When sold in the 1940's, several structural changes were made to the home, including the conversion of a room Codman used for X-rays into a kitchen. A back staircase was also torn down and replaced by an elevator. The single-family home has since been converted into a series of two-floor duplexes. The Codman retirement/vacation home at Green Street in Ponkapoag no longer exists. In a beautiful wooded section on the border of Canton and Milton, Massachusetts, the home and several neighboring ones were torn down in the late 1950's to make room for Route 128, the beltway around Boston (now part of I-95). In a 1936 Canton (MA) Real Estate Valuation, the Codman's holdings were listed as a house on Green Street, then worth $4,650, a barn valued at $500, land of 26½ acres on Green and Royal Street valued at $9,850, and an additional 10 acres of land on E/S Green Street worth $3,600. The total valuation was $18,600.

it would have been easy for Katy Codman to live a very comfortable life, merging into higher Boston society, and accomplishing little of her own. Such was not the case.

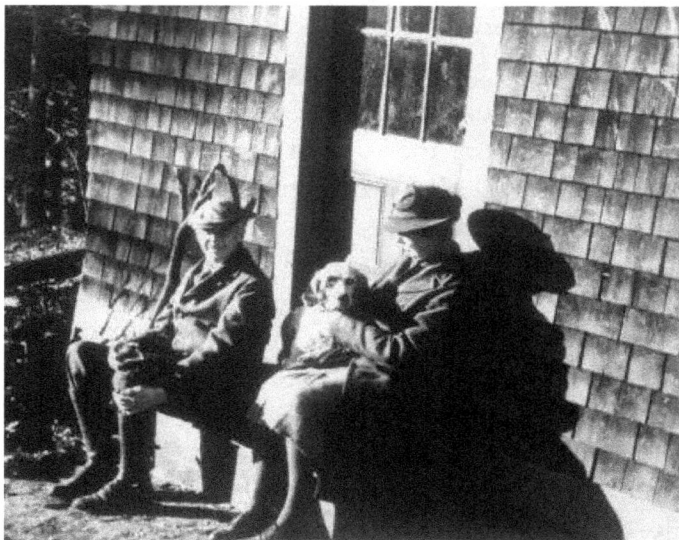

Figure 20—Katherine and Amory Codman, after a day of hunting, in later life. (Courtesy Francis A. Countway Library of Medicine, Rare Books and Special Collections Department)

Katy Codman achieved very little lasting fame during her lifetime but she became prominent in the women's suffrage movement after the turn of the century, and the women with whom she worked, and with whom she promoted this movement, became very famous indeed. She also became an important supporter of nursing education and lent financial assistance to the Simmons School of Public Health Nursing, which opened in 1918 under the leadership of Ann Harvey Strong. A letter from Simmons College to Mrs. Codman documented this, "I beg to acknowledge receipt of your cheque for $4,000 being a gift to Simmons College to pay the salary of Professor (Miss) Strong for two years."[479] Katy eventually became Secretary and President of the

---

479CA 8/157.

Instructive District Nursing Association of Boston.[480] Her only known published journal article discussed that association and its efforts in lending assistance to the victims of a fire near Boston; it was entitled: "District Nursing After the Chelsea Fire."[481]

Katy's two closest friends were Alice Hamilton (1869-1971) and Emily Balch (1867-1961), two of the outstanding women of that era. Less is known about her relationship with Emily Balch, who was a sociologist and a leader of the women's movement for peace during and after World War I. Miss Balch graduated from Bryn Mawr in Pennsylvania and eventually began teaching at Wellesley in 1897. She was a delegate to the 1915 International Congress of Women and help found the Women's International League for Peace and Freedom of which she was Secretary-Treasurer from 1919 to 1922, and again from 1934 to 1935. For her efforts on behalf of the women's movement and the peace movement, in 1946 she became the first American woman to receive the Nobel Peace Prize, which she shared jointly with John Raleigh Mott (1865-1955). Katy Codman apparently became friendly with Emily Balch via the marriage of Katy's sister, Lucy Rockwell Bowditch, to Dr. Franklin Greene Balch. In Katy Codman's will, dated 1935, she gave some of her real estate holdings to Lucy Rockwell Balch and to her niece, Katherine Balch.[482]

Much more is known about the relationship between Katy Codman and Alice Hamilton, thanks to Hamilton's autobiography as well as a biography by Barbara Sicherman.[483] Alice Hamilton (1869-1971) was a prominent woman physician, which was quite rare for the time. She received her medical degree from the University of Michigan in 1893, and later specialized in occupational medicine and the study of

---

480CA 8/157; and Neuhauser article, p. 9.

481Codman KB. District nursing after the Chelsea fire. *Charities and the Commons*, 21: 970-973, 13 February 1909.

482CA 8/180. I have been unable to determine the exact relationship between Lucy Rockwell Balch and Emily Balch. Franklin Balch, the husband of Lucy Rockwell Bowditch, was not Emily Greene Balch's brother, so it is likely they were cousins.

483Sicherman B. *Alice Hamilton: A Life in Letters.* (Harvard University Press, Cambridge, Massachusetts and London, England, 1984).

industrial toxicology. She was also a leader of the women's movement and somewhat of a radical Socialist.

Hull House was one of the first Socialist communes in North America. It was established by Jane Addams (1860-1935) and Ellen Gates Starr (1859-1940) in Chicago in 1899. Alice Hamilton was a major supporter of Hull House and lived there during her early years in practice. She practiced in Chicago from 1897 until 1919 at which time she was appointed Assistant Professor in Industrial Medicine at the School of Public Health at Harvard.

It is not known for certain if Alice Hamilton and Katy Codman knew each other well before Hamilton arrived Boston. However, they must certainly have had some contact via the women's movement because Alice Hamilton moved into the Codman house at 227 Beacon Street upon her arrival in Boston on 21 September 1919. While she was living in Boston, from 1919 to 1935, the Codman house was her residence. In 1933, she also rented an apartment at Codman's old hospital at 15 Pinckney Street, still owned by the Codmans at that time.

Sicherman noted that Hamilton and Katy Codman became friends and political associates and describes Katy "a woman of buoyant spirit and easy grace who became one of Alice Hamilton's closest friends and a co-worker in radical causes, among them birth control and abolition of capital punishment."[484] Hamilton obviously had a deep affection for Katy Codman, as demonstrated by her letter to Katy Codman, dated 27 February 1920:

> **Bryn Mawr College**
> **Friday morning**
> **[February 27, 1920]**
> **Dearest Lady,**
> I hope you will remember to miss me, you know you promised to and I am counting on it. I wish I had it in me to tell you just how grateful I am to you for this winter but I cannot. I think you have the gift of kindness, it seems to come without any effort and without the least trace of fussing. All through these

---

484Sicherman, p. 245.

months I am quite sure you have never failed to do the kindest possible thing, the quite unnecessary thing often, and yet you never made me feel—in spite of my natural suspiciousness—that you were bothering about me a bit. It has been a happy winter because of you. It would have been a nice one and an interesting one anyway, I should have liked Boston and found people new and pleasantly different, but it is you that have made it really happy and given me a warm feeling when I think back on it all, and made me feel I belong in a niche, instead of being just pasted on the outside. I suppose you have done this sort of thing to lots of people before—you betray a practiced hand, but indeed you never did it to one who was more grateful than I am.

Yours always
Alice H.

Katy Codman was frequently of great help to Hamilton, one example of which is given in a letter from Hamilton to another friend, "There was one on the physical examination of children who apply for working papers, and finally a two-day hearing in the biggest room in the State House, on the Child-Labor amendment. Katy stayed through both days of that but I couldn't so I got most of it from her."[485] Another letter from Hamilton, discussing a Socialist commune, also mentioned their mutual friend, Emily Balch, "Finally Elizabeth Balch, Emily's sister, decided to join the colony and is going to fit herself as a cheesemaker at an agricultural school."

Backed by her friends, Katy Codman served as a major influence in the attempts to free the famed Massachusetts anarchists, Sacco and Vanzetti, who were tried and convicted of murder in one of the most renowned crimes in Bay State history.

On 15 April 1920 in South Braintree, Massachusetts, just south of Boston, a paymaster and a security guard were shot to death by two robbers, who escaped in a getaway car. Several weeks later the

---

485Sicherman, p. 282.

investigation turned to two Italian immigrants, who barely spoke English, Nicola Sacco and Bartolomeo Vanzetti. Sacco and Vanzetti were foreigners and anarchists who had fled to Mexico to avoid serving in the U.S. Army during World War I and they both had been armed when arrested. There was little evidence to connect them to the crime in South Braintree, but they were brought to trial in Dedham, Massachusetts on 31 May 1921, in what would became the most famous trial in modern Massachusetts history.

Many well-known people supported their case, including Albert Einstein, Thomas Mann, the poet Edna St. Vincent Millay and, in an article in *The Atlantic Monthly*, Professor Felix Frankfurter, a future Associate Justice of the U.S. Supreme Court, attacked the trial and the judge who oversaw it, Webster Thayer. All to no avail. Sacco and Vanzetti proclaimed their innocence until their death by electrocution on 23 August 1927. Sacco commented, "I am so convinced to be right that if you execute me two times, and if I could be reborn those other two times, I would live again to do what I have already."[486]

Katy Codman and Alice Hamilton were incensed by the convictions of Sacco and Vanzetti, believing, as did many, that they were innocent and had been framed. One of their friends was Elizabeth Glendower Evans, who served as a rallying point for the cause, and did much to publicize the case. It was she who interested Felix Frankfurter in the trial. Katy Codman did more than simply lend a tacit verbal backing, even going so far as to visit the men in prison. She also visited and lent moral support to Sacco's wife, Rose. Katy's efforts were described by Alice Hamilton in a letter,

> **The Frankfurters were there, and Katy Codman and Margaret Shurtleff who has for the last two months taken turns with Katy in visiting the men twice a week and in seeing after Rose Sacco. Katy has been a dear about it and of course the feeling of those three women was not abstract as ours was, but personal, for they have all grown fond of both men.**

486Wallechinsky D. *The People's Almanac Presents The Twentieth Century: The Definitive Compendium of Astonishing Events, Amazing People, and Strange-But-True Facts.* Boston: Little Brown, 1995, p. 116.

> **We were together till the end, some others joining from time to time and bringing news from State House and Defense Committee. They were planning how to secure the bodies—of two men living then—it seemed too ghastly. We had meant to go back on an afternoon train but Katy begged me to stay and keep Mrs. Evans from trying to get into the jail for goodby or even going to the Defense Committee, for she was so wrought up no one knew what might happen after the pleasant excitement of signing checks to bail out the pickets was over.[487]**

There is nothing in the Codman Archives, or Katy Codman's personal papers,[488] which mention any interest Amory Codman had in the trial.

There is little to say about the relationship of Katy and Amory Codman. There are very few mentions in Amory's papers concerning Katy, and in letters to her friends, Katy only discusses Amory in passing. There is no mention of how they interacted in each other's lives. Codman's letters do not mention Katy helping in any way with his professional life. However, there is nothing to suggest that theirs was a troubled marriage in any way. There are no skeletons here. There were no other women in Amory Codman's life, and despite the fact that Katy's good friends had close ties to what was then a radical women's movement, there is nothing in her letters to suggest that Katy's relationship with Balch and Hamilton was anything but platonic. Without children, there are no close relatives who remember either of them, and can tell us anything of their relationship. We know nothing of Katy's or Amory's thoughts about children, and if they would have liked to have had them. Their marriage was not an obvious one of convenience, but there are also no hints of passion in their letters, although perhaps this only reflected the era in which they lived. We would like to know more, but it has not been left to us, and we are only left to speculate.

487Sicherman, p. 306.

488Mrs. Codman's papers are held at the Radcliffe Library in Cambridge, Massachusetts.

Katherine Putnam Bowditch Codman survived her husband by 21 years, dying on 1 March 1961 in their family home at 227 Beacon Street. Her obituary noted at the time of her death that she left 61 nieces and nephews, grand-nieces and grand-nephews, and great-grand-nieces and great-grand-nephews. It described her as a "philanthropist who was an ardent worker for the suffrage of women and for the abolition of capital punishment."

What of the philosophical processes that shaped Ernest Amory Codman? Surely, he was a highly intelligent man given to much introspection and certainly, he had to have a well-defined philosophy, as do most men of such bent. He gives us a great hint of this in the Preface to his *The Shoulder*, which is appropriately labeled, "An Autobiographic Preface."

An Autobiographic Preface

The prefaces in medical books, particularly in those that concern new fields, are often too brief and impersonal. If an author has conscientiously labored to present his material in clear English, properly punctuated and painstakingly illustrated for the benefit of the reader, surely he deserves to be allowed to indulge himself in his preface. Let him try his sense of humor, however heavy it may be, let him ride his hobbies, relate his favorite anecdotes, tell his life history or otherwise endeavor to please himself. Despise these amusements if you must, but do not forget that they are the normal pleasures of the average man, especially if he is over sixty. No one is obliged to read a preface, but in it the author should introduce himself to the reader and give him a glimpse of his own personality, amusements and intellectual processes.[489]

489Preface, p. v.

In this Preface he devotes two sections to describing his philosophy and religion during various times of his life. During his childhood he noted his philosophy as "Unable to agree with the doctrine of the Trinity."[490] From 1889 to 1896, while a Harvard student, his philosophy was summarized as "life is a joke, etc."[491] But he eventually listed his final philosophy as having evolved into something which is more typical of how we view him, "Have discovered that I am not happy unless working most of the time for what I believe is for the general good, preferably for the third and fourth generation." [492]

At the end of the Preface, written near the end of his life, Codman fully summarized his philosophical outlook:

> **Although seeing no clear reasons for belief in, or worship of, a deity, and having no expectation of an after-life, I find little intellectual difficulty in explaining to myself a desire to take what is usually called a moral point of view. I am satisfied with recognition of the fact that a happy and satisfactory life is impossible, unless one has the sense of being of service to others. The normal individual cannot evade this conclusion, for heredity from countless generations has given him a trial instinct to appease.**
>
> **It is so instinctive to wish to be popular with, rather than despised by one's own generation, that great philosophic effort must be made to satisfy this tribal urge in substituting appreciation after death for present wealth or honor. But if the prophet is confident of the value of his service, he may keep his equanimity in spite of the jeers of his contemporaries. Although the End Result Idea may not achieve its entire fulfillment for several generations, I hope to be as content when dying as any soldier on the battlefield, who, although he may have fought for**

490Chart.

491*Ibid.*

492*Ibid.*

quite the wrong side, feels the glow of patriotism, or as many an old financial baron, breathing his last in his fourposter, convinced that he has left his children protected from a wicked world. Honors, except those I have thrust on myself, are conspicuously absent on my chart, but I am able to enjoy the hypothesis that I may receive some from a more receptive generation.[493]

Codman also described his own philosophy many times in letters which are contained in the Codman Archives. He was not bashful about expressing his own feelings, as we have seen earlier numerous times. He discussed much of the essence of his philosophy in his thoughts about World War I. In the Codman Archives there is a seven-page typewritten manuscript, dated 12 April 1917, in which he discussed the war in Europe, and in which he stated, "I believe that truth is superior to patriotism and even friendship. I want no country which denies me the right to express what I believe to be the truth, and I want no friends who deny me the same privilege. I freely acknowledge that I am often mistaken in my efforts to find what is true, but I also insist that my friends may be. There is a distinction between action and discussion."[494]

Codman was against the war, but apparently not completely opposed to it as evidenced by a letter he sent from Paris to Richard Cabot on 26 December 1918.

Your work and interest to date do not seem to me a whit less important than mine over here. You're trying to maintain an advanced civilization. The American army is trying to defend that same civilization. Nothing gives me more satisfaction over here than to remember that you and your wife and my wife and other good citizens are punching away at the enemies

---

493Preface, pp. xxxvii-xxxviii

494CA 10/199.

of civilization, disease and bad doctoring, ignorance
and thoughtlessness at home[495]

In another letter to Cabot he again described his religion and his
philosophy, "I am an agnostic and I have no moral standards beyond
my habits and tastes than your professor of ethics at a great university
so it is a little absurd for me to tell you that malicious gossip of that
kind is wrong."[496]

Though he maintained that he did not believe in a deity, Codman
was raised an Episcopalian, and as noted in Chapter One, his
grandfather was a well-known Unitarian minister. As he grew and
became more educated, however, he became less religious. There is a
chart in the Preface in which he described his religion from 1891 to 1898
as "that of a Harvard student of the period," while his final religion in
that chart is listed as "believe that if we worked for the general good,
for one day in seven, we should need no religion."[497]

Another source of Codman's philosophizing are the reports of the
Class of 1891 from Harvard College. All Harvard College classes have
typically produced a class report, yearly for ten years after graduation,
and then every five years. The reports describe what the graduates of
the class were doing at that time and allow them to write a short
summary of their lives, in which many of the students have used the
opportunity to divulge a bit about themselves. In the 1899 report,
Codman mentioned, "Since then have practiced medicine at 104 Mount
Vernon Street, Boston. Am perfectly content to continue."

In the Twenty-Year Report of 1911, he described himself thusly,

**Since the last class report there has been no change
in my ways of life. I have continued to try to be a better
surgeon than I am known to be. The public has not yet
discovered me so I feel that my lifelong endeavor has
been a success. There are many men in the class of '91**

495CA 1/7.

496CA 1/7, letter of 6 June 1929, Codman to Cabot.

497Preface, p. vi.

who make more money but there are very few who really enjoy their work as much as I do, and I know of no one else who has sense enough to go fishing and shooting as much.

As to the request of the secretary for 'books you have written', etc., these must remain in the medical limbo where they belong. My medical papers may be appreciated by a future generation but I cannot give them away to this. The only position of 'small Honor and Trust' which I hold is that of 'Assistant Visiting Surgeon to the Massachusetts General Hospital.' This is sometimes considered a position of Honor and Trust, but in reality it is a peculiar form of licensed graft which the reforming public has not yet awakened to. I can at least say that working from the inside out I hope to get ahead of the reforming public."[498]

His final comment above predated his Boston Medical Library Meeting by four years but, obviously, anticipated it. He considered his position at the Mass General as "licensed graft," as he knew he was but the recipient of the ostrich's Golden Eggs. Her earlier comments about "the public has not yet discovered me ..." obviously have some reference to his lack of recognition for his End Result Idea.

The next report, issued in 1916 as the Silver Report (25 years) of the class, further described his problems with the Massachusetts General Hospital and the End Result Idea, and also included more of his philosophy concerning the war.

I have continued to have as my main interest in life the Massachusetts General Hospital and, as explained in a previous report, I have tried to eradicate certain abuses which have existed at that institution for a number of years. Thus far I have had partial success, even though I have resigned as a member of the staff

---

498Harvard College, Class of 1891. *Secretary's Report, No. V.* Cambridge: Privately printed, 1911, p. 48.

>in order to bring to the attention of the Trustees one of
>the most evident reasons for the fact that the
>institution has been eclipsed by the Mayo Clinic at
>Rochester, Minnesota.
>
>I have pro-German sympathies and am therefore at
>present not popular in this community, but believe
>that after a time the American public will come out of
>its present hysterical trance.[499]

It was a time, 1916, during which Codman was not popular with many people, for far more reasons than simple pro-German sympathies.

What was Codman like personally? Obviously he irritated a great number of people. But the personal comments from those who knew him seemed to support that he could be a great friend to his close acquaintances, and was well liked by those around him. In his obituary in the *New England Journal of Medicine*, John Homans noted, "If Codman seemed at times to violate good taste or even ethics, he did so with the idea of attacking sham and smugness, the horrors of his life. He never said hard things of those who disagreed with him, only of those whose motives he felt to be unworthy and even then, he never attacked individuals."[500]

One of Codman's students was Dr. Carter [Redd] Rowe (né 1906), who later become one of the foremost shoulder surgeons of his generation. In a lecture he gave at the first International Conference on Surgery of the Shoulder, he described his encounters with Codman as follows:

>I had seen Dr. Codman from afar as a student. I
>first met him when I was an orthopaedic resident at
>the MGH in 1937. He had been called in to see a

499Harvard College, Class of 1891. *Twenty-Fifth Anniversary Report: 1891-1916*. Norwood, MA: Plimpton Press, 1916, pp. 67-68.

500Homans, p. 296.

patient in the Phillips House with a tumor of the shoulder. It was my lot to present this patient to Dr. Codman. I remember him as a quiet, gentle person, with steady, penetrating eyes. One quickly sensed integrity, intelligence, and self-confidence. His faithful English Setter accompanied him, settling down quietly in the corner of the patient's room while Dr. Codman interviewed and examined the patient. He reassured the patient and said my observations were very helpful, thus revealing his subtle humor.

Dr. Henry Marble, one of our early hand surgeons at the MGH and an associate of Dr. Codman's, told me the story of his summons one day to Dr. Codman's office because "Dr. Codman has a bone to pick with you." With trepidation, he arrived at Codman's office, wondering what he had done, or had not done. Within a few minutes, Dr. Codman's secretary accompanied him into Dr. Codman's office where a table had been set with two beautifully cooked partridges awaiting him. Dr. Codman said, "Henry, I thought you would enjoy picking a few bones with me." Henry would tell this with delight and never-failing amusement.

Every orthopaedic student and practicing orthopaedic surgeon should browse through Codman's classic book, The Shoulder. One will be impressed with the depth and accuracy of his evaluation of the shoulder and of its mechanical function. His long and discouraging effort to persuade his surgical colleagues and the MGH to accept his "End Result Idea" is also presented, often with a touch of humor. Of particular note are the preface and the epilogue of his book, which contain interesting aspects of this philosophy, including his recollections of grouse hunting in his study of hospital efficiency. He loved hunting and fishing and suggested that everyone should spend a selected period of time at

**intervals, relaxing and enjoying one's hobbies. There
is a hint of Mark Twain in Codman. His subtle humor
and nimble mind are impressive.**[501]

Codman was described as lovable by Quinby who went shooting
with him often as a young man. And during those hunting trips,
Quinby noted the affection that many people held for Codman,
commenting, "It was remarkable how these native people of humble
origin clearly loved this man." He summed up his feelings about
Codman during his description of the typical way that they returned
from various hunting trips, "As his Franklin wheezed down the drive,
I knew that I had had the time of my life with one of the finest men I
ever met. I had not heard him say an unkind word about any person. I
warmly welcomed such trips that were all too rare and believe there
are very few still alive who were privileged to have hunted with this
man."[502] (Figure 21)

501Rowe CR. *Lest We Forget.* (Dublin, NH: William L. Bauhan Publisher, 1996)

502Quinby, p. 4.

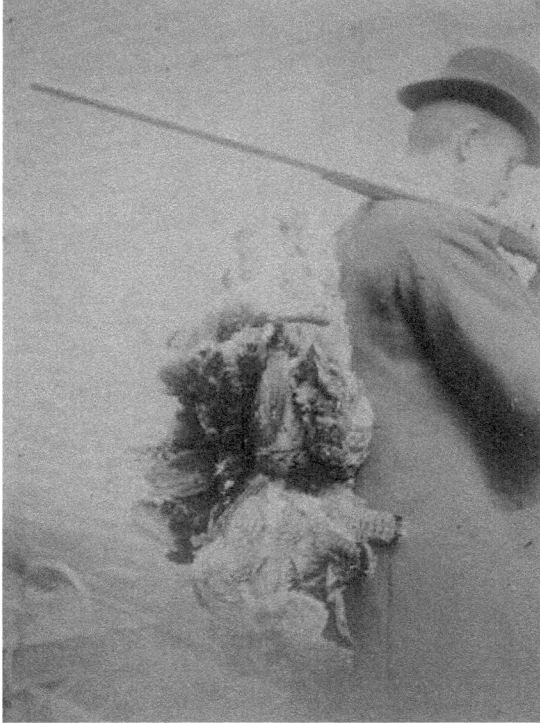

Figure 21—Codman, returning with the day's catch—a common occurrence. (Courtesy Francis A. Countway Library of Medicine, Rare Books and Special Collections Department)

Thus, though he may have been difficult professionally, personally Codman was apparently well liked by those who knew him well. The final word on his true personality must be left to Homans, "It was impossible to resist his fundamental goodness and charm."[503]

503Homans, p. 299.

CHAPTER 13
FINAL YEARS AND RETROSPECTIVE

For the whole world is the sepulchre of famous men; and their story is not graven only on stone over their native earth, but lives on far away, without visible symbol, woven into the stuff of other men's lives.

Pericles, *Funeral Oration to the Athenian Dead*, quoted by Thucydides in *The History of the Peloponnesian War*, book II, section 43.

Codman finished his book on the shoulder in 1934, at the age of 64, publishing the summary of his life's work on shoulder injuries. It is the work for which he has been best remembered by the medical world, although he would certainly have preferred that he be remembered for his work on the End Result Idea, and it is likely that future generations will judge him for that contribution.

In his last decade, Codman settled into the role of elder statesman at the Massachusetts General Hospital. By the early 1920's, he had reconciled somewhat with his old hospital and training ground, and in 1925, Mass General gave him an office from which he could conduct his Registry of Bone Sarcoma studies. In 1929 he was appointed to the Consulting Staff of the Massachusetts General Hospital, a position he held until his death.[504] We would like to know more, but details of his reconciliation with the MGH are not given to us in the Codman Archives.

---

[504]Moore FD. Surgical biology and applied sociology: Cannon and Codman fifty years later. *Harvard Med Alumni Bull*, Jan/Feb 1975, p. 17.

He continued to see occasional patients on a consultation basis, mostly shoulder problems or patients with bone sarcoma. He continued to run the Registry of Bone Sarcoma and consult, without charge, on any case of a bone tumor sent to him. He also spoke occasionally, and even after the publication of his last book, continued to contribute a few papers to medical journals. Most of these were talks or papers befitting that of an elder statesman, usually requested review papers summarizing his life's work.

In May 1934 he chaired a symposium entitled "The Treatment of Primary Malignant Bone Tumors," at the Memorial Hospital in New York, in which he discussed papers given by several other experts on the topic. A paper summarizing the symposium was published in January 1935 in the *American Journal of Surgery*. Codman later spoke at a cancer symposium in Philadelphia on 23 October 1936 in which he gave a talk entitled "The Treatment of Giant Cell Tumors Near the Knee Joint." The publication of this talk became his last paper on bone sarcoma that was published in February 1937 under the title "Treatment of Giant Cell Tumors About the Knee, A Study of 153 Cases Collected by the Registry of Bone Sarcoma of the American College of Surgeons."[505] He followed this later in the year with a historical review of rotator cuff tears which was published in the *Journal of Bone and Joint Surgery*, "Rupture of the Supraspinatus—1834 to 1934."[506] His final published paper appeared in the *American Journal of Surgery* in December 1938 and was entitled, "Rupture of the Supraspinatus."[507] These last two papers reviewed his studies on the shoulder and were essentially short synopses of material that he had published in *The Shoulder*.

Codman's personal life also saw a change in the 1920s. He and Katy had lived in Boston all their married life, since 1904 at 227 Beacon Street. However in 1911 the Codmans had purchased their retirement home on Green Street in Ponkapoag, southwest of Boston. From 1915 to 1935 it served mostly as a vacation home, but during the '20s Amory

---

505SGO, 64 (2A): 495-496, February 1937.

506*J Bone Joint Surg*, 19(3): 643-652, 1937. This is the only paper that Codman ever had published in the *Journal of Bone and Joint Surgery*, now regarded as the leading journal of orthopedics.

507*Amer J Surg*, 42: 603-626, December 1938.

Codman began to spend more time there. In his last few years he spent most of his time at Ponkapoag, only venturing back to Boston for special consultations or work at Mass General. Katy remained mostly at 227 Beacon Street. (Figures 22-23) As described earlier, it is uncertain how close the marriage was.

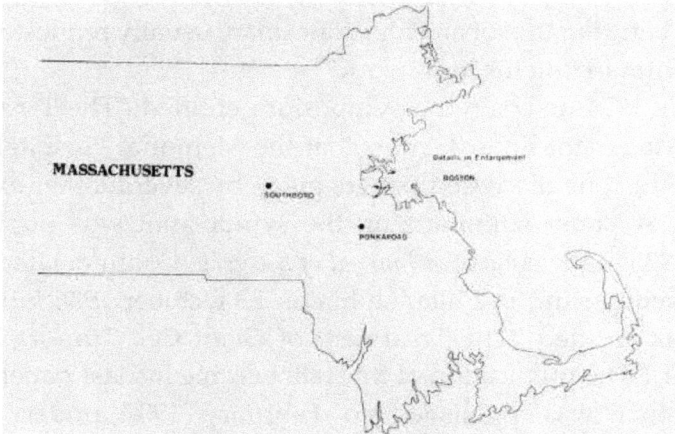

Figure 22—Map of Massachusetts showing the landmark sites in Codman's life: Boston—where he was born and spent most of his life and career; Southborough—where he attended grade school and high school; and Ponkapoag—where he had a retirement home and eventually died.
(Courtesy Bill Mallon, M.D. Collection)

Codman also spent his last decade hunting and fishing, as described earlier in more detail. He even played golf occasionally, having taken up that sport after his return from World War I. He was a member of the Hoosick-Whisick Club in Canton, Massachusetts, a nine-hole course near Ponkapoag. Amory Codman was also a member of the Somerset Club and Union Club, both elite clubs frequented by many Boston Brahmins. But he could not enjoy that privilege much near the end, as Codman withdrew both memberships in 1933, possibly due to financial problems that would haunt much of his last decade.

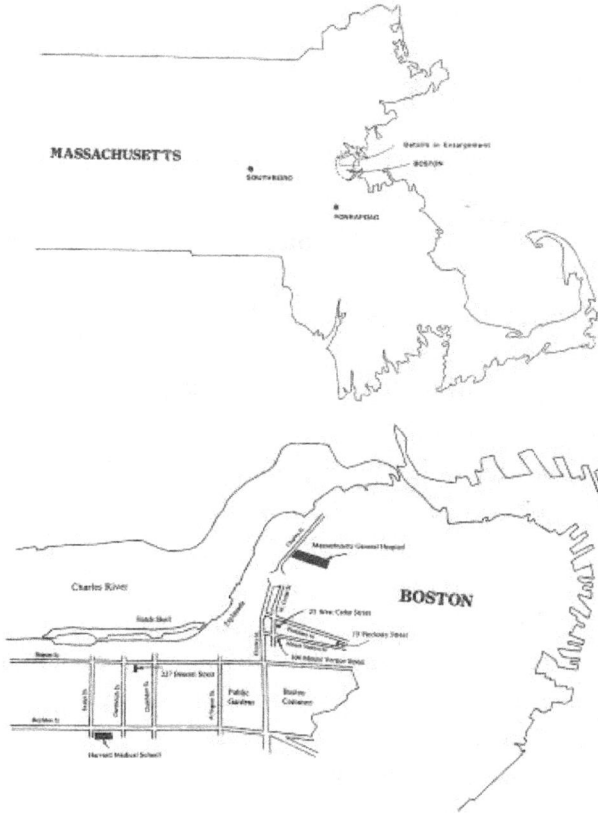

Figure 23—Enlargement of Boston from the map in Figure 16, showing further landmark sites in Codman's life: 23 West Cedar Street—his parent's home, where he was born; 104 Mount Vernon Street—where he lived during medical school (at his brother John's home) and where he and Katherine lived during the early years of their marriage after John's death; Harvard Medical School—where he attended medical school; Massachusetts General Hospital—where he spent the first 19 years of his surgical practice; 15 Pinckney Street—the location of the Codman Hospital; and 227 Beacon Street—where he and Katherine Codman lived from 1905 until their respective deaths in 1940 (Amory) and 1961 (Katherine). (Courtesy Bill Mallon, M.D. Collection)

Codman and Harvey Cushing continued their friendship they had begun almost 45 years previously. By the 1930s, Cushing was at Yale, but still they corresponded frequently.

> **8 December 1937**
> **Dear Amory:**
> I haven't heard from you for an age and don't even know whether you are still living at 227 Beacon Street or not; but I do know that you are alive and flourishing for I have just this minute read during my lunch your altogether delightful article on "Fishing with J. L." Such a picture of the man it gives! How it would make him chuckle! It is the most perfect sort of obituary tribute that one could possibly imagine.
> Why don't you and Katie motor down here sometime when Spring comes and Connecticut shows what she can do with the dogwood and other things? There are trout streams around here also that might interest you; but you will have to dig your own worms unless Kate chooses to do so, which I am sure she gladly would. I think the last and perhaps only time we went fishing together was off the Mayo boat on the Mississippi—altogether too many years ago.
> With love to you both, I am always affectionately yours,
> **Harvey Cushing**[508]

The so-called golden years were difficult for Amory Codman. He was not in good health and suffered with his final illness, malignant melanoma, for three or four years before succumbing. Even before this, the financial difficulties that beset him much of his life were becoming more and more acute. In his collected papers he wrote of them many times. By the last decade of his life, he and Katy were living mostly off of her inherited money, which, because this was during the peak of the depression, had greatly depreciated in value.

508CA 2/24.

In 1933 Codman's bankers wrote him, asking him to start paying off the loans on his various properties, noting that few payments had been made in the last few years. He wrote them back on 4 June 1934, as follows:

> **Katie has enough income to support us both in quiet comfort if I retire and give up 227 [Beacon St.] to the bank. I have furnished most of her support for all these years and she might be happy to have me as a chauffeur and general helper than as a senile practitioner who is an expense. I would not feel so very badly about asking for money to buy fish hooks and cigarettes now and then, but I already do feel very badly about helping my relatives out. My brother is 73 and has lost every cent and has recently been sick, and is not yet strong. My sister is 74 and unable to plan her own life. Her income is only $100 a month. As you know, John and Constance never know whether they can pay the next month's bills. Rosamonde and Ruth have other prospects. Billy is not on my mind.**[509]

He received a letter from the Franklin Savings Bank in which they insisted that he pay down the mortgage on 227 Beacon Street and Codman replied, "My wife has a small, diminishing income, but it is sufficient to pay the mortgage on 227 Beacon Street, and the taxes. I should advise you to let well enough alone, so long as she sees fit to live in the city. If you foreclosed on this mortgage you would only bring on the foreclosure of my other properties and I doubt you would be doing best for your stockholders if you undertook to take over this property."[510] Several letters went back and forth between Codman and the Franklin Savings Bank concerning the mortgage on 227 Beacon Street as well as letters to the First National Bank of Boston in which he attempted to get a mortgage rate reduction from both banks to enable

---

509CA 8/178.

510CA 8/176.

him to maintain the properties.[511] They were eventually able to keep their house at 227 Beacon Street. (Figure 24A-B)

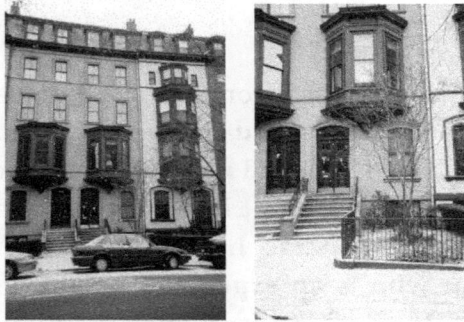

Figure 24A-B—Codman's home at 227 Beacon Street, a typical Back Bay Boston brownstone. It is entered by the right-hand door of the two adjacent doors and occupies five stories. (Courtesy Marcia Scott, M.D.)

In 1934 Codman wrote a distant relative of his, Walter Briggs, and commented further on his financial difficulties.

> Walter, you have so many troubles of your own that I hesitate to write you about mine. However, you may be willing to help me out, therefore we have a common interest in leaving something to Ruth and Rosamonde.
>
> As a family you know we are completely bust. William has nothing at all, John is keeping up the firm and doing a lot of business but is barely able to make enough to take care of his wife and two children. Constance is doing all the work for her four children and Ned is almost useless. My sister, Annie's income, is reduced to $100 a month and she has to live at small boarding houses, making rather frequent changes.
>
> My proposition is this, that you should put in some cash to enable me to remodel 15 Pinckney Street, and

> that the property be run by John in the form of a trust for my sister, Annie, during her lifetime and then for the benefit of Rosamonde and Ruth, and their children. In general you know the property and I will send you, within a few days, a syllabus which John has gotten up to show to the bank as an argument for having them advance $25,000 provided we put it into repair.[512]

This was never done.

By 1939 Codman had to know that his time was getting short. He was, by then, suffering from malignant melanoma, a deadly skin cancer. His early X-ray experiments exposed him to huge amounts of radiation, and Cushing had intimated that Codman's experiments had harmed his health. But there is no known association between X-radiation and malignant melanoma. Perhaps his many days hunting and fishing, out in the sun for long hours, were responsible, as there is known to be an association between malignant melanoma and large amounts of exposure to ultraviolet radiation. However, Codman's heritage probably played the most significant role—fair-skinned, reddish-blonde hair, a definitive Celtic appearance. People of this background are known to be at increased risk for skin cancers, including malignant melanoma. But this is speculative; a definite cause for his final illness cannot be deduced.

On 14 July 1939 his lawyer (and also his nephew), Leonard Andrew Wheeler, Jr. wrote him suggesting that he make out a new will because of the recent deaths of his sister and brother (Anna and William Codman). Codman made out the new will on 25 September 1939 leaving everything to his wife, which is what eventually occurred, as Katy Codman survived until 1961. The will also stated that if his wife predeceased him all of his estate would go to his niece, Constance Codman Brooks (wife of Edward Brooks of Brooklyn). He also willed his entire medical library to be given to the Massachusetts General Hospital including any copies of his book, *The Shoulder*, which were unsold at his death. A few months after his will was made out, he made

---

512CA 8/181.

inquiries about headstones for a grave at the Forest Hills Cemetery in Jamaica Plain, Massachusetts.

Ernest Hemingway once said that all true stories, if followed to their conclusion, end in death. Codman likely would have paraphrased this to read, "For all patients, the ultimate End Result is always death." For Ernest Amory Codman the ultimate End Result came on Saturday, 23 November 1940, at his home in Ponkapoag, from complications of malignant melanoma. His final words and thoughts have not been recorded. If they were of a personal nature, possibly they were of his wife, Katy, or perhaps of some pleasant day spent in the woods or ponds, hunting and fishing with his dogs. If they were of a professional nature, they were undoubtedly about the End Result Idea. Perhaps he thought of that January day in 1915 at the Boston Medical Library when his promising career effectively imploded. If so, it is certain that he did not regret it.

His funeral took place on Monday, 25 November 1940 at 3:00 P.M. It was held in the Story Chapel in the Mt. Auburn Cemetery in Cambridge, one of the Boston area's largest cemeteries. He is buried there in the Bowditch plot. It is not known if his financial condition near the end necessitated this. Perhaps the headstone at the Forest Hills Cemetery was too expensive? But his grave does not bear his name, as he rests either in or near a large mausoleum—it actually cannot be determined. The only name at the mausoleum base is "Bowditch."

Within the week obituaries appeared in the Boston[513] and Canton papers.[514] They were brief, occupying only five short paragraphs each. They described his education, his medical practice, his work on bone tumors, his study of shoulder problems, and that he left Katy as his only survivor.

And thus the circle never quite made it back around. A favored son of Boston, with the scientific and educational background found in few doctors in his era, early on he had it all—until he decided that his calling was to reform the medical world in which he lived. But the calling nearly destroyed his professional career, and nearly ruined him

---

513*Boston Herald*, 25 November 1940.

514*Canton Journal*, 29 November 1940, p. 1.

financially as well. Had the circle been completed, had life been fair, at the end he would have been recognized for his valiant attempts at medical reform. But the circle stopped only at an unmarked grave and obituaries in which the End Result Idea was never mentioned. (Figure 25)

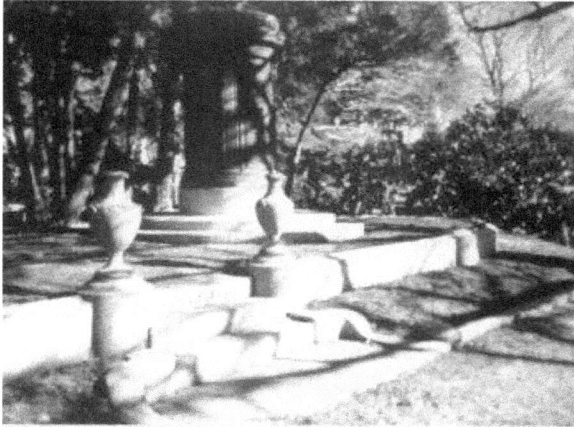

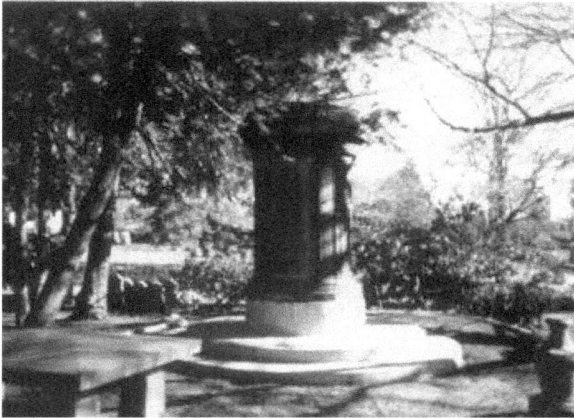

Figure 25—The final End Result. Two views of the mausoleum which is the final resting place of Ernest Amory Codman. It is a part of the Bowditch family cemetery plot. His name is not to be found on it. (Courtesy Bill Mallon, M.D. Collection)515

515 In 2012-13, the American Cancer Society, the American Medical Association, the American Shoulder and Elbow Surgeons, and the Department of Orthopaedics at Harvard Medical School donated funds to erect a headstone on Codman's grave, after obtaining permission from Mount Auburn Cemetery and Codman's heirs. The headstone is scheduled to be placed in the spring of 2014.

But after his death, Ernest Amory Codman was not quickly forgotten, and hindsight has treated him well. Edward Martin had predicted that his epitaph would read, "EAC—killed by his colleagues."[516] Shortly after his death, however, both the American College of Surgeons (ACS) and the Massachusetts General Hospital issued short published tributes to his memory and his career, sending them both to Katy Codman. The ACS tribute was as follows:

ERNEST AMORY CODMAN

December 30, 1869 - November 23, 1940

The Board of Regents of the American College of Surgeons, at a meeting held in Chicago on February 16, 1941, adopted the following resolution:

Whereas, Dr. Ernest Amory Codman of Boston, Massachusetts, a Founder of the American College of Surgeons, and a member of the Board of Governors of said College, has contributed in an extremely important manner to its work, especially through the establishment and conduct of the Registry of Bone Sarcoma, and

Whereas, this Registry of Bone Sarcoma not only introduced a new co-operative method of scientific study on a large scale but made possible definite advances in the knowledge of a subject concerning which much ignorance had prevailed, and as a result of which many human lives have undoubtedly been saved, and

Whereas, it is recognized that the success of the Registry of Bone Sarcoma was overwhelmingly due to the scientific zeal and self-sacrificing labors of Dr. Codman, and

Whereas, Dr. Codman passed from this earth November 23, 1940,

---

516CA 2/33. Also quoted in Reverby, p. 170.

Therefore, Be It Resolved by the Regents of the American College of Surgeons at their regular meeting held in Chicago on February 16, 1941, that an expression of their appreciation of the work of Dr. Codman be spread upon the minutes of the said meeting and that a copy of this resolution be sent to his widow, Katharine [sic] Bowditch Codman, with an expression of their deepest sympathy.

Irvin Abell, M.D.
Chairman, Board of Regents

An illuminated memorial honoring Dr. Codman has been transmitted to his family.[517]

There is no mention of the End Result Idea in the above tribute. But the Trustees of the Massachusetts General Hospital, with whom he had battled in his early years, did not forget. They adopted the following resolution at their meeting of 13 December 1940.

Dr. Ernest Amory Codman, 1869-1940

East Surgical House Officer, 1895
Surgeon to Out-Patients, 1900
Assistant Visiting Surgeon, 1907
Resigned, 1914
Board of Consultation, 1929
Champion of truth; original in thought; firm in his convictions, and willing to sacrifice personal place and standing to achieve what he believed to be right. To him rightfully belongs the credit for conceiving and effecting many policies which have contributed to the improvement and advancement of surgery and to the renown of this Hospital. Through his efforts the General Executive Committee was formed, the policy of Special Assignments accepted, the practice of advancement solely upon the basis of seniority

517*Bull Amer Coll Surg*, no bibliographic information available. Found in CA 10/209.

abandoned, and a Follow-up and End-Result system adopted. He showed early promise of originality and energy. As a House Officer, together with Harvey Cushing, he compiled the first recordings of the administration of anesthetics and "Ground out on the old static machine the first faint x-ray picture of a hand ever taken here."

As a surgeon Dr. Codman will be remembered primarily for his work on duodenal ulcer, for his book on 'The Shoulder', and for the institution of the Registry of Bone Sarcoma.

Mankind, Medicine, and the Massachusetts General hospital are his debtors.

Yours very truly,
Reginald Gray
Secretary.[518]

Shortly thereafter, a longer obituary was jointly published in the *New England Journal of Medicine* and in the *Communications of the Massachusetts Medical Society*, both presumably written by John Homans, his hunting and fishing companion. The almost encomiastic obituary ended with the following paragraph:

Amory Codman had many devoted friends in many walks of life. No one could associate with him intimately without coming under the spell of his enthusiasm, his squareness and the attractive whimsical streak which, in all but his most strenuous moments, took the sharp edge off his intensity. In everyday life he was affectionate, thoughtful, fair, a good companion. His was a strong character, remarkably free from pretense and affectation, uncompromising, of a sort much needed in this day. He should be counted one of New England's great

518CA 2/38.

figures, a man who has left a deep mark and has deserved well of posterity, for whom he labored.[519]

Within a few years, the End Result Idea was recognized in a book on the history of medicine by Haagensen and Lloyd:

> The man who was largely responsible for forcing surgeons to adopt proper record systems and institute proper clinic follow ups was a Boston surgeon named E. A. Codman. A man of truly heroic candor, he sacrificed his own surgical career to put across his conviction of the importance of knowing the end results of surgical treatment. It was in 1910 that he turned the major share of his efforts to this purpose. The climax came in 1914 with his resignation from the staff of Massachusetts General following a burst of devastating publicity. But his colleagues knew he was right about his end result idea, and although they excluded him from their circle, they adopted the principle within a short time, and the Massachusetts General became one of the first hospitals to adopt necessary changes in the case record system and to institute a systematic follow up of patients.[520]

Shortly before Codman's death, Dr. Frederic Washburn, director of the MGH from 1908-34, and his contemporary with whom he had frequently battled over instituting the End Result Idea at that hospital, wrote of Codman in notes that he left us in his own copy of *The Shoulder*:

> New England has been fortunate in producing in each generation a few men who stand out from the crowd because of their original thinking. They have sometimes been of the stuff of which martyrs are

---

519Homans J. *New Engl J Med*, 224(7): 299, 13 February 1941.

520CA 8/159, from Haagensen CD, Lloyd WB. *One Hundred Years of Medicine*. New York: Sheraton House, 1943.

made. A few centuries ago they would have been burned at the stake, would have gloried in it and have sought the opportunity to make the sacrifice. Egotism is usually a characteristic of these men. Yet but for them the world's progress would be infinitely slower, and many important advances would have been delayed and perhaps never have eventuated. My friend Amory Codman is one of these men.

He has courageously accomplished much good. It is seldom that a man's ideas are carried out in the exact way which he proposes. If, as did Amory Codman, he calls attention to a situation that needs improvement, makes a reluctant and conservative organization examine its weaknesses and take steps to remove them, he should feel the satisfaction of accomplishment. I still believe that if Dr. Codman had stayed within the fold of the Massachusetts General Hospital, he would have seen his reforms largely accomplished, for other forces than his were also at work. But that wasn't his way. His dramatic resignation and the meeting at the Medical Library undoubtedly hastened the change under way at the Hospital. The formation of the General Executive Committee of the Staff in 1912 made possible special assignments in Surgery. The contributions to the advancement of Surgery made at our hospital in the last twenty years have been accomplished largely because of these special assignments. Follow-up work has been carried out in many groups of cases. Perhaps not just as Dr. Codman would have done it. It has been of great value.[521]

So it was obvious that Codman was not forgotten by his peers. But now, with the benefit of almost 60 years of reflection since his death, how important was he to the advancement of medical science? His life's

521 Washburn FA, pp. 433-434

contributions can be considered in six different fields: 1) anesthesiology, 2) radiology, 3) general surgery, 4) bone sarcoma, 5) shoulder surgery, and 6) the End Result Idea.

Anesthesiology

Amory Codman and Harvey Cushing were the first doctors to publish what they called "ether charts," which we know today as the anesthesia record, in which the patient's vital signs and other details of the anesthesia during surgery are recorded. It was a very important contribution. Monitoring the patient during anesthesia foreshadowed Codman's attempt to improve medical science by applying the scientific method to anesthesia. By monitoring the patient he could see when and where things went, or were going, wrong, and how the patient's care could be improved in the case of poor results. Though not exactly the End Result Idea, it presaged his interest in better monitoring of the patient in every way.

The ether charts were an important breakthrough, although they were still a fairly small one in the history of anesthesiology. In addition, it is almost certain that such a method of monitoring the patient would have been developed within a few years by someone else, had Codman and Cushing not developed it on their own.

Radiology

Amory Codman began his career after medical school essentially as a radiologist, then called a "skiagrapher," and one of his early appointments was as the first skiagrapher to the Boston Children's Hospital. He performed numerous experiments on the early use of X-rays in surgery and in the diagnosis of disease, notably using fluoroscopy for the evaluation of gastrointestinal disorders. He also published an outstanding archive of plates of normal X-rays of the joints of the body in varying positions.

Codman became an expert on the early use of radiology, and especially on the dangers of X-ray burns resulting from the extremely high radiation doses then in use. But, after his first decade of practice, he rarely concentrated on radiology as a separate science, using it only to further his advances in abdominal surgery, shoulder surgery, and orthopedic oncology. He later commented that his plates of normal X-rays of the joints were kept at the Warren Museum, and were so full of dust that probably nobody had looked at them since he had donated them to the Warren Museum.[522]

Though now little remembered for his radiologic work, it actually appears that Codman's contributions to radiology were highly valued during his life. In late 1927 he received a letter from the Secretary-Treasurer of the New England Roentgen Ray Society informing him, "It gives him great pleasure to inform you that at the annual meeting of the New England Roentgen Ray Society you were unanimously elected a member of the Society. This was done in recognition of the extremely valuable and important findings which you contributed in the early days of roentgenology."[523]

General Surgery

Codman <u>was</u> a general surgeon. Although he became most famous for advances he made to the study of orthopaedic surgery, notably on the shoulder and bone sarcoma, he began his career as a general surgeon. He wrote papers on general surgical topics at least until the 1920s and in the era in which he lived, when specialization was much less common than it is today, he always considered himself a general surgeon with an orthopaedic emphasis.

Codman's most significant work in general surgery was in his study of duodenal ulcers, a problem that gave him personal grief much of his life. On this topic he made important, although probably not landmark, contributions. Some of his papers were anticipated by earlier work done by the Mayo brothers in the United States and by Lord Moynihan in England. Still, he was recognized as one of the nation's experts on this problem which, in that era, was considered somewhat rare.

Bone Sarcoma

Although Codman's contributions to the above three specialties of medicine, anesthesiology, radiology, and general surgery were important, if not outstanding, he can be considered one of the most

---

522Preface, pp. ix-x.

523CA 3/60.

significant figures in the history of the remaining three fields of medicine in which he concentrated.

He was certainly the first surgeon to make important studies of bone sarcoma. Prior to Codman, all the work in this field was done by pathologists, notably Dr. James Ewing and Dr. James Bloodgood and, at that time, surgeons served only to amputate limbs after the tumors were discovered.

Codman began the Registry of Bone Sarcoma effectively by himself, only enlisting Drs. Ewing and Bloodgood to help him because of their knowledge of pathology. His papers and his book on bone sarcoma are the absolute early outstanding works in the field. They were the first to present a systematic method of classification and nomenclature for bone sarcomata. Like many early aspects of medicine, however, they are of little use today, having largely been supplanted by discoveries of more recent years with the advancement of medical science. Still, Codman's early advances stood as the platform upon which later orthopaedists and pathologists built, in order to further our knowledge of bone sarcoma.

To Codman, his work on bone sarcoma was something more. After he had been ostracized by the Boston medical community and found it difficult to practice medicine, his work on bone sarcoma served as an example of using the End Result Idea to study the outcome of medical interventions. In the 1920s, it was all he had left, and all he could do to attempt to perpetuate the End Result Idea.

Shoulder Surgery

Codman began the last sentence of his Preface to *The Shoulder* with, "Now start in and read the best book there is on the human shoulder (it is the only one) ..."[524] It was the first book ever written solely about the shoulder (in English) and it might still be the best.

In the field of shoulder surgery, Ernest Amory Codman bestrides the orthopaedic world like a Colossus. His early papers on the rotator cuff, written beginning in 1906, would still stand up well today in discussions of the clinical diagnosis and treatment of rotator cuff pathology. His book on the shoulder, written in 1934, could still be used

---

524Preface, p. xl.

today by an aspiring shoulder surgeon as an excellent text to learn about problems of the shoulder. Codman's prescience concerning problems of the shoulder was astounding, as has been well described earlier. Rowe, himself an outstanding shoulder surgeon, noted of him, "Although many surgeons have contributed to surgery of the shoulder, no investigator has revealed the shoulder in its entirety as has Codman."[525]

Between the 1950s and 1980s, Dr. Charles S[umner] Neer, II (né 1917) of New York established himself as the foremost shoulder surgeon in North America. He dominated this niche of orthopedic surgery during this time, and his contributions to the field were legion. Neer developed the first effective system for shoulder arthroplasty; he developed a new operation for certain types of shoulder instability; he popularized the use of an antero-inferior acromioplasty to relieve the pain from rotator cuff tendinitis; and he developed the classification system in current use for fractures about the shoulder.

Neer did not surpass Amory Codman, but only furthered the work which he had begun. Some of Neer's work, notably that on fracture classification and rotator cuff problems, is built upon ideas first developed by Codman, but Codman and Neer must be considered the two absolute giants of the field of shoulder surgery. Their only rival among orthopaedists concentrating on a single joint is Sir John Charnley (1911-1982) of England, whose work was on the hip, and whose primary contribution was the development of total hip arthroplasty.

End Result Idea

But if Codman is one of the two or three leading orthopaedic surgeons of this century in the field of shoulder surgery and bone sarcoma, even those contributions are dwarfed by his work on outcome studies, or as he called it, the End Result Idea. It was the single great idea of his life, and his attempt to implement it and change medicine was the great quest of his life. He failed, and one could even say he failed miserably, possibly due to the foibles of his own personality.

525Rowe CR. Codman—His Influence on the Development of Surgery of the Shoulder, In: *Shoulder Surgery*, I Bayley, L Kessel, eds.. Berlin: Springer-Verlag, 1982., p. 1.

There are probably other, possibly even more important reasons why he failed. McGuire discussed several of these in his thesis, mentioning the fact that World War I interrupted his crusade, that the Halifax disaster effectively closed the Codman Hospital, that a lack of money prevented implementation of many of his ideas, and that the public of that era did not perceive a need for the End Result Idea. He also noted that physicians of that era rejected the system because of a fear that outcomes study would erode their professional autonomy. McGuire stated, "Although Codman's personality played a significant role in the outcome of the crusade, the profession refused the message, not the messenger."[526]

Reverby concurred, noting, "But even if Codman had been a less acerbic character, more willing to compromise, it is perhaps less speculative to assume that the end of the story would have been the same, given the ideological ascendancy of physicians at the time."[527] Both McGuire and Reverby seem to say the same thing—few physicians disagreed with Codman's ideas, but they were simply not willing to accept such changes to their own practices, for many reasons. It was an era in which seemingly only one eccentric Boston surgeon was espousing the need to do outcome studies, and they did not share his enthusiasm that they were necessary.

But, in a larger sense, Codman did not fail. Eighty-plus years after the meeting at the Boston Medical Library, the study of outcomes, or End Results, has become all the rage in modern medicine. In his own time, it was too revolutionary for him to be appreciated. Yet Codman was not seeking recognition for his work. He wanted to improve medicine, and he realized that his efforts may not bear fruit for some time, as has been shown to be true. He predicted this when he ended his book on the shoulder with: "However, if my work or my writing succeed in bringing about the establishment of an End Result System of Organization in our hospitals, even a few years earlier than it would otherwise have arrived, I shall have left to the children of my great

---

526McGuire KJ. pp. 98-102.

527Reverby, p. 171.

nieces and nephews, more than a money value, although they will share it with all the other heirs of the world."[528]

In referring to Codman's contributions, Dr. George Ward, a gynecologist at the Women's Hospital of the Cornell University Medical Center in New York, stated, "I wish to take this opportunity to pay tribute to Dr. Codman by expressing my great appreciation of the wonderful work and great good that he had accomplished by fearless insistence ... on end result study in our hospitals today. He has been the means of saving many lives, much suffering and much money ..."[529]

Future implementation of the End Result Idea, now termed "Outcomes Study," is almost a given by American medicine today. Third-party payors, hospital administrators, lawyers, and even patient advocacy groups are now demanding that doctors study and publish the outcomes of their interventions. Dr. Arnold Relman, former editor of the *New England Journal of Medicine*, has termed this "The Third Revolution in Medical Care." He described the first era as "The Era of Expansion," lasting from the turn-of-the-century until the 1960s, followed by the "The Era of Cost Containment." The current era, "The Third Revolution," is described as "The Era of Accountability."[530] Codman would surely feel justified. Perhaps it would be better termed "The Era of Codman."

Possibly the best short summary of Codman's life has been given us by Carter Rowe, in the dedication to his own book, also entitled *The Shoulder*, "This book is dedicated to Ernest Amory Codman, a man of intellect, courage, conviction, controversy, and irrepressible honesty. He was a surgeon far ahead of his time, whose legacy to the medical world has been the establishment of the 'End-Result Idea' for doctors and hospitals, the initiation of the Registry of Bone Sarcoma, and the

---

528Epilogue, p. 29.

529Neuhauser, p. 319; referencing Ward GG. The value and need for more attention to end results and follow-up in hospitals today. *Bull Amer Coll Surg*, 8: 29-34, 1924.

530Relman AS. The third revolution in medical care. *New Engl J Med*, 319(18): 1220-1222, 3 November 1988.

publication of his classic book, *The Shoulder*, in 1934, from which came the inspiration for this book."[531]

Codman was far ahead of his time, so far, in fact, that he is little remembered today. In an excellent article celebrating the career of Ernest Amory Codman, Donabedian discussed the neglect with which Codman's contributions have been treated. He opened with the following, "I intend to summon from a shadowy past someone who should have been recognized always as a towering figure in the history of our field. ... I hope to celebrate the man, making amends, in my small way, for the neglect he has so long unjustly suffered. ... [The End Result Idea] led him to disgrace, notoriety, isolation, and near financial ruin. It also set him, as I hope to show, on the road to immortality."[532] He concluded with the cogent remark, "In his views of the nature of the hospital, of its social responsibility, and of its accountability to a more exigent public, Codman seems more a man of our time than of his."[533] He was.

Six fields of medicine. In three of them he was an important contributor to the advancement of medical science, in two of them he was an absolute giant in the field, and in one he was a revolutionary who was so far ahead of his time that his accomplishments and desires could not, or would not, be appreciated by his peers. Any doctor of the 20th century making the contributions which Codman made in one or two fields would be long remembered. To have propagated such advances in three or four separate fields of medicine would be a stunning accomplishment. But significant advances in six separate fields of medicine? It is hard to comprehend, difficult to understand, and almost unfathomable. As Berwick noted, "Codman looked ahead. He looked, indeed, beyond us. Seventy-eight years ago he began his life's work; forty-eight years ago he died. Are we ready for him yet?"[534]

Are we ready for this Surgeon of the '90's? His medical career was born in the 1890s, he is now remembered more in the 1990s, but the

---

531 Rowe CR. *The Shoulder*. New York: Churchill Livingstone, 1988. Dedication page.

532 Donabedian, pp. 233-235.

533 *Ibid.*, p. 246.

534 Berwick, p. 266.

appreciation due him may not come for 100 more years, until the 2090s. In Amory Codman's lifetime, respect came but appreciation never did. In fact, his efforts to reform medical science brought him mostly ridicule, poverty, and censure. Remember, that at his death, the newspaper obituaries mentioned only two of the six fields to which he contributed—bone sarcoma and shoulder surgery. (Figure 26)

The End Result Idea was never mentioned.

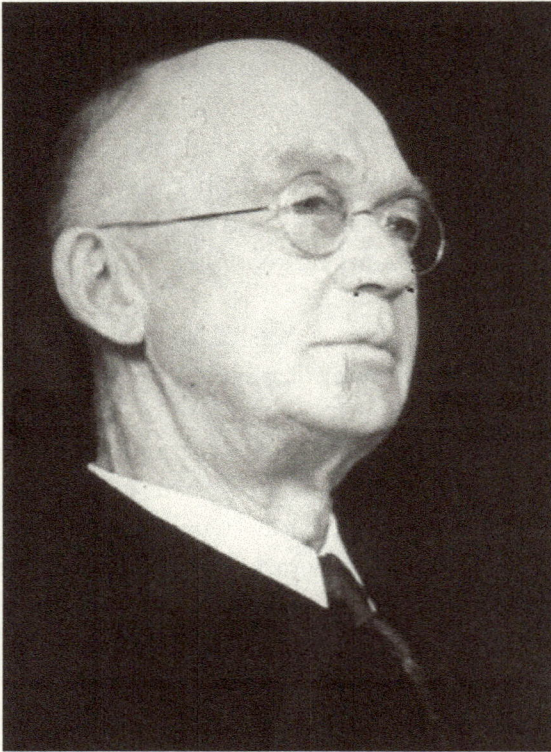

Figure 26—The last known surviving photograph of Amory Codman. (Courtesy Francis A. Countway Library of Medicine, Rare Books and Special Collections Department)

APPENDIX I

CODMAN'S EPONYMIC FAME

Codman has been remembered in the medical literature and language by eight eponyms which bear his name, although only five are seen with any regularity. The five main eponyms are discussed within the main text of the biography, but they must be sought out, therefore, I have chosen to provide a separate listing of the eponyms with their definitions and sources. Not all of these are listed in the main medical dictionaries. Following each eponym, I have listed the name of medical dictionaries in which it can be found. Full bibliographic references for those dictionaries are listed under "Sources Consulted."

Of note, the main medical book listing eponyms, *Dictionary of Medical Eponyms* (2nd ed., BG Firkin, JA Whitworth, eds.; New York: Parthenon, 1996), does not list <u>any</u> eponyms containing Codman's name. Two main medical dictionaries, *Mellon's Illustrated Medical Dictionary* (3rd ed.; New York: Parthenon, 1993), and *Taber's Cyclopaedic Medical Dictionary* (16th illustrated ed., Philadelphia: F. A. Davis, 1989), also do not list any Codman eponyms.

Of note, Codman's Exercises and Codman's Paradox are not listed in any of the standard dictionaries, but they are definitely known to all orthopaedic surgeons, especially those sub-specializing in shoulder surgery.

Codman is also remembered by a recently established award given his name. This is described below as well.

Though the current trend is to avoid eponyms in medical terminology, they still proliferate. If I could propose one further eponymic tribute to Codman, one which he would surely appreciate the most, it would be that outcome studies be termed "Codman's Studies."

Codman's Tumor: Codman's tumor is more properly known as a chondroblastoma, and specifically as a chondroblastoma of the proximal humerus. This is a benign tumor of cartilaginous origin, which usually occurs in the former epiphyses of long bones of the skeleton. Codman first described it in his 1931 paper which was entitled "Epiphyseal Chondromatous Giant Cell Tumors of the Upper End of the Humerus." In 1942, Jaffe and Lichtenstein first termed this a chondroblastoma, the name which survives today. The first references to the term Codman's Tumor occur in 1947 and 1949 in works by Coley: "Benign central cartilaginous tumors of bone," by Bradley L. Coley, M.D. and Anthony J. Santoro, M.D., published in *Surgery*, 22(3): 411-423, September 1947, and the book, *Neoplasms of Bone* by Bradley L. Coley (New York: Paul Hoeber, 1949), in which, in the chapter on "Benign Chondroblastoma of Bone," Coley sub-titled it "Codman's Epiphyseal Chondromatous Giant Cell Tumor." A possible earlier reference is in an article entitled "Codman Tumors, So-Called Bone Sarcomas," written by C. Bonne, and published in *Nederl. Tijdschr. v. geneesk*, 78: 3236-3243, 14 July 1934. However, this article appears to discuss all sarcomas in general, labeling them as Codman's tumors because of his early work on this topic. Also of note, a chondroblastoma is benign, and thus is not a sarcoma. [Gould, Stedman's]

Codman's Triangle: Codman's Triangle is a radiographic sign seen mostly in malignant bone sarcomas, in which the rapid growth of the tumor elevates the periosteum overlying the metaphysis, creating a calcified line angling away from the diaphyseal shaft. Occasionally, this angle is filled in at the top, near the physis, by further calcification, creating a triangular-shaped elevation of periosteum visible on the radiograph. Codman's Triangle is pathognomonic of an aggressive malignant tumor of bone. It can be seen in many such lesions, however, and does not make the specific diagnosis, although it is mentioned most commonly in association with osteosarcoma. Codman first described this, although somewhat vaguely, in his chapter in Keen's textbook of surgery, *Surgery: Its Principles and Practices* (Philadelphia: W. B. Saunders, editions between 1909-1919), entitled "The Use of X-ray and Radium in Surgery." He later discussed it in his book *Bone Sarcoma,* although he mentioned it in there reference to Ewing's sarcoma. No true first reference for the eponym can be found. The earliest reference I could find to it is in Coley's book, *Neoplasms of Bone* (by Bradley L. Coley. New York: Paul Hoeber, 1949, p. 238), in which he states, " … described by Codman and often referred to as Codman's Triangle." [Butterworth's, Dorland's, Gould, Stedman's]

Codman's Exercises: Codman's exercises are now usually termed "pendulum exercises," or "Codman's pendulum exercises." They are used frequently today as a method of shoulder rehabilitation and therapy. They are performed by the patient leaning forward at the waist, supporting the body with the good arm on a table or post, and allowing the injured arm and shoulder to hang down naturally from the shoulder, creating an approximate angle of 90° with the thorax. From this position the arm is moved in gentle pendulum motions. This exercise works by allowing active motion but eliminating the effect of gravity. In addition, shoulder pain is often relieved in this position because the humeral head is flexed on the glenoid and the rotator cuff disappears posteriorly behind the acromion, rather than impinging upon it. Codman first described this exercise in the article "Abduction of the Shoulder. An Interesting Observation in Connection With Subacromial Bursitis and Rupture of the Tendon and Supraspinatus," which was published in the *Boston Medical and Surgical Journal,* (166(24): 890-891, 13 June 1912), although he called them "stooping exercises." In the article, he made the following points concerning these exercises, "When a person stands with the knees straight and the fingertips close to the floor, the humerus is abducted on the scapula by gravity alone without muscular effort." He went on further, "In treatment, too, this observation can be utilized by beginning the mobilization of very acute cases and postoperative cases by simply having them lean the body forward with the arm hanging instead of making an attempt at abduction against gravity in the usual way." He also recommended use of this exercise on all shoulders with rotator cuff problems, "Finally let me say this, that, simple as to which this point I call attention is, its proper appreciation by the medical profession will materially help to relieve the suffering and hasten the recovery of *all* stiff and painful shoulders. Obvious and trivial as it may seem, I am sure that from now on it will prove assistance in *every* shoulder case and should become of daily use in *every* hospital clinic." Codman was correct. The exercise is included by almost all orthopaedic surgeons today in their shoulder rehabilitation program. [Not described in any current medical dictionaries.]

Codman's Sign: Codman's sign refers to a sign of physical examination of the shoulder in which the painful shoulder will be painful during a certain arc of elevation, but after reaching a certain point, when the rotator cuff has passed underneath the acromion and is no longer mechanically impinging upon it, the pain will subside and further elevation of the arm will be pain-free. This today is often referred to as a "Painful Arc Syndrome," in the European literature, and describes what in the United States is often termed the "Impingement Syndrome." Of note, the three definitions given in Butterworth's, Dorland's, and Stedman's are not exactly the same, and actually can be confusing in the interpretation of this sign, especially so because it is often confused with another examination finding in patients with subacromial bursitis, Dawbarn's Sign, which is more consistently described in medical dictionaries. The three given definitions of Codman's Sign are as follows: Butterworth's—for rupture of the supraspinatus tendon: the arm can be passively abducted without pain but active abduction in the middle range of the movement is either impossible or painful; Dorland's—in rupture of the supraspinatus tendon, the arm can be passively abducted without pain, but when support of the arm is removed and the deltoid contracts suddenly, pain occurs again; and Stedman's—in the absence of rotator cuff function, hunching of the shoulder occurs when the deltoid muscle contracts. Stedman's and Dorland's both define Dawbarn's Sign, almost similarly, as follows: Dorland's—in acute subacromial bursitis, when the arm is at the side palpation over the bursa causes pain, but when it is abducted this pain disappears; and Stedman's—pain of subacromial bursitis disappears when the arm is abducted. [Butterworth's, Dorland's, Stedman's]

Codman's Paradox: Codman's Paradox is described in his book on *The Shoulder*, in Chapter II: "Normal Motions of the Shoulder Joint." On page 43, he notes that "And now we come to a curious paradox which I have only recently observed, although I have studied the motions of the shoulder for years. You can prove that the completely elevated arm is in either extreme external rotation or in extreme internal rotation." He then describes this proof, and on page 44, Figure 29 has a stick-figure demonstration of the proof. The paradox is incorrect, but, similar to Zeno's famous paradoxes, it takes some rather difficult mathematical reasoning to prove the error in Codman's reasoning. This has only recently been published.535 [Not described in any current medical dictionary.]

Codman's Bursa; Codman's Bursitis; Codman's Bursal Incision: All three of these are listed only in *Butterworth's Medical Dictionary* (2nd edition). The definitions given are as follows: Codman's Bursa — the subacromial bursa; Codman's Bursitis - subacromial bursitis; Codman's Bursal Incision — an incision used for the removal of Codman's (subacromial) bursa and extending 5 cm. (2 in.) forward from the acromioclavicular joint. I have never heard these eponyms in modern discussion of shoulder surgery. They are not listed in any current books on the shoulder, nor are they routinely used in the *Journal of Shoulder and Elbow Surgery*, by the American Shoulder and Elbow Surgeons, nor in shoulder articles in the standard orthopaedic journals. [Butterworth's]

The Ernest A. Codman Award: This award was first given out in 1997 and is sponsored by the Joint Commission on Accreditation of Healthcare Organizations (JCAHO), with support and cooperation from Pfizer, Inc. The purpose of the award is described as follows: "The Ernest A. Codman Award recognizes health care organizations that use

---

535 Mallon WJ. On the hypotheses that determine the definitions of gleno-humeral joint motion: with resolution of Codman's pivotal paradox. *J Shoulder Elbow Surg*, 21(12): December 2012.

process and outcomes measures to improve organization performance and, ultimately, the quality of care provided to the public. Named for the physician regarded in health care as 'the father of outcomes measurement,' the Ernest A. Codman Award seeks both to recognize exemplary achievements in the effective use of performance measures and to expand knowledge and encourage the use of performance measurement to improve the quality of health care."[536] The Codman Award is open to any JCAHO-accredited organization with a current accreditation status of "Accreditation with Recommendations for Improvement" or better.[537] The first award was given in 1997 and was won by the Middletown Regional Hospital in Middletown, Ohio for its hospital performance improvement efforts.

One would hope that the award could be renamed in the future as either the "Ernest Amory Codman Award" or the "E. Amory Codman Award," reflecting Codman's personal use of his middle name.

---

[536]JCAHO, *Brochure on the "The 1997 Ernest A. Codman Award."*Oakbrook Terrace, IL: JCAHO, 1998, p. 6.

[537]*Ibid,,* p. 7.

APPENDIX II

CHRONOLOGY OF CODMAN'S LIFE

All biography can be written in two basic methods—either chronologically or topically. I have mostly chosen the topical approach in this biography, though not strictly, because many of Codman's important contributions overlapped during periods of his life, and a strict chronologic approach would have made it very difficult to follow the full importance of each these contributions. However, this appendix includes a detailed chronology of the life of Ernest Amory Codman, M.D., for the readers who desire it.

1821—William Coombs Codman, Amory Codman's father, is born.

1836—Elizabeth Hurd, Amory Codman's mother, is born.

1 May 1859—Anna Gertrude Codman, Amory's sister, is born

6 August 1860—William Coombs Codman, Jr., Amory's older brother, is born.

16 January 1863—John Codman, Jr., the younger of Amory's brothers, is born.

8 April 1869—Harvey Williams Cushing, who would become the first great neurosurgeon, and Amory Codman's closest friend, is born in Cleveland, Ohio.

30 December 1869—Ernest Amory Codman born in Boston. His parents, William Coombs Codman and Elizabeth Hurd Codman, live at 23 West Cedar Street.

1876—Begins attending elementary school at The Fay School in Southborough, Massachusetts, a private boarding school.

1881—Begins attending junior high school at Saint Mark's School, an exclusive private boarding school in Southborough, Massachusetts. He will remain there through high school.

Summer 1885—Takes a hunting and fishing trip to Virginia with his brother, John Codman, shortly after John's graduation from Harvard.

April-May 1887—Takes a hunting and fishing trip to North Carolina with his brother, John, missing two months of school shortly before graduation.

June 1887—Graduation from St. Mark's Academy. He is given The Founder's Medal as the top student at graduation.

September 1887—Begins attending Harvard College.

November 1889—Codman is presented with his first dog, Dick, a Gordon Setter, by Mrs. Outram Barys.

19 June 1891—Graduates *cum laude* from Harvard College.

Summer 1891—Hunting in Nova Scotia and at Chebeaque Island, a small island off the coast of Maine.

September 1891—Begins attending Harvard Medical School on the corner of Boylston and Exeter Streets in Boston. Receives a Bullard Scholarship and a Shattuck Scholarship.

Sep-Oct 1891—Hunting in New Hampshire and Vermont.

1892-1893—Travels and studies in Europe in England, France, Switzerland, Italy, Austria, and Egypt, visiting surgical clinics while there. In Vienna, he is first introduced to the concept of the subacromial bursa at a clinic run by Eduard Albert.

9 October 1894—Dick, his first dog, runs away, and is never found.

1894-1895—While a 4th-year medical student, Codman serves his internship on the surgical service at the Massachusetts General Hospital. During this period, he and his best friend, Harvey Cushing, begin developing "ether charts," the first known example of the anesthesia record during surgery.

26 June 1895—Graduates from Harvard Medical School.

3 October 1896—Codman's mother, Elizabeth Hurd Codman, dies.

1 May 1897—Reads a paper to the Committee on the Bullard Fellowship of the Harvard Medical School on "Experiments on the application of the roentgen rays to the study of anatomy." This is later

published in the *Journal of Experimental Medicine* and is Codman's first published paper.

31 August 1897—John Codman, Jr., Amory's younger brother, dies of heart disease.

5-24 September 1897—A New Brunswick hunting and fishing trip with Bob Barlow.

6 April 1898—Reads a paper before the Surgical Section of the Suffolk District Medical Society on "A Case of Actinomycosis."

November 1898—Becomes engaged to Katherine Putnam Bowditch.

Late 1898-early 1899—Hunting trip to Wyoming with brother,William.

Summer 1899—Hunting and fishing trip out West during which Codman served as a personal physician to W. Cameron and Waldo E. Forbes.

16 November 1899—Marries Katherine Putnam Bowditch in Chestnut Hill, Massachusetts.

19 March 1900—Reads a paper before the Boston Society for Medical Improvement on "A study of the x-ray plates of one hundred and forty cases of fracture of the lower end of the radius."

11-29 Oct 1901—Hunting trip to Woodstock, Vermont and Meriden and Charlestown, New Hampshire.

25 December 1901—Codman makes a pre-operative diagnosis of a perforated duodenal ulcer and operates on the patient, saving him, and stimulating his own interest in that problem.

15 January 1902—Reads a paper before the Clinical Section of the Suffolk District Medical Society on "Acute perforation of a malignant ulcer of the pylorus resembling a case of acute appendicitis."

April 1902—Reads a paper before the Clinical Meeting of the Medical Board of the Massachusetts General Hospital on "A resume of the results of Dr. FB Harrington's service from June to Oct. 1, 1900, as seen in the following June or later."

15 October 1902—He buys Peter, his next dog

2 February 1903—Reads a paper before the Johns Hopkins Medical Society on "The use of the X-ray in surgery."

25 April 1903—Reads a paper before the Annual Meeting of the Suffolk District Medical Society "The formation of loose cartilages in the knee joint."

11 July 1903—Formation of the American Society of Clinical Surgery with Codman elected as a charter member.

13-14 Nov 1903—Codman attends the first meeting of the American Society of Clinical Surgery in Philadelphia (13th) and Baltimore (14th).

1903—William Coombs Codman, Amory Codman's father, dies. The exact date is not known.

9 March 1904—Was scheduled to read a paper before the Worcester District Medical Society on "Some points on the diagnosis and treatment of certain neglected minor surgical lesions," but his talk was omitted due to lack of time.

4 November 1904—First mention of Ponkapoag occurs in the Codman hunting diary when he notes that he hunted in Ponkapoag behind Joe Crocker's.

1904—Reads a paper before the Nova Scotia Medical Society on "The use of the X-ray in the diagnosis of diseases of the bone."

5 April 1905—Reads a paper before the Section for Surgery of the Suffolk District Branch of the Massachusetts Medical Society on "Report of results in nontraumatic surgery of brain and spinal cord. Observations upon the actual results of cerebral surgery at the Massachusetts General Hospital."

26 October 1905—Codman performs a bone transference operation, moving the fibula to replace a resected osteomyelitic segment of tibia.

24 January 1906—Reads a paper before the Surgical Section of the Suffolk District Medical Society on "A report of recurrent spontaneous gangrene of the index finger: Successive amputations of the phalanges: Abatement of the process after excision of a portion of the radial nerve and stretching of the median nerve."

16 March 1906—Reads a paper before the Academy of Medicine at Cleveland on "On stiff and painful shoulders. Subdeltoid Bursitis: The anatomy of the subdeltoid or subacromial bursa and its clinical importance."

3 February 1907—Reads a paper before the Suffolk District Medical Society on "Bone transference. Report of a case of operation after the method of Huntington."

1907—Undergoes exploratory laparotomy for lifelong abdominal complaints.

5 February 1908—Reads a paper before the Suffolk District Medical Society on "A case of intra-vesical cyst of the ureter: dilatation of ureter with very slight dilatation of the renal pelvis and containing twenty-eight movable calculi; bacteriuria; alkalinuria; phosphaturia."

13 March 1908—Reads a paper before the Clinical Meeting of the Medical Board of the Massachusetts General Hospital on "Chronic obstruction of the duodenum by the root of the mesentery."

9 June 1908—Reads a paper before the annual meeting of the Massachusetts Medical Society on "Bursitis subacromialis, or periarthritis of the shoulder-joint. Subdeltoid bursitis."

Jun-Oct 1908—Codman saw patients this summer at a clinic in Cohasset, Massachusetts.

10 April 1909—Reads a paper before the New Bedford Medical Society, "On the surgical significance of pus, blood and bacteria in the urine."

14 April 1909—Reads a paper before the Worcester District Medical Society, "On the importance of distinguishing simple round ulcers of the duodenum from those ulcers which involve the pylorus or are above it."

11 March 1909—Codman performs an operative repair of the rotator cuff on a 52-year-old woman (J. A.). This is the first known repair of the rotator cuff and will be published as such on 18 May 1911.

15 June 1909—Reads a paper before the annual meeting of the Massachusetts Medical Society on "The diagnosis of ulcer of the duodenum."

Summer 1909—European trip during which he visits Belgrade, Serbia and Paris, France. He hunts in both places.

14 January 1910—Reads a paper before the Clinical Meeting of the Medical Board, Massachusetts General Hospital on "Case of mesenteric thrombosis; resection of intestine; end-to-end anastomosis. Recovery."

28 June-7 July 1910—Meeting in London of Clinical Congress of Surgeons of North America. Codman and Edward Martin make plans to form the American College of Surgeons and a sub-committee of the College, the Committee for Hospital Standardization.

July-September 1910—While in England, Codman undergoes a gastro-jejunostomy by Berkeley, Lord Moynihan at the Leeds Council Infirmary for a duodenal ulcer. He was noted to be hunting at Fetterness in Scotland on 10 September 1910 and returned to America near the first of October.

10 January 1911—Codman performs his second repair of a rotator cuff tear, this one on a 40-year-old man (D.R.). This, and his first case, will be published on 18 May 1911.

25 March 1911—Codman presents his first two patients who had undergone rotator cuff repair to the Interurban Orthopaedic Club.

18 May 1911—Codman published the first description in English of a repair of the rotator cuff in the *Boston Medical and Surgical Journal*.

August 1911—Resigns his full-time position at the Massachusetts General Hospital.

November 1911—Codman opens his own private hospital at 15 Pinckney Street in Boston, less than ¼-mile from the Massachusetts General Hospital. With 12 beds, he hopes to use the hospital to demonstrate his own use of the End Result Idea.

7 December 1911—Reads a paper before the Waltham Medical Club on "Diagnosis of diseases of the stomach and intestines by the x-ray."

11-16 Nov 1912—Third Annual Session of the Clinical Congress of Surgeons of North America at which the Committee for Standardization of Hospitals was established, with Codman as chairman.

14 May 1913—In Thomson Hall, at 8:30 PM, Codman reads a paper before the Philadelphia County Medical Society on "The product of a hospital." The talk is somewhat controversial and is not well-received by all the doctors in attendance.

10 June 1913—Reads a paper before the annual meeting of the Massachusetts Medical Society on "Observations on a series of ninety-eight consecutive operations for chronic appendicitis."

27 August 1913—Reads a paper before the American Hospital Association on "Money spent on hospitals is for cure of patients: follow-up system the only way to determine value of institution's services-accounts must include death and disability, which are wasted effort."

February 1914—Codman publishes his first paper discussing the End Results of his own efforts at the Codman Hospital, in "Money spent on hospitals is for cure of patients: follow-up system the only way to determine value of institution's services-accounts must include death and disability, which are wasted effort," based on his talk of 27 August 1913.

March 1914—Codman resigns from the Massachusetts General Hospital (MGH) in protest against the seniority system for senior surgeons. The day after his resignation, he supposedly re-applies for the position of Chief of the Surgical Service on the basis that his results are better than all the other surgeons at the MGH, though that is less definite.

24 April 1914—Codman presents two monographs to the Massachusetts General Hospital on the results of his own surgery on the shoulder and duodenum, entitled, "Abstracts And References To Hospital Records Of The Cases Hitherto Operated On By Dr. Codman For Lesions About The Shoulder Joint. Bibliography," and "Abstracts and End Results Reports in Reference to the Hospital Records of the Cases Hitherto Operated on by E. A. Codman for Lesions of the Stomach and Duodenum."

10 May 1914—Publication of his first monograph on the End Results at the Codman Hospital, *A Study in Hospital Efficiency. As Demonstrated by the Case Report of the First Two Years of a Private Hospital.*

December 1914—Selected by the Central Committee on Credentials of the American College of Surgeons to serve as a member of the Committee on Credentials for Massachusetts.

21 December 1914—Codman turns down the appointment in a reply letter to Dr. Franklin Martin.

6 January 1915—Codman chairs the meeting of the Suffolk District Surgical Society at the Boston Medical Library. It is an incendiary

meeting in which he unveils his famous cartoon of the ostrich kicking out golden eggs to the professors of the Massachusetts General Hospital. He is asked to step down as chairman of the society in response to the furor raised at the meeting.

19 October 1915—Publication of his second monograph on the End Results at the Codman Hospital, *A Study in Hospital Efficiency: As Demonstrated by the Case Report of the First Two Years of a Private Hospital.*

27 December 1915—Codman resigns as Chairman of the Committee on Hospital Standardization of the American College of Surgeons.

22 January 1916—Reads a paper before the Harvard Medical Society of New York on "The dividing line between medical charity and medical business."

19-20 October 1917—Codman spoke in Chicago at the Gold Room of the Congress Hotel at a meeting of the American College of Surgeons Hospital Standardization Program-Joint Session of International and State Committees on Standards. His speech was given at 2:30 p.m. on October 19th and was called "Case Records and Their Value" in the section on "What the Profession of Medicine Wants in Hospitals.

7 December 1917—Two army munition ships, the *Imo* and the *Mont Blanc*, collide in the harbour of Halifax, Nova Scotia, destroying a large part of the city in the largest man-made explosion prior to World War II and atomic weapons.

8 December 1917—Codman immediately closes his hospital in Boston and travels to Halifax to help care for the sick and injured from the explosion.

19 December 1917—He returns from Halifax after 10 days treating the injured.

1917—Publication of his first real book, giving the End Results at the Codman Hospital after five years of service, *A Study in Hospital Efficiency. As Demonstrated by the Case Report of the First Five Years of a Private Hospital.* There is some confusion as to the exact publishing date, which is not listed in the book.

8 June 1918—Reads a paper before the American Surgical Association on "The treatment of malignant peritonitis of ovarian origin."

29 July 1918—Codman received his commission for appointment in the Medical Officers Reserve Corps.

Fall 1918—mid-1919—Codman serves in the U.S. Army, in Delaware, Virginia, and Kentucky, talking care of many victims of the influenza pandemic of 1918.

21 September 1919—Alice Hamilton, a close friend of Katy Codman, and an early leader of the feminist movement, moved into the Codman house at 227 Beacon Street.

11 November 1919—Reads a paper before the Springfield Academy of Medicine on "Intestinal obstruction."

October 1921—Reads a paper before the Clinical Congress of American College of Surgeons in Philadelphia on "Pathological fractures."

October 1921—Codman, James Ewing, and Joseph Bloodgood present the idea of the Registry of Bone Sarcoma to the American College of Surgeons. The idea is accepted and the Registry is made a standing committee of the College.

20 November 1922—Entry for this date in Codman hunting diary opens by noting it is, "Jenny's first season." Jenny was his new dog.

Dec 1922 - Jan 1923—Takes a southern hunting trip with Katherine and several friends, visiting and hunting in Delaware, North Carolina, South Carolina, Georgia, and Florida.

3-6 September 1924—Reads a paper before the American Roentgen Ray Society, Swampscott, Massachusetts on "The nomenclature used by the registry of bone sarcoma."

1925—Publication of his book on the Registry of Bone Sarcoma, *Bone Sarcoma: An Interpretation of the Nomenclature Used by the Committee on the Registry of Bone Sarcoma of the American College of Surgeons.*

11 June 1927—Elected an honorary member of the New England Roentgen Ray Society for his early contributions to the field of radiology.

1928—He begins writing his book *The Shoulder*.

25 January 1928—Reads a paper before the Suffolk District Medical Society on "The application of pathology to surgical problems."

13-17 October 1930—Reads two papers before the Clinical Congress of the American College of Surgeons, Philadelphia, one on "Rupture of the supraspinatus tendon," and the other on "Epiphyseal chondromatous giant cell tumors of the upper end of the humerus."

16 March 1932—Codman is involved in an automobile accident outside Harvard Medical School, when two boys run in front of his car, and he hits one of them, William McDonald of Roxbury, who is, fortunately, not seriously injured.

June-August 1933—Amory and Katherine Codman take a trip to Ireland, during which time Amory hunts in many different counties of Ireland.

1934—Publication of *The Shoulder: Rupture of the Supraspinatus Tendon and Other Lesions In or About the Subacromial Bursa*.

25 May 1934—Reads a paper before the New York Memorial Hospital on "Symposium on the treatment of primary malignant bone tumors. The Memorial Hospital conference on the treatment of bone sarcoma."

19-23 October 1936—Reads a paper before the Cancer Symposium of the Clinical Congress of the American College of Surgeons, Philadelphia on "Treatment of giant cell tumors about knee. A study of 153 cases collected by the registry of bone sarcoma of the American College of Surgeons."

Spring 1937—Anna Codman, Amory's only sister, dies.

17 March 1938—Dr. Edward Martin, a close friend of Codman's, and probably the biggest supporter of his End Result Idea, dies in Philadelphia.

9 May 1938—Codman's surviving brother, William Coombs Codman, Jr., dies.

7 October 1939—Harvey Cushing dies in New Haven, Connecticut.

January 1940—Codman is presented with a gold medal by the American Academy of Orthopaedic Surgery (AAOS) for his work on bone sarcoma and for his presentation on that topic at the AAOS Annual Meeting in Boston.

23 November 1940—Ernest Amory Codman, M.D. dies of malignant melanoma at his retirement home in Ponkapoag, Massachusetts.

25 November 1940—Codman's funeral takes place at 3:00 P.M., with a service at the Story Chapel in the Mt. Auburn Cemetery in Cambridge, Massachusetts, where he is buried—his name does not appear on the mausoleum in which he rests.

1 March 1961—Katherine Putnam Bowditch Codman dies.

APPENDIX III

ERNEST AMORY CODMAN, M.D.—*CURRICULUM VITÆ*

Following is a complete listing of Codman's published literature. It is listed chronologically, as all the articles have Codman as either first or, in most cases, only author. The search began with the chart in the Preface to *The Shoulder*, but unfortunately, that chart was missing almost half his published articles. He also included a bibliography of his published works in his first book, *A Study in Hospital Efficiency*, but that also omitted a few of his early papers. The gaps were filled by the use of *Index Medicus* (1891-1926), *Quarterly Cumulative Index to [Current] Medical Literature* (1916-1926), and after their merger, *Quarterly Cumulative Index Medicus* (1927-1944), for the years 1891-1944. It should be noted that none of the above five sources contains all his published works, and that all the sources were necessary to compile the following list. To be certain of all references, sources, and page numbers, I have been able to obtain and examine <u>all</u> of his published literature for use in this biography.

Journal Articles
1. Codman EA. Experiments on the application of the roentgen rays to the study of anatomy. *J Exp Med*, <u>3(3)</u>: 383-391, 3 March 1898. [Report by the author to the Committee on the Bullard Fellowship of the Harvard Medical School, 1 May 1897.]
2. Codman EA. A case of actinomycosis. *Boston Med Surg J*, <u>139(6)</u>: 134-135, 11 August 1898. [Read before the Surgical Section of the Suffolk District Medical Society, 6 April 1898.]

3. Codman EA. A study of the x-ray plates of one hundred and forty cases of fracture of the lower end of the radius. *Boston Med Surg J*, <u>143(13)</u>: 305-308, 27 Sep 1900. [Read before the Boston Society for Medical Improvement, 19 March 1900.]

4. Codman EA. Comment to paper read by Dr. J. L. Goodale on "Retropharyngeal abscess." *Boston Med Surg J*, <u>144(5)</u>: 116, 31 January 1901.

5. Codman EA. Acute perforation of a malignant ulcer of the pylorus resembling a case of acute appendicitis. *Boston Med Surg J*, <u>146(9)</u>: 228-230, 27 February 1902. [Read before the Clinical Section of the Suffolk District Medical Society, 15 January 1902.]

6. Codman EA. A study of the cases of accidental x-ray burns hitherto recorded. *Philadelphia Med J*, <u>9(10)</u>: 438-442, 8 March 1902.

7. Codman EA. A study of the cases of accidental x-ray burns hitherto recorded. *Philadelphia Med J*, <u>9(11)</u>: 499-503, 15 March 1902.

8. Codman EA. A resume of the results of Dr. [FB] Harrington's service from June to Oct. 1, 1900, as seen in the following June or later. *Boston Med Surg J*, <u>146(20)</u>: 515-517, 15 May 1902. [Read before the Clinical Meeting of the Medical Board of the Massachusetts General Hospital, April 1902.]

9. Codman EA. The use of the X-ray in surgery. *Johns Hopkins Hosp Bull*, <u>14(146)</u>: 120-124, May 1903. [Read before the Johns Hopkins Medical Society, 2 February 1903, and also before the Nova Scotia Medical Society in early 1904.] (Abstract also published in *Nova Scotia Med Bull*, <u>16</u>: 269, June 1904.)

10. Codman EA. Clinical meeting of the staff of the Massachusetts General Hospital, Feb. 20, 1903. *Boston Med Surg J*, <u>149(4)</u>:101-102, 23 July 1903. [Codman presented three cases: 1) Traumatic rupture of kidney; nephrectomy; recovery. 2) Osteo-chondroma of posterior surface of pubes; excision; recovery; no recurrence in a year and a half. 3) Intussusception in a man of twenty-four; resection of the intestine; recovery.]

11. Codman EA. The formation of loose cartilages in the knee joint. *Boston Med Surg J*, 149(16): 427-428, 15 October 1903. [Read at the Annual Meeting of the Suffolk District Medical Society, 25 April 1903.]

12. Codman EA. Report of a bone cyst of a digital phalanx. *Boston Med Surg J*, 150(8): 211-212, 25 February 1904.

13. Codman EA. Some points on the diagnosis and treatment of certain neglected minor surgical lesions. *Boston Med Surg J*, 150(14): 371-374, 7 April 1904. [Was to be read at the meeting of the Worcester District Medical Society on 9 March 1904, but omitted due to lack of time.]

14. Codman EA. Results of Dr. FB Harringtons service - 1 June → 1 October 1900. *Boston Med Surg J*, 150(23): 618-622, 9 June 1904.

15. Codman EA. Remarks on the resume of Dr. F. B. Harrington's service for the year 1902. *Boston Med Surg J*, 151(3): 74-75, 21 July 1904.

16. Codman EA. The use of the X-ray in the diagnosis of diseases of the bone. *Canada Lancet*, 38: 128-132, 1904-1905. (Also published in *Maritime Medical News*, 16: 295-299, 1904.) [Read before the Maritime Medical Association, July 1904.]

17. Codman EA. A method of rhinoplasty illustrated by plastic operation for rodent ulcer on the face. *Boston Med Surg J*, 152(10): 275-278, 9 March 1905.

18. Codman EA, Chase HM. The diagnosis and treatment of fracture of the carpal scaphoid and dislocation of the semilunar bone: With a report of thirty cases. [Part I]. *Ann Surg*, 41(3): 321-362, March 1905.

19. Codman EA. The use of the X-ray in the post-operative treatment of cancer in the mouth. *Boston Med Surg J*, 152(15): 424-425, 13 April 1905.

20. Codman EA, Chase HM. The diagnosis and treatment of fracture of the carpal scaphoid and dislocation of the semilunar bone. With a report of thirty cases. [Part II]. *Ann Surg*, 41(6): 863-902, June 1905. (Abstract of this report and the one of March 1905 in *Annals of Surgery* was also published in *Publ Mass Genl Hosp*, 1: 102-104, 1906.)

21. Codman EA. Report of results in nontraumatic surgery of brain and spinal cord. Observations upon the actual results of cerebral surgery at the Massachusetts General Hospital. *Boston Med Surg J*, 153(3): 74-76, 20 July 1905. [Read at a meeting of the Section for Surgery of the Suffolk District Branch of the Massachusetts Medical Society in conjunction with the Boston Medical Library, 5 April 1905.]

22. Codman EA. A case of amputation at the shoulder joint for infection with Welch's gas-producing bacillus. Recovery. *Boston Med Surg J*, 154(10): 270-271, 8 March 1906.

23. Codman EA. Removal of a clasp pin from the right bronchus and a hairpin from the bladder. *Boston Med Surg J*, 154(10): 271, 8 March 1906.

24. Codman EA. On stiff and painful shoulders. The anatomy of the subdeltoid or subacromial bursa and its clinical importance. Subdeltoid bursitis. *Boston Med Surg J*, 154(22): 613-620, 31 May 1906. [Read before the Academy of Medicine at Cleveland, 17 March 1906.]

25. Codman EA. A report of recurrent spontaneous gangrene of the index finger: Successive amputations of the phalanges: Abatement of the process after excision of a portion of the radial nerve and stretching of the median nerve. *Boston Med Surg J*, 155(2): 33-36, 12 July 1906. [Read at the Surgical Section of the Suffolk District Medical Society (Library Meeting), 24 January 1906.]

26. Codman EA. On the bier treatment of infections and septic wounds of the extremities. *Boston Med Surg J*, 155(16): 434-435, 18 October 1906. [Also published in *Publ Mass Genl Hosp*, 1(3): 63-67, 1907.]

27. Codman EA. On stiff and painful shoulders. Subdeltoid bursitis: the anatomy of the subdeltoid or subacromial bursa and its clinical significance. *Ohio State Med J*, 2(2): 55-68, 15 August 1906. [Read before the Academy of Medicine of Cleveland, 16 March 1906.]

28. Codman EA. Observations on six cases of acute perforating ulcer of the duodenum. *Boston Med Surg J*, 158(7): 217-219, 13 February 1908.

29. Codman EA. Case of bullet wound of the brain; successful removal of the bullet. *Boston Med Surg J*, 158(7): 228-229, 13 February 1908.

30. Codman EA. Remarks upon intussusception, with a suggestion for a new method of operation upon cases in which reduction is not possible. *Boston Med Surg J*, 158(14): 439-446, 2 April 1908.

31. Codman EA. Chronic obstruction of the duodenum by the root of the mesentery. *Boston Med Surg J*, 158(16): 503-510, 16 April 1908. [Prepared for the Clinical Meeting of the Medical Board of the Massachusetts General Hospital, 13 March 1908.]

32. Codman EA. A case of intra-vesical cyst of the ureter: dilatation of ureter with very slight dilatation of the renal pelvis and containing twenty-eight movable calculi; bacteriuria; alkalinuria; phosphaturia. *Boston Med Surg J*, 158(22): 828-831, 28 May 1908. [Read at the meeting of the Suffolk District Medical Society in conjunction with the Boston Medical Library, 5 February 1908.]

33. Codman EA. Bursitis subacromialis, or periarthritis of the shoulder-joint [Subdeltoid bursitis]. *Boston Med Surg J*, 159(17): 533-537, 22 October 1908. (See also final article in series for other publication and presentation data.)

34. Codman EA. Bursitis subacromialis, or periarthritis of the shoulder-joint [Subdeltoid bursitis]. *Boston Med Surg J*, 159(18): 576-582, 29 October 1908. (See also final article in series for other publication and presentation data.)

35. Codman EA. Bursitis subacromialis, or periarthritis of the shoulder-joint [Subdeltoid bursitis]. *Boston Med Surg J*, 159(19): 615-616, 5 November 1908. (See also final article in series for other publication and presentation data.)

36. Codman EA. Bursitis subacromialis, or periarthritis of the shoulder-joint [Subdeltoid bursitis]. *Boston Med Surg J*, 159(20): 644-648, 12 November 1908. (See also final article in series for other publication and presentation data.)

37. Codman EA. Bursitis subacromialis, or periarthritis of the shoulder-joint [Subdeltoid bursitis]. *Boston Med Surg J*, 159(21): 677-681, 19 November 1908. (See also final article in series for other publication and presentation data.)

38. Codman EA. Bursitis subacromialis, or periarthritis of the shoulder-joint [Subdeltoid bursitis]. *Boston Med Surg J*, 159(22): 723-726, 26 November 1908. (See also final article in series for other publication and presentation data.)

39. Codman EA. Bursitis subacromialis, or periarthritis of the shoulder-joint [Subdeltoid bursitis]. *Boston Med Surg J*, 159(23): 756-759, 3 December 1908. (Entire series of above seven [7] articles also published in *Commun Mass Med Soc*, 21: 277-359, 1908; and in *Publ Mass Genl Hosp*, 2(2): 521-591, October 1909.) [Entire series of above seven (7) articles read before the Massachusetts Medical Society, 9 June 1908.]

40. Codman EA. Bone transference. Report of a case of operation after the method of Huntington. *Ann Surg*, 49(6): 820-823, June 1909. [Read before the meeting of the Suffolk District Medical Society, 3 February 1907.] (Also published in *Publ Mass Genl Hosp*, 2: 592-597, 1909.)

41. Codman EA. On the surgical significance of pus, blood and bacteria in the urine. *Boston Med Surg J*, 161(6): 177-183, 5 August 1909. [Read before the New Bedford Medical Society, 10 April 1909.]

42. Codman EA. On the importance of distinguishing simple round ulcers of the duodenum from those ulcers which involve the pylorus or are above it. *Boston Med Surg J*, 161(10): 313-318, 2 September 1909 (See also final article in series for other publication data.)

43. Codman EA. On the importance of distinguishing simple round ulcers of the duodenum from those ulcers which involve the pylorus or are above it. *Boston Med Surg J*, 161(11): 351-355, 9 September 1909. (See also final article in series for other publication data.)

44. Codman EA. On the importance of distinguishing simple round ulcers of the duodenum from those ulcers which involve the

pylorus or are above it. *Boston Med Surg J*, <u>161(12)</u>: 399-403, 16 September 1909. [Entire series of three (3) articles read before the Worcester District Medical Society, 14 April 1909.] (Entire series of above three [3] articles also published in in *Publ Mass Genl Hosp*, <u>3</u>: 35-82, 1910. In addition, a pre-publication abstract of the series was given in the *Boston Med Surg J*, <u>160(17)</u>: 550, 29 April 1909.)

45. Codman EA. The diagnosis of ulcer of the duodenum. *Boston Med Surg J*, <u>161(22)</u>: 767-774, 25 November 1909. (See also final article in series for other publication and presentation data.)

46. Codman EA. The diagnosis of ulcer of the duodenum. *Boston Med Surg J*, <u>161(23)</u>: 816-822, 2 December 1909. (See also final article in series for other publication and presentation data.)

47. Codman EA. The diagnosis of ulcer of the duodenum. *Boston Med Surg J*, <u>161(24)</u>: 853-857, 9 December 1909. (See also final article in series for other publication and presentation data.)

48. Codman EA. The diagnosis of ulcer of the duodenum. *Boston Med Surg J*, <u>161(25)</u>: 887-891, 16 December 1909. (Entire series of above four [4] articles also published in *Commun Mass Med Soc*, <u>22</u>: 465-548, 1909; and in *Publ Mass Genl Hosp*, <u>3</u>: 83-143, 1910.) [Entire series of above four (4) articles read at the annual meeting of the Massachusetts Medical Society, 15 June 1909.]

49. Codman EA. Case of mesenteric thrombosis; resection of intestine; end-to-end anastomosis. Recovery. *Boston Med Surg J*, <u>162(11)</u>: 355-357, 17 March 1910. [Read at a clinical meeting of the Medical Board, Massachusetts General Hospital, 14 January 1910.] (Also published in *Publ Mass Genl Hosp*, <u>3</u>: 146-149, 1910.)

50. Codman EA. Depressed fracture of the malar bone. A simple method of reduction. *Boston Med Surg J*, <u>162(16)</u>: 532, 21 April 1910. [Also published in *Publ Mass Genl Hosp*, <u>3</u>: 144-145, 1910.]

51. Codman EA. Complete rupture of the supraspinatus tendon. Operative treatment with report of two successful cases. *Boston Med Surg J*, <u>164(20)</u>: 708-710, 18 May 1911.

52. Codman EA. Progress in surgery. Duodenal ulcer. *Boston Med Surg J*, <u>165(2)</u>: 54-59, 13 July 1911.

53. Codman EA. "On stiff and painful shoulders" as explained by subacromial bursitis and partial rupture of the tendon of the supraspinatus. *Boston Med Surg J*, 165(4): 115-120, 27 July 1911.

54. Codman EA. Comment on S. W. Goddard's article on "surgical treatment of pyloric stenosis, with report of cases." *Boston Med Surg J*, 165(13): 479-483, 28 September 1911.

55. Codman EA. Diagnosis of diseases of the stomach and intestines by the x-ray. *Boston Med Surg J*, 166(5): 155-159, 1 February 1912. [Read before the Waltham Medical Club, 7 December 1911.]

56. Codman EA. Abduction of the shoulder. An interesting observation in connection with subacromial bursitis and rupture of the tendon of the supraspinatus. *Boston Med Surg J*, 166(24): 890-891, 13 June 1912.

57. Codman EA. Observations on a series of ninety-eight consecutive operations for chronic appendicitis. *Boston Med Surg J*, 169(14): 495-502, 2 October 1913. [Read at the annual meeting of The Massachusetts Medical Society, 10 June 1913.] (Also published in *Commun Mass Med Soc*, 24(1): 227-250, 1913.)

58. Codman EA. Our little balloons. Some observations on gas and ptosis. *Boston Med Surg J*, 169(15): 540-542, 9 October 1913.

59. Codman EA, Chipman WW, Clark JG, Kanavel AB, Mayo WJ. Standardization of Hospitals: Report of the committed appointed by the Clinical Congress of Surgeons of North America. *Trans Clin Cong Surg North Amer*, 4: 2-8, November 1913.

60. Codman EA. Comments in discussion section of article by JA Hornsby, "Standardization of Hospitals." *Trans Am Hosp Assoc*, 15: 183-190, 1913.

61. Codman EA. Committee for hospital standardization. *Surg Gyn Obst*, 18(Suppl): 8-12, January 1914.

62. Codman EA, Sheldon RF. The prognosis of sarcoma of the testicle. *Boston Med Surg J*, 170(8): 267-269, 19 February 1914

63. Codman EA. Money spent on hospitals is for cure of patients: follow-up system the only way to determine value of institution's services-accounts must include death and

disability, which are wasted effort. *Modern Hosp*, 2(2): 87-88, February 1914. [Read before the American Hospital Association, 27 August 1913.]

64. Codman EA. The product of a hospital. *Surg Gyn Obst*, 18(4): 491-496, April 1914. [Read before the Philadelphia County Medical Society, 14 May 1913] (Reprinted in *Arch Pathol Lab Med*, 114: 1106-1111, November 1990.)

65. Codman EA. A study in hospital efficiency as represented by product. *Trans Am Gynec Soc*, 39: 60-100, 1914.

66. Codman EA. Report of committee for hospital standardization. *Surg Gyn Obst*, 22(1): 119-120, January 1916. [*In:* Transactions of the Clinical Congress of Surgeons of North America.]

67. Codman EA. The dividing line between medical charity and medical business. *Medical Record*, 89: 868-872, 13 May 1916. [Read before the Harvard Medical Society of New York on 22 January 1916.]

68. Codman EA. A wise preliminary to the adoption of any compulsory health insurance act. *Boston Med Surg J*, 176(12): 435-438, 22 March 1917.

69. Codman EA. Uniformity in hospital morbidity reports. *Boston Med Surg J*, 177(9): 279-283, 30 August 1917.

70. Codman EA. Comments to Robert L. Dickinson article on "Hospital organization as shown by charts of personnel and powers and functions." *Bull Taylor Society*, 3(5): 4, October 1917. [Dickinson article and Codman comments presented before The Taylor Society in New York, 8 December 1916.]

71. Codman EA. The value of case records in hospitals. *Modern Hosp*, 9: 426-428, December 1917. [Read at the Hospital Standardization Session of the American College of Surgeons, Chicago, 19-20 October 1917.]

72. Codman EA. Case-records and their value. *Bull Am Coll Surg*, 3(1): 24-27, 1917. [Presented at the Conference on Hospital Standardization Joint Session of Committees on Standards, Chicago, 19-20 October 1917.]

73. Codman EA. The treatment of malignant peritonitis of ovarian origin. *Ann Surg*, 68: 338-346, 1918. [Read before the American

Surgical Association, 8 June 1918.] (Also published in *Trans Am Surg Assoc*, 36: 483-494, 1918.)

74. Codman EA. Intestinal obstruction. *Boston Med Surg J*, 182(17): 420-424, 22 April 1920. [Read before the Springfield Academy of Medicine on 11 November 1919.]

75. Codman EA. Intestinal obstruction. *Boston Med Surg J*, 182(18): 451-458, 29 April 1920. [Read before the Springfield Academy of Medicine on 11 November 1919.]

76. Codman EA. The registry of cases of bone sarcoma. *Surg Gyn Obst*, 34(3): 335-343, March 1922.

77. Codman EA. The registry of bone sarcoma and medical human nature. *Boston Med Surg J*, 187(6): 208-211, 10 August 1922.

78. Codman EA. Bone sarcoma; prevalence in Massachusetts. *Boston Med Surg J*, 187(15): 543-544, 12 October 1922.

79. Codman EA. Pathological fractures. *Surg Gyn Obst*, 34: 611-613, May 1922. [Read before the Clinical Congress of American College of Surgeons, Philadelphia, October 1921.]

80. Codman EA, Pool EH. The analysis of end-results: Joint discussion. *Surg Gyn Obst*, 36: 138-140, 1923. (Also published in *Bull Amer Coll Surg*, 8: 15-17, 1923.)

81. Codman EA. The method of procedure of the registry of bone sarcoma. *Surg Gyn Obst*, 38: 712-721, May 1924.

82. Codman EA. A new instrument to be called the registry of bone sarcoma scissors. *Surg Gyn Obst*, 39: 127-128, July 1924. (Also published in *Boston Med Surg J*, 190(17): 710, 24 April 1924.)

83. Codman EA. The nomenclature used by the registry of bone sarcoma. *Am J Roentgenology Radium Ther*, 13(2): 105-126, February 1925. [Read at the Twenty-Fifth Annual Meeting, American Roentgen Ray Society, Swampscott, Mass., 3-6 September 1924.]

84. Codman EA. The pathology and treatment of lesions in and about the shoulder joint. *Indust Doct*, 4(8): 121-131, 1926.

85. Codman EA. Registry of bone sarcoma: Part I—Twenty-five criteria for establishing the diagnosis of osteogenic sarcoma; Part II—Thirteen registered cases of "five year cures" analyzed

according to these criteria. *Surg Gyn Obst*, <u>42</u>: 381-393, March 1926.

86. Codman EA. Obscure lesions of the shoulder; rupture of the supraspinatus tendon. *Boston Med Surg J*, <u>196(10)</u>: 381-387, 10 March 1927.

87. Codman EA. The application of pathology to surgical problems. *New Engl J Med*, <u>198(7)</u>: 330-332, 5 April 1928. [Read before the Suffolk District Medical Society, 25 January 1928.] [Note: *Boston Medical and Surgical Journal* became the *New England Journal of Medicine* in late 1927.]

88. Codman EA. John Wheelock Elliott, M.D. *New Engl J Med*, <u>198(19)</u>: 994-1004, 28 June 1928. [An obituary by Codman on Elliott.]

89. Codman EA, Akerson IB. The pathology associated with rupture of the supraspinatus tendon. *Ann Surg*, <u>93(1)</u>: 348-359, 19 January 1931.

90. Codman EA. Rupture of the supraspinatus tendon. *Surg Gyn Obst*, <u>52(2A)</u>: 579-586, 15 February 1931. [Presented at the Conference on Traumatic Surgery, read before the Clinical Congress of the American College of Surgeons, Philadelphia, 13-17 October 1930.]

91. Codman EA. Epiphyseal chondromatous giant cell tumors of the upper end of the humerus. *Surg Gyn Obst*, <u>52(2A)</u>: 543-548, 15 February 1931. [Presented in the Symposium on Cancer, read before the Clinical Congress of the American College of Surgeons, Philadelphia, 13-17 October 1930.]

92. Codman EA. Symposium on the treatment of primary malignant bone tumors. The Memorial Hospital conference on the treatment of bone sarcoma. *Am J Surg*, <u>27</u>: 3-6, January 1935. [Presented at the Memorial Hospital, New York, 25 May 1934.]

93. Codman EA. Treatment of giant cell tumors about knee. A study of 153 cases collected by the registry of bone sarcoma of the American College of Surgeons. *Surg Gyn Obst*, <u>64(2A)</u>: 485-496, February 1937. [Presented in the Cancer Symposium, before the Clinical Congress of the American College of Surgeons, Philadelphia, 19-23 October 1936.]

94. Codman EA. Rupture of the supraspinatus—1834-1934. *J Bone Joint Surg*, <u>19(3)</u>: 643-652, July 1937.
95. Codman EA. Fishing with J. L. *Recreation*, <u>31(9)</u>: 521-525, 582, December 1937.
96. Codman EA. Rupture of the supraspinatus. *Amer J Surg*, <u>42(3)</u>: 603-626, December 1938.

Published Correspondence

1. Codman EA. Correspondence. Radiograph of fetal arm. *Boston Med Surg J*, <u>134(13)</u>: 327, 26 March 1896.
2. Codman EA. Correspondence. A reversed radiograph. *Boston Med Surg J*, <u>134(18)</u>: 450, 30 April 1896.
3. Codman EA. Correspondence. An important improvement in radiography. *Boston Med Surg J*, <u>134(21)</u>: 522-523, 21 May 1896.
4. Codman EA. Correspondence. Practical medical use of the X-ray. *Boston Med Surg J*, <u>135(2)</u>: 50-51, 9 July 1896.
5. Codman EA. Correspondence. The cause of burns from X-rays. *Boston Med Surg J*, <u>135(24)</u>: 610-611, 10 December 1896.
6. Codman EA. Correspondence. No practical danger from the X-ray. *Boston Med Surg J*, <u>144(8)</u>: 197, 21 February 1901.
7. Codman EA. Correspondence. Diagnosis of subdeltoid bursitis. *Boston Med Surg J*, <u>154(26)</u>: 750, 28 June 1906.
8. Codman EA. Correspondence. Registry of bone sarcoma. *Boston Med Surg J*, <u>186(5)</u>: 161, 2 February 1922.
9. Codman EA. Correspondence. Registry of bone sarcoma. *Boston Med Surg J*, <u>186(10)</u>: 335, 9 March 1922.
10. Codman EA. Correspondence. Registry of bone sarcoma. *Boston Med Surg J*, <u>186(13)</u>: 441-442, 30 March 1922.
11. Codman EA. Correspondence. Registry of bone sarcoma. *Boston Med Surg J*, <u>186(14)</u>: 489, 6 April 1922.
12. Codman EA. Correspondence. Registry of bone sarcoma. *Boston Med Surg J*, <u>186(14)</u>: 489, 6 April 1922.
13. Codman EA. Correspondence. A tribute to Dr. Lawrie Byron Morrison. *New Engl J Med*, <u>206</u>: 276-277, 1933.

Book Chapters

1. Codman EA. "The use of X-ray and radium in surgery," pp. 1143-1179. Chapter LXXXIII, Volume V. In: Keen WW, *Surgery:*

Its Principles and Practices. Philadelphia: Saunders, 1909, 1910, 1911, 1912, 1914, 1916, and 1919.

2. Codman EA. "The X-ray in surgery," pp. 1004-1015. Chapter CLIV, Volume VI. In: Keen WW, *Surgery: Its Principles and Practices*. Philadelphia: Saunders, 1909, 1910, 1911, 1912, 1914, 1916, and 1919.

Books

1. Codman EA. *A Study in Hospital Efficiency. As Demonstrated by the Case Report of the First Two Years of a Private Hospital*. 1st edition privately published by Codman on 10 May 1914, printed by Thomas Todd Co. 2nd edition privately published by Codman on 19 October 1915, printed by Thomas Todd Co.

2. Codman EA. *A Study in Hospital Efficiency. As Demonstrated by the Case Report of the First Five Years of a Private Hospital*. Boston: Thomas Todd Co., 1918-1920. Reprinted edition - Oakbrook Terrace, IL: Joint Commission on Accreditation of Healthcare Organizations, 1995. (The reprinted edition contains three supplementary essays on Codman not contained in the original book.) (The publishing dates of the original book are not certain. No date is listed in the book. In the Preface to *The Shoulder*, Codman appears to give the date as 1919, although he calls the book, *"The End Result Hospital."* Dates listed in *Index Medicus* are 1918 in the January 1919 edition, 1919 in the June 1919 edition, and 1920 in the January 1921 edition. There were probably various printings.)

3. Codman EA. *Bone Sarcoma: An Interpretation of the Nomenclature Used by the Committee on the Registry of Bone Sarcoma of the American College of Surgeons.*. New York: Paul B. Hoeber, Inc., 1925. (There were likely several printings. The March 1926 edition of *Index Medicus* listed the book as 93 pages, the June 1926 edition listed it as 107 pages, while the September 1926 edition listed it as 104 pages.)

4. Codman EA. *The Shoulder: Rupture of the Supraspinatus Tendon and Other Lesions In or About the Subacromial Bursa*. Boston: Thomas Todd Co., 1934. 1st Reprinted Edition— Brooklyn: G. Miller & Co., 1965. 2nd Reprinted Edition—

Malabar, FL: Robert E. Krieger, 1984. 3rd Reprinted Edition—
New York: The Classics of Surgery Library, Gryphon Editions,
1991. (The 2nd reprinted edition contains a foreword by
Anthony F. DePalma, M.D. not contained in the original
edition. I have the original edition and the Krieger edition, but
have never found a copy of the edition published by Miller in
1965. The Classics of Surgery edition is a direct re-print but a
small summary of Codman's life has been inserted as a small
pamphlet.)

SOURCES CONSULTED

In addition to all of Codman's own works (see Appendix Three), all of the following sources were used in the compilation of this biography.

1. Albert E. **Diagnöstik der Chirugischer Krankheiten**. Vienna: Alfred Holder, 1893.
2. Barzansky B, Gevitz N, eds. **Beyond Flexner: Medical Education in the Twentieth Century**. New York: Greenwood Press, 1992.
3. Beatty J. **The Rascal King**. Reading, MA: Addison-Wesley, 1992.
4. Beecher HK. The first anesthesia records (Codman, Cushing). Surg Gyn Obst, 71: 689-693, 1940.
5. Berwick DM. E. A. Codman and the rhetoric of battle: a commentary. Milbank Quarterly, 67(2): 262-267, 1989.
6. Beveridge WI. **Influenza: The Last Great Plague. An Unfinished Story of Discovery**. New York: Prodist, 1978.
7. Bird MJ. **The Town that Died**. Halifax, Nova Scotia: Nimbus Publishing Limited, 1995. (Originally published by Toronto: McGraw-Hill Ryerson, 1967.)
8. **Blakiston's Gould Medical Dictionary**. 4th edition. New York: McGraw-Hill, 1979.
9. Bloom BS. Does it work? The outcomes of medical interventions. Int J Tech Assessment in Health Care, 6: 326-332, 1990.

10. Book Review of **L'Épaule**, by Antoine Basset and Jacques Mialaret. Paris: Masson et. Cie, 1934. In: J Bone Joint Surg, <u>17(1)</u>: 243-244, January 1935.

11. Book Review of **The Shoulder: Rupture of the Supraspinatus Tendon and Other Lesions in or About the Subacromial Bursa**. In: J Bone Joint Surg, <u>16(3)</u>: 745-746, July 1934.

12. Book Review of **The Shoulder: Rupture of the Supraspinatus Tendon and Other Lesions in or About the Subacromial Bursa**. In: Surgery, Gynecology & Obstetrics, <u>60(1)</u>: 130, January 1935.

13. "Bowditch, Charles Pickering," In: **Dictionary of American Biography**, Volume II, p. 492. New York: Scribners, 1929.

14. "Bowditch, Charles Pickering," In: **The National Cyclopædia of American Biography**, <u>20</u>: 290-291. New York: James T. White & Co., 1943.

15. "Bowditch, Henry Ingersoll," In: **Dictionary of American Biography**, Volume II, pp. 492-494. New York: Scribners, 1929.

16. "Bowditch, Henry Pickering," In: **Dictionary of American Biography**, Volume II, pp. 494-496. New York: Scribners, 1929.

17. "Bowditch, Nathaniel," In: **Dictionary of American Biography**, Volume II, pp. 496-498. New York: Scribners, 1929.

18. Burkhead WZ, Habermeyer P. The rotator cuff: a historical review of our understanding. In: **Rotator Cuff Disorders**, WZ Burkhead, Jr., ed., pp. 8-13. Baltimore: Williams & Wilkins, 1996.

19. **Butterworth's Medical Dictionary**. 2nd edition. M Critchley, ed. London: Butterworth, 1978.

20. "Cabot, Richard Clarke," In: **National Cyclopædia of American Biography**, <u>A</u>: 223-224. New York: James T. White & Co., 1930.

21. "Cartoon by Physician Makes Stir," Boston Post, 18 January 1915, pp. 1, 3.

22. "Cartoon Raises Surgeons' Ire," Boston Daily Globe, 18 January 1915, pp. 1, 5.

23. Christoffel T. Medical care evaluation: an old new idea. J Med Ed, <u>51</u>: 83-88, 1976.

24. "Clark, John Goodrich," In: **National Cyclopædia of American Biography**, 21: 63-64. New York: James T. White & Co., 1931.

25. "Dr. Codman, Bone Specialist, Dies at His Home Here," In: Canton Journal, 29 November 1940, p. 1.

26. "Dr. Codman Rites Today: Noted Bone Surgeon Died in Ponkapoag," In: Boston Herald. 25 November 1940.

27. "Codman, Ernest Amory," In: **The National Cyclopædia of American Biography**, 30: 66-67. New York: James T. White & Co., 1943.

28. "Codman, John," In: **Dictionary of American Biography**, Volume IV, p. 259. New York: Scribners, 1930.

29. Codman KB. "District nursing after the Chelsea fire," In: Charities and the Commons, 31: 970-973, 13 February 1909.

30. "Codman, Richard," In: **The National Cyclopædia of American Biography**, 22: 132-133. New York: James T. White & Co., 1932.

31. Codman EA. "The situation at the Y.M.C.A. Hospital on the evening of December 14, 1917, with a brief statement concerning the use of the Y.M.C.A. Building since the accident on Dec. 6th. Dr. Codman's connection with the Hospital." In: Harris DF. "Report of the Halifax Medical Commission." Unpublished document held at the Public Archives of Nova Scotia, Call Number MG36c, #118-119.

32. Coley BL. **Neoplasms of Bone and Related Conditions: Their Etiology, Pathogenesis, Diagnosis, and Treatment**. New York: Paul B. Hoeber, 1927.

33. Coley BL, Santuro A. Benign central cartilaginous tumors of bone. Surgery, 22(3): 411-423, September 1947.

34. Committee for Standardization of Hospitals [of the American College of Surgeons]. Minimum standard for hospitals, Bull Am Coll Surg, 8: 4, 1924.

35. Crosby AW, Jr. "The Influenza Pandemic of 1918," In: **History, Science, and Politics: Influenza in America 1918-1976**, June E. Osborn, ed. New York: Prodist, 1977.

36. "Curley, James Michael," In: **National Cyclopædia of American Biography**, A: 431-432, . New York: James T. White & Co., 1930.

37. "Cushing, Harvey Williams," In: **Dictionary of American Biography**, Supplement Two. pp. 137-140. New York: Scribners, 1958.

38. "Cushing, Harvey Williams," In: **National Cyclopædia of American Biography**, 32: 402-404. New York: James T. White & Co., 1945.

39. Davis L. **Fellowship of Surgeons: A History of the American College of Surgeons**. Springfield, IL: C. C. Thomas, 1960.

40. Dickinson RL. Hospital efficiency from the standpoint of a hospital surgeon, Boston Medical and Surgical Journal, 172(21): 775-778, 27 May 1915. Abstract of paper read by Dickinson at the Boston Medical Library Meeting of 6 January 1915.

41. "Dickinson, Robert Latou," In: **National Cyclopædia of American Biography**, 39: 485-486, New York: James T. White & Co., 1954.

42. "Doctor-Critic Stirs Wrath," Boston Herald, 18 January 1915, p. 9.

43. Donabedian A. The end results of health care: Ernest Codman's contribution to quality assessment and beyond. Milbank Quarterly, 67(2): 233-256, 1989. [Revised and expanded version of speech made at the Harvard School of Public Health on 15 November 1988.]

44. **Dorland's Illustrated Medical Dictionary**. 28th edition. Philadelphia: WB Saunders, 1994.

45. Firkin BG, Whitworth JA. **Dictionary of Medical Eponyms**. 2nd edition. New York: Parthenon, 1996.

46. Flexner A. **Medical Education in the United States and Canada: Report to the Carnegie Foundation for Advancement of Teaching**. New York: Merrymount Press, 1910.

47. Fulton J. **Harvey Cushing: A Biography**. Springfield, IL: C. C. Thomas, 1946.

48. Gilbreth FB. Hospital efficiency from the standpoint of the efficiency expert, Boston Medical and Surgical Journal, 172(21):

774-779, 27 May 1915. Abstract of paper read by Gilbreth at the Boston Medical Library Meeting of 6 January 1915.

49. "Gilbreth, Frank Bunker," In: **National Cyclopædia of American Biography**, 26: 401-402. New York: James T. White & Co., 1937.

50. Goldthwait JE. An anatomic and mechanical study of the shoulder-joint, explaining many of the cases of painful shoulder, many of the recurrent dislocations, and many of the cases of brachial neuralgias or neuritis. Am J Ortho Surg, 6: 579-606, 1909.

51. "Goldthwait, Joel Ernest," In: **National Cyclopædia of American Biography**, 49: 207-208, New York: James T. White & Co., 1966.

52. Griscom JT, Teele RL. Radiology at Children's Hospital in Boston: a history. Amer J Roentgenology, 161: 887-891, 1993.

53. "Halifax," In: **Encyclopedia Canadiana**, 5: 62-63. Toronto: Grolier of Canada, 1972.

54. "Hamilton, Alice," In: **National Cyclopædia of American Biography**, G: 107-108. New York: James T. White & Co., 1946.

55. Hamilton A. **Exploring the Dangerous Trades: The Autobiography of Alice Hamilton, M.D.** Boston: Little Brown, 1943.

56. Harris DF. "Report of the Halifax Medical Commission." Unpublished document held at the Nova Scotia Public Archives. (Contains Codman's report of his work in Halifax — see above reference under Codman.)

57. **Harvard Annual Report: 1886—1890**. Cambridge: Harvard University, 1891.

58. **Harvard Annual Report: 1890—1894**. Cambridge: Harvard University, 1895.

59. **Harvard Annual Report: 1894—1896**. Cambridge: Harvard University, 1897.

60. Harvard College, Class of 1891. **Secretary's Report, No. 3**. Cambridge: Privately printed, 1899.

61. Harvard College, Class of 1891. **Secretary's Report, No. V**. Cambridge: Privately printed, 1911.

62. Harvard College, Class of 1891. **Twenty-Fifth Anniversary Report: 1891-1916**, pp. 67-68. Norwood, MA: Plimpton Press, 1916.

63. Harvard College, Class of 1891. **50ᵗʰ Anniversary of the Class of 1891**. Camrbidge: Privately printed, 1941.

64. "He stood 8 feet tall but was invisible," MGH News. February 1972.

65. Henry RS. **The Armed Forces Institute of Pathology: Its First Century 1862-1962**. Washington: United States Government Printing Office, 1964.

66. Homans J. Obituary: Ernest Amory Codman (1869-1940). New Engl J Med, 224(7): 296-299, 13 February 1941.

67. "Howard, Herbert Burr," In: **Who Was Who in America**. Vol. 3, p. 593. Chicago: Marquis Who's Who, 1960.

68. Jaffe HL, Liechtenstein L. Benign chondroblastoma of bone: a re-interpretation of the so-called calcifying or chondromatous giant cell tumor. Amer J Path, 18(6): 969-991, 1942.

69. JCAHO. "Voluntary accreditation: its value and evolution in a changing health care environment," In: **Committed to Quality: An Introduction to the Joint Commission on Accreditation of Healthcare Organizations**. Oakbrook Terrace, Illinois: JCAHO, 1985, 1987, 1988, and 1990.

70. JCAHO. Brochure on "The 1997 Ernest A. Codman Award," Oakbrook Terrace, Illinois: JCAHO, 1998.

71. "Kanavel, Allen Buckner," In: **National Cyclopædia of American Biography**, 28: 17. New York: James T. White & Co., 1940.

72. Kaufman M, Galishoff S, Savitt TL, eds. **Dictionary of American Medical Biography**. Westport, CT: Greenwood Press, 1984.

73. Kolodny A. **Bone Sarcoma: The Primary Malignant Tumors of Bone and The Giant Cell Tumor**. Chicago: Surgical Publishing Company of Chicago, 1927. (Contains dedication to Codman)

74. Küster E. Ueber Bursitis subacromialis (periarthritis humero-scapularis). Archiv Klin Chir, 67: 1013-1021, 1902.

75. Lembcke PA. Evolution of the medical audit. J Amer Med Assoc, <u>199(8)</u>: 111-118, 1967.

76. "Martin, Edward," In: **National Cyclopædia of American Biography**, <u>33</u>: 420-421. New York: James T. White & Co., 1947.

77. "Mayo, Charles Horace," In: **National Cyclopædia of American Biography**. <u>30</u>: 2-3, 1943.

78. "Mayo, William James," In: **National Cyclopædia of American Biography**. <u>30</u>: 1-2, 1943.

79. McGuire KJ. **The End Results System: Ernest Amory Codman and the Origins of Accountability in American Medicine, 1910-1934**. B.A. Thesis, Princeton University, 1993.

80. McLendon WW. Ernest A. Codman, MD (1869-1940), the end result idea, and The Product of a Hospital. Arch Pathol Lab Med, <u>114</u>: 1101-1104, November 1990.

81. **Mellon's Illustrated Medical Dictionary**. 3rd edition. New York: Parthenon, 1993.

82. Metson, G. **The Halifax Explosion, December 6, 1917**. Toronto: McGraw-Hill Ryerson, Ltd., 1967.

83. Millenson ML. **Demanding Medical Excellence: Doctors and Accountability in the Information Age**. Chicago: Univ. of Chicago Press, 1997.

84. Moore FD. Surgical biology and applied sociology: Cannon and Codman fifty years later. Harvard Med Alumni Bull, <u>49(3)</u>: 12-21, Jan/Feb 1975. [Address presented to the Boston Surgical Society on the occasion of the award of the Henry Jacob Bigelow Medal, 5 November 1973.]

85. Moss AJ. Codman and the chondroblastoma. Research paper written 28 June 1956 as project at the Harvard Medical School. Copy of paper contained in the Codman Archives at the Countway Medical Library, Harvard Medical School.

86. "Mrs. Codman, 90, Doctor's Widow, Philanthropist," Boston Herald, 2 March 1961.

87. Mulley AG Jr. E. A. Codman and the end results idea: a commentary. Milbank Quarterly, <u>67(2)</u>: 257-261, 1989.

88. Murray TJ. Medical aspects of the disaster: the missing report of Dr. David Fraser Harris, pp. 229-244. In: **Ground Zero**, see below under Ruffman and Howell for publishing data.

89. Neer CS II. Displaced proximal humeral fractures. Part I: classification and evaluation. J Bone Joint Surg, <u>52-A(6)</u>: 1077-1089, 1970.

90. Neer CS II. Displaced proximal humeral fractures. Part II: treatment of three-part and four-part displacement. J Bone Joint Surg, <u>52-A(6)</u>: 1090-1103, 1970.

91. Neer CS II. Impingement lesions. Clin Orthop, <u>173</u>: 70, 1983.

92. Neer CS II. **Shoulder Reconstruction**. Philadelphia: W. B. Saunders, 1990.

93. Neuhauser D. Ernest Amory Codman, M.D., and end results of medical care. Int J Tech Assessment Health Care, <u>6</u>: 307-325, 1990.

94. Neuhauser D. "Introduction: Ernest Amory Codman and the end results of medical care." In: **Codman: A Study in Hospital Efficiency. As Demonstrated by the Case Report of the First Five Years of a Private Hospital**, Oakbrook Terrace, IL: Joint Commission on Accreditation of Healthcare Organizations, 1996. pp. 7-47. (This introduction to a reprinted edition of Codman's book is an updated version of Neuhauser's earlier article, with more complete footnote documentation.)

95. **The New Encyclopædia Britannica**. 15th edition. 30 vols. Chicago/London: Encyclopædia Britannica, Inc., 1978.

96. O'Leary DS. A concept in search of fulfillment. J Med Assoc Georgia, <u>76</u>: 569-572, August 1987.

97. Osborn JE, ed. **History, Science, and Politics. Influenza in America 1918-1976**. New York: Prodist, 1977.

98. Peltier LF. "Ernest Amory Codman 1869-1940," In: Codman EA. **The Shoulder: Rupture of the Supraspinatus Tendon and Other Lesions In or About the Subacromial Bursa**. 3rd Reprinted Edition—San Francisco: Norman Publishing, to be published 1999.

99. Quinby WC "Recollections of Grouse Hunting with Amory Codman," In: **Codman, A Study in Hospital Efficiency.**

Oakbrook Terrace, Illinois, Joint Commission and Accreditation of Health Organizations, 1996. pp. 1-6.

100. Rathbun JB, McNab I. The microvascular pattern of the rotator cuff. J Bone Joint Surg, 52-B(3): 540-553, 1970.

101. Ratshesky AC. **Report of the Halifax Relief Expedition, December 6 to 15, 1917**. Boston: Wright and Potter Printing Company, 1918.

102. Relman AS. The third revolution in medical care. New Engl J Med, 319(18): 1220-1222, 3 November 1988.

103. Reverby S. Stealing the golden eggs: Ernest Amory Codman and the science and management of medicine. Bull History Med, 55: 156-171, 1981.

104. Roberts JS, Coale JG, Redman RR. A history of the joint commission on accreditation of hospitals. J Am Med Assoc, 258(7): 936-940, 21 August 1987.

105. Rowe CR. "Codman—his influence on the development of surgery of the shoulder," In: **Shoulder Surgery**, I. Bayley and L. Kessel, eds.. Berlin: Springer-Verlag, 1982. [Lecture given at the First International Conference for Surgery of the Shoulder, London, 1981.]

106. Rowe CR. **Lest We Forget**. Dublin, NH: William L. Bauhan Publisher, 1996.

107. Rowe CR, ed. **The Shoulder**. New York: Churchill Livingstone, 1988. Dedication page to Ernest Amory Codman.

108. Ruffman A and Howell CD, eds. **Ground Zero: A Reassessment of the 1917 Explosion in Halifax Harbour**. Halifax, Nova Scotia: Nimbus Publishing Limited, 1994. Co-published with Gorsebrook Research Institute for Atlantic Canada Studies at Saint Mary's University, Halifax, Nova Scotia.

109. Shumacker HB Jr. **History of The Society of Clinical Surgery**. Indianapolis: Benham Press, Inc., 1977.

110. Sicherman, Barbara. **Alice Hamilton: A Life in Letters**. Cambridge, MA: Harvard University Press, 1984.

111. Simmons CC. Ernest Amory Codman. 1869-1940. Trans Am Surg Assoc, 59: 611-613, 1941.

112. Simmons CC. The follow-up system. Boston Med Surg J, 177(9): 275-279, 30 August 1917.

113. Snodgrass LE. **Observations on "The Shoulder": A Book Review**. Philadelphia: Westbrook Publishing Co., 1938.

114. **Stedman's Medical Dictionary**. 25th edition. Baltimore: Williams & Wilkins, 1990.

115. **Taber's Cyclopedic Medical Dictionary**, 16th illustrated ed. Philadelphia: F. A. Davis, 1989.

116. Taylor FW. **Principles of Scientific Management**. New York: W. W. Norton, 1911.

117. "Taylor, Frederick Winslow," In: **National Cyclopædia of American Biography**. 23: 47-48. New York: James T. White & Co., 1933.

118. Vindex, School newspaper at Saint Mark's School in Southborough, Massachusetts. Editions of January 1886; April 1886; October 1886; and April 1887.

119. Wallechinsky D. **The People's Almanac Presents The Twentieth Century: The Definitive Compendium of Astonishing Events, Amazing People, and Strange-But-True Facts**. Boston: Little Brown, 1995.

120. "Dr. Walter W. Chipman," Obituary In: The New York Times, 5 April 1950, p. 31.

121. Washburn FA. **The Massachusetts General Hospital: Its Development, 1900—1935**. Boston: Houghton-Mifflin, 1939.

122. **Webster's Third New International Dictionary**. 17th edition. 3 vols. Chicago/London: G. & C. Merriam, Co., 1976.

123. Wesselhoeft W. Hospital efficiency from the standpoint of hospital trustees, Boston Med Surg J, 172(21): 778-779, 27 May 1915. Abstract of paper read by Wesselhoeft at the Boston Medical Library Meeting of 6 January 1915.

124. "Wesselhoeft, Walter," In: **National Cyclopædia of American Biography**, 18: 359-360, New York: James T. White & Co., 1922.

125. Wheatley SC. **The Politics of Philanthropy: Abraham Flexner and Medical Education**. Madison, WI: Univ. of Wisconsin Press, 1988.

126. Wilson PD. Complete rupture of the supraspinatus tendon. J Am Med Assoc, 96: 433-438, 1931.

127. Wrege CD. The efficient management of hospitals: pioneer work of Ernest Codman, Robert Dickinson, and Frank Gilbreth, 1910-1918. Proc Acad Mgt, 114-118, 1980.

128. Wrege CD. Medical men and scientific management: a forgotten chapter in management history. Rev Business Econ Res, 18: 32-47, 1983.

PERSONAL CORRESPONDENCE

1. Hill AJdV. Letter to Author of 15 December 1994.
2. McGuire KJ. Letter to Author of 7 February 1997.
3. Moore FD. Letter to Author of 16 December 1996.
4. Murray TJ. Letter to Author of 16 December 1996.
5. Neuhauser D. Letter to Author of 6 January 1997.
6. Neuhauser D. Letter and review comments to Author of 17 March 1997.
7. Noble N. Letter to Author of 9 February 1997.
8. Quinby WC. Letter to Author of 26 December 1996.
9. Rasetti MA. Letter to Author of 20 December 1994.
10. Reverby S. Letter to Author of March 1997.
11. Rowe CR. Letter to Author of January 1997.
12. Ruffman A. Letter to Author of 6 January 1997.
13. Scott M. Letter to Author of 28 January 1997.
14. Shedore L. Letter to Author of 24 October 1996.
15. Twitchell EB. Letter to Author of 3 February 1997.
16. Wolfe RJ. Letters to Author of 12 October 1993 and 3 March 1995.

THE CODMAN ARCHIVES

Codman's papers are held in a series of 11 boxes in the Rare Book Collections of the Francis A. Countway Library of Medicine at the Harvard Medical School. These papers were consulted in detail for the preparation of this biography. References to them in the footnotes are listed as "CA #/#", which refers to "Codman Archives, Box #/Folder #. I am not able to reproduce the inventory listing in its entirety, but the following is an overview of what is contained in the 11 boxes.

Box 1, Professional correspondence and related materials relating to the American College of Surgeons and the Committee on Standardization of Hospitals, and to the Clinical Congress of Surgeons of North America. Letters included in this folder are from John Bowman, LeRoy Broun, Richard C. Cabot, Henry S. Pritchett of the Carnegie Foundation, Walter Chipman, John Clark. Included herein is the Manual of Hospital Standardization and the Report of the Committee on Standardization of Hospitals.

Box 2 Professional correspondence and related materials, much of it related to the Committee on Standardization of Hospitals. Letters included in this folder are from Morris Cooke, George Crile, Harvey Cushing, Robert Dickinson, S. S. Goldwater, John Hornsby, Allen Kanavel, G. Paul LaRoque, Edward Martin, William Mayo, and the Massachusetts General Hospital.

Box 3 Professional correspondence and related materials, much of it relating to the Meeting at the Boston Medical Library. Letters included in this folder are from Albert Ochsner, C. Sherman Peterkin, the Philadelphia County Medical Society, Frederick Shattuck, M. P. Smithwick, Stephen Tracy, Walter Wesselhoeft, Samuel Woodward, and the Suffolk County Medical Society. Also included is general correspondence and some letters from patients.

Box 4 Correspondence relating to hospital standardization and the End Result Idea, including various hospital annual reports. Included herein are the brochures on "A Study in Hospital Efficiency" as well as various chart, cards, and forms.

Box 5 Various correspondence, first relating to the Codman Hospital, then to the book on the shoulder. There is also material from late in his life on bone sarcoma and some late correspondence concerning the anesthesia record.

Box 6 Various professional correspondence, including some typewritten papers from Codman.

Box 7 Personal correspondence and related materials, including letters to/from his parents while at Saint Mark's School, and during his travels in the 1890s. Other correspondence includes letters to/from his sister Anna Codman, and friends Lawrence Brooks, and the Forbes family.

Box 8 Personal correspondence, much of it financial relating to his difficulties in his last decade. His wills are included herein and correspondence re his burial headstone.

Box 9 Personal correspondence, much of it relating to his hunting and fishing. His hunting diary is included in this box. A separate diary for 1899 and engagement books for 1921 and 1931 are also in this box.

Box 10 Various personal correspondence and related material. Some typed articles written by Codman are in this box. Obituaries and posthumous articles about Codman are in this box as well.

Box 11 Photographs.

ABBREVIATIONS USED

Certain sources are used very frequently in the footnotes. Because of this, I have used the following abbreviations in the footnotes to refer to these frequently mentioned sources.

BMSJ = Boston Medical and Surgical Journal

Bone Sarcoma = Codman EA. **Bone Sarcoma: An Interpretation of the Nomenclature Used by the Committee on the Registry of Bone Sarcoma of the American College of Surgeons.**. New York: Paul B. Hoeber, Inc., 1925. All page references to this book refer to this original edition. It is very rare, but there has been no reprinted edition.

CA #/# = Codman Archives, Box #/Folder #

Chart = Refers to the chart contained on p. vi of the Preface to Codman's shoulder book. See "Preface" below for full bibliographic details.

Epilogue = Codman EA. "An Epilogue: The Ethics of Advertising by the Medical Profession," In: **The Shoulder: Rupture of the Supraspinatus Tendon and Other Lesions In or About the Subacromial Bursa**. Boston: Thomas Todd, 1934. pp. 1-29. All page references to this book refer to the original edition. Please note that the Epilogue page numbers begin at #1, at the end of the main section of the book.

Homans = Homans J. Obituary: Ernest Amory Codman (1869-1940). New Engl J Med, 224(7): 296-299, 13 February 1941.

Preface = Codman EA. "An Autobiographic Preface," In: **The Shoulder: Rupture of the Supraspinatus Tendon and Other Lesions In or About the Subacromial Bursa**. Boston: Thomas

Todd, 1934. pp. v-xl. All page references to this book refer to the original edition. In the text, all reference to "the Preface" refer to this source.

SGO = Surgery, Gynecology & Obstetrics

Shoulder = Codman EA. **The Shoulder: Rupture of the Supraspinatus Tendon and Other Lesions In or About the Subacromial Bursa.** Boston: Thomas Todd, 1934. pp. 1-513. All page references to this book refer to the original edition.

SHE = Codman EA. **A Study in Hospital Efficiency. As Demonstrated by the Case Report of the First Five Years of a Private Hospital.** Boston: Thomas Todd Co., 1917-1920. Reprinted edition—Oakbrook Terrace, IL: Joint Commission on Accreditation of Healthcare Organizations (JCAHO), 1995. Because of the extreme rarity of the original, all page references in this case refer to the reprinted edition by the JCAHO. I have, however, used my own original copy to confirm the consistency of all quotes used.

ABOUT THE AUTHOR

BILL MALLON is an orthopaedic surgeon, primarily working on the shoulder and upper extremity. Dr. Mallon practices with Triangle Orthopaedic Associates in Durham, NC where he served as Medical Director from 2002-2011. Since 2008 Mallon has served as the Editor-in-Chief of the *Journal of Shoulder and Elbow Surgery*, and is the current President-Elect of the American Shoulder and Elbow Surgeons (ASES), assuming the Presidency in October 2014. Prior to going to medical school, he was a professional golfer, who played on the PGA Tour from 1975-79, ranking in the top 100 money winners in 1976 and 1977. He has written extensively on orthopaedic injuries, and on the Olympic Games and sports, with over 30 books on those topics.

Book List

Orthopaedics for the House Officer. Baltimore: Williams & Wilkins, 1990. (with MM McNamara and JR Urbaniak)

Feeling Up to Par: Medicine from Tee to Green. Philadelphia: F. A. Davis, 1994. (with CN Stover and JR McCarroll)

The Golf Doctor. New York: Macmillan, 1996. (with Larry Dennis)

Ernest Amory Codman: The End Result of a Life in Medicine. Philadelphia: Elsevier, 1999.

Quest for Gold: The Encyclopaedia of American Olympians. NY: Leisure Press, 1984. (with Ian Buchanan)

The Olympics: A Bibliography. New York: Garland Publishing, 1984.

The United States National Championships in Track & Field Athletics 1876-1985. Indianapolis: The Athletics Congress, 1986. (with Ian Buchanan)

The Olympic Record Book. New York: Garland, 1988.

The Golden Book of the Olympic Games. Milan: Vallardi, 1993. (with Erich Kamper)

The Guinness International Who's Who of Sports. London: Guinness, 1993. (with Peter Matthews and Ian Buchanan)

Historical Dictionary of the Olympic Movement. Lanham (MD): University Press, 1995. (with Ian Buchanan [first three editions], Jeroen Heijmans [fourth edition]) (four editions through 2011)

The 1896 Olympic Games. Jefferson (NC): McFarland, 1997. (with Ture Widlund)

The 1900 Olympic Games. Jefferson (NC): McFarland, 1997.

The 1904 Olympic Games. Jefferson (NC): McFarland, 1998.

The 1906 Intercalated Olympic Games. Jefferson: McFarland, 1998.

The 1908 Olympic Games. Jefferson (NC): McFarland, 2000. (with Ian Buchanan)

The 1912 Olympic Games. Jefferson (NC): McFarland, 2001. (with Ture Widlund)

The 1920 Olympic Games. Jefferson (NC): McFarland, 2002. (with Tony Bijkerk)

Historical Dictionary of Golf. Lanham (MD): Scarecrow Press, 2011. (with Rand Jerris)

Historical Dictionary of Cycling. Lanham (MD): Scarecrow Press, 2011. (with Jeroen Heijmans)

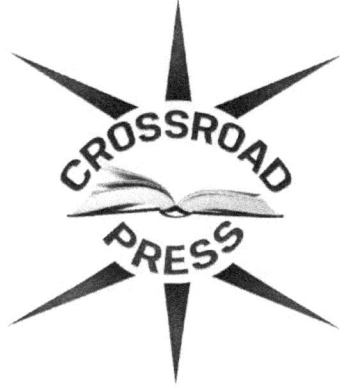

Curious about other Crossroad Press books? Stop by our website:
http://crossroadpress.com
We offer quality writing
in digital, audio, and print formats.

Subscribe to our newsletter on the website homepage and receive a
free eBook.